PULMONARY EMBOLISM

PULMONARY EMBOLISM

Paul D. Stein, M.D.

Henry Ford Heart and Vascular Institute
Detroit, Michigan

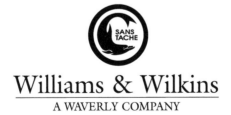

Williams & Wilkins
A WAVERLY COMPANY

BALTIMORE • PHILADELPHIA • LONDON • PARIS • BANGKOK
BUENOS AIRES • HONG KONG • MUNICH • SYDNEY • TOKYO • WROCLAW

MidTown

Editor: Sharon R. Zinner
Managing Editor: Tanya Lazar
Production Coordinator: Peter J. Carley
Book Project Editor: Robert Magee
Designer: Ellen Zanolle
Cover Designer: Ellen Zanolle
Illustration Planner: Peter J. Carley, Jennifer Jett
Typesetter: Port City Press, Inc.
Printer: Port City Press, Inc.
Binder: Port City Press, Inc.

Printed in the United States of America

First Edition,

Library of Congress Cataloging-in-Publication Data
Stein, Paul D.
   Acute pulmonary embolism / by Paul D. Stein. — 1st ed.
     p. cm.
   Includes bibliographical references and index.
   ISBN 0–683–07996–4
   1. Pulmonary embolism.   I. Title.
   [DNLM: 1. Pulmonary Embolism. WG 420 S819a 1997]
RC776.P85S74   1997
616.2'49—dc20
DNLM/DLC
for Library of Congress
                   96–20423
                      CIP

To purchase additional copies of this book, call our customer service department at **(800) 638-0672** or fax orders to **(800) 447-8438.** For other book services, including chapter reprints and large quantity sales, ask for the Special Sales department.

Canadian customers should call **(800) 268-4178,** or fax **(905) 470-6780.** For all other calls originating outside of the United States, please call **(410) 528-4223** or fax us at **(410) 528-8550.**

Visit Williams & Wilkins on the Internet: **http://www.wwilkins.com** or contact our customer service department at **custserv@wwilkins.com.** Williams & Wilkins customer service representatives are available from 8:30 am to 6:00 pm, EST, Monday through Friday, for telephone

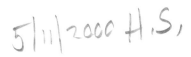

Dedication

This book is dedicated to the memory of the late Lewis Dexter, M.D.

Preface

The purpose of this monograph is to present detailed information on the prevalence, diagnosis, management and prognosis of acute pulmonary embolism. Much of the data were derived from continuing analysis of the database of the Prospective Investigation of Pulmonary Embolism Diagnosis (PIOPED). Most, but not all, of the data presented have been published in peer review journals. The book is meant to be a useful resource for physicians with an interest in specific aspects of the syndrome. This monograph presents in-depth data to give a readily available resource for the basis of reaching a bedside impression based on simple laboratory tests. This monograph also describes the literature upon which a probability assessment of ventilation-perfusion lung scans can be made, the validity and complications of pulmonary angiography, and the basis for noninvasive strategies of diagnosis and management. I have tried to present sufficient data to be scientifically useful but have excluded many of the statistics to allow the text to flow and be readable.

Pulmonary embolism is a vibrant field, and data continues to accrue with respect to its prevention, diagnosis and management. This book was begun several years ago, but delayed because of the rapid acquisition of new information from the PIOPED database.

Topics addressed in this monograph are selected. Some topics of importance related to the prevention of acute pulmonary embolism are discussed only in passing because they are described in detail elsewhere. Symposia that cover some of the topics described only briefly in this book have been published since this book was begun. Attention is called to the following symposia:

Thromboembolic Disease, I, II, and III, edited by Paul D. Stein and Russell D. Hull. Progress in Cardiovascular Disease 1994;36:417–447, 1994;37:1–25, and 1994:59–93.

Venous Thromboembolism, edited by Victor F. Tapson, William J. Fulkerson and Herbert A. Saltzman. Clinics in Chest Medicine 1995;16:229–392.

Fourth ACCP Conference on Antithrombotic Therapy, edited by James E. Dalen and Jack Hirsh. Chest 1995;108 (Suppl):225S–522S.

Pulmonary Embolism, edited by Paul D.Stein. Seminars in Respiratory and Critical Care Medicine 1996;17:1–99.

Some recent books on pulmonary embolism or with a large amount related to it are the following:

Hull RD, Pineo GF, editors. Disorders of Thrombosis. WB Saunders Co., Philadelphia, 1996.

Goldhaber SZ, editor. Prevention of Venous Thromboembolism. Marcel Dekker Inc., New York, 1993.

Hull RD, Pineo G, Raskob G, editors. Venous Thromboembolism: An Evidence-Based Atlas. Futura Publishing Co., Mount Kisco, NY, 1996.

Recruitment for PIOPED started in January 1985 and concluded in September 1986. Six clinical centers as well as a data and coordinating center participated: Duke University, Henry Ford Hospital, Massachusetts General Hospital, University of Michigan, University of Pennsylvania, Yale University and the Maryland Medical Research Institute. The investigation was the product of the devoted effort of many physicians, nurses, and non-physician scientists, and representatives of the National Heart Lung and Blood Institute. The investigators formed a collaborative nucleus of physicians interested in the field. For many investigators, their collegiality has continued and broadened into deep friendship. Data have been spread outside of this collaborative group. Networks of collaboration with groups not involved with PIOPED have developed. The international community has become involved with the data, and a sense of camaraderie has developed with many groups, even though their approaches to pulmonary embolism may be diverse. In every instance there has been a gentlemanly effort to acquire factual information,. Herbert A. Saltzman, M.D., deserves particular recognition for maintaining the PIOPED data repository in good order at Duke University and for continuing to facilitate ready access to the data.

Several friends and colleagues deserve special thanks and recognition. Gerald W. Henry, M.S. worked long and hard on the computerized PIOPED database and collaborated with me while he was an undergraduate and graduate student. He continues to work with me while a medical student at Wayne State University. He is a brilliant worker. Bruce Relyea, M.D., has filled in for Jerry and has been a devoted and respected colleague and friend.

Alexander Gottschalk, M.D., collaborated with me on most of the investigations related to ventilation-perfusion scintigraphy. He supplied many of the illustrations of ventilation-perfusion lung scans and proof-read those he did not supply. Alex has been a dear friend, and I enjoyed our 10 p.m. telephone calls to discuss our various investigations. At 12 a.m. the calls often would switch to Russell D. Hull, M.B.B.S., M.Sc., which was convenient because Calgary is three hours earlier than Detroit. Our thoughts ranged widely, and useful collaboration was derived based on his approach to the diagnosis of deep venous thrombosis and the PIOPED data on pulmonary embolism.

Joanne Husovski, associate managing editor at Williams & Wilkins, was a big help and a friendly and strong support. Marilyn E. Nack was available to provide occasional secretarial assistance when needed. My wife, Janet, and family kindly tolerated the time I spent with this book, and I appreciate that a great deal.

Finally, I recall with gratitude the late Lewis Dexter, M.D., to whom this book is dedicated. Dr. Dexter made fundamental contributions to cardiology. He was the first to position a catheter in the pulmonary artery. His research led to the development of diagnostic cardiac catheterization. He performed research in the pathophysiology and diagnosis of acute pulmonary embolism.

Contents

Part **III**

Ventilation-Perfusion Lung Scan

Part **IV**

Pulmonary Angiography

Part **V**

Diagnosis in Particular Patient Populations

P a r t **VI**

Strategies of Diagnosis and Management

P A R T

Prevalence and Prognosis

CHAPTER 1

Prevalence in a General Hospital

The prevalence of pulmonary embolism varies according to the age and morbidity of the population studied. An assessment of the prevalence of pulmonary embolism depends on the method employed for evaluation and may include any of the following, alone or in combination: clinical diagnosis, ventilation-perfusion lung scan diagnosis, angiographic diagnosis, or autopsy. Each diagnostic method, in turn, depends on the completeness of the survey of the population and the care with which the diagnostic studies were performed. For example, with routine examination at autopsy, 12% of patients were found to have pulmonary embolism, but with meticulous examination of the contralateral lung of the same patients, after inflation and fixation of the lung, some evidence of pulmonary embolism was found in 52% (1). Dalen and Alpert estimated that 15% of deaths in acute general hospitals were because of pulmonary embolism and 25% of deaths in nursing homes or chronic hospitals were as a result of pulmonary embolism (2).

Dalen and Alpert (2) define pulmonary embolism as a major contributing factor in death if the clinical and pathologic data indicate that the patient would not have succumbed to his or her underlying disease if pulmonary embolism had not occurred. Pulmonary embolism as the primary cause of death in patients in a general hospital without other potentially lethal disease was observed in 7% of autopsies (1,3). An additional 7 to 10% of deaths at autopsy had pulmonary embolism as a major contributing factor (1,3). Pulmonary embolism, based on autopsy data, therefore, was a sole or major contributing cause of death in 15% of adult patients dying in a general hospital (2).

The circumstances associated with the collection of data for the national collaborative investigation, Prospective Investigation of Pulmonary Embolism Diagnosis (PIOPED), provided an opportunity to estimate the prevalence of acute pulmonary embolism in a participating general hospital (Henry Ford Hospital, Detroit, MI) during the period of recruitment (4). In PIOPED, patients with a clinical suspicion of acute pulmonary embolism consented to undergo obligatory angiography if the ventilation-perfusion lung scan was abnormal (5). More patients than usual, therefore, underwent pulmonary angiography during the period of participation in PIOPED. In addition, the data from PIOPED showed the frequency of acute pulmonary embolism among patients with ventilation-perfusion lung scans that were interpreted as high, intermediate, or low probability for pulmonary embolism, or nearly normal. This permitted an estimate of the prevalence of pulmonary embolism among patients in whom ventilation-perfusion scans were reported and no further tests were obtained. During the 21-month period of recruitment for PIOPED, among patients 18 years of age or older, there were 51,645 admissions to Henry Ford hospital and 2235 deaths.

In patients in whom a pulmonary angiogram was not obtained because they declined or were ineligible for randomization for angiography, pulmonary embolism was assessed from ventilation-perfusion lung scans. Based on observations of the validity of ventilation-perfusion scans in PIOPED, pulmonary embolism was assumed to be present in 87% of patients with ventilation-perfusion scans interpreted as high probability for pulmonary embolism (5). Based on the same data, pulmonary embolism was estimated to be present in 30% of patients with intermediate probability scans, 14% of patients with low probability scans, and 4% of patients with nearly normal ventilation-perfusion scans (5).

THE AUTOPSY DIAGNOSIS OF ACUTE PULMONARY EMBOLISM

Reports of all autopsies of patients 18 years of age or older at Henry Ford Hospital during the 21-month period of recruitment for PIOPED were reviewed for the presence of pulmonary embolism (4). Autopsies were performed in 404 of 2235 (18%) patients who died. Pulmonary embolism was considered to be present if any antemortem thromboemboli were identified.

Hospital records were reviewed in all patients in whom pulmonary embolism was found at autopsy. Pulmonary embolism was interpreted as causing death if emboli were found in the central pulmonary arteries at autopsy and death was not otherwise explained, or if death was associated with acute cardiopulmonary arrest or rapidly progressing respiratory failure. Pulmonary embolism was considered to have contributed to death if the clinical and pathologic data indicated that the patient would not have succumbed to the underlying disease at that time if pulmonary embolism had not occurred. Pulmonary embolism was considered incidental if thromboemboli were observed only in peripheral branches of the pulmonary arteries, and if the clinical course was essentially unaffected by the pulmonary embolism. This was often a qualitative assessment and the opinion of the prosector was considered to be valid. None of the patients at autopsy had postmortem angiography of the lungs or inflation and fixation of the lungs before dissection.

The estimated prevalence of acute pulmonary embolism in 51,645 patients admitted to the hospital was 1.0% (4). The distribution of diagnoses by pulmonary angiography, ventilation-perfusion scans, and autopsy is shown in Table 1–1. Pulmonary embolism in patients admitted to the hospital, based on extrapolated data from autopsy, was estimated to have caused or contributed to death in 0.2% of cases. Pulmonary embolism severe enough to cause clinical manifesta-

Table 1-1.   PULMONARY EMBOLISM AMONG 51,645 HOSPITALIZED PATIENTS 18 YEARS OF AGE OR OLDER

Method of Diagnosis	PE (%)
Pulmonary angiography	104 (0.2)
High probability VQ scans*	45 (0.1)
Non-high probability VQ scans**	71 (0.1)
Autopsy, PE caused or contributed to death and not diagnosed antemortem (extrapolated)***	106 (0.2)
Autopsy, PE incidental (extrapolated)	200 (0.4)
Total	526 (1.0)

* Assumes 87% pulmonary embolism among 52 patients with high probability ventilation-perfusion scans.
** Assumes pulmonary embolism in 30% with intermediate ventilation-perfusion, 14% with low probability ventilation-perfusion, and 4% with nearly normal ventilation-perfusion.
*** Extrapolation based on 18% autopsy rate.
PE = pulmonary embolism

Total pulmonary embolism that caused or contributed to death, irrespective of whether the diagnosis was suspected antemortem, based on extrapolation data from autopsy, was 122 (0.2%).

Modified from Stein PD, Henry JW (4) and reproduced with permission.

Table 1-2.   AUTOPSY PATIENTS 18 YEARS OF AGE OR OLDER (n=404)

	Caused Death PE (%)	Contributed to Death PE (%)	Incidental PE (%)	Total PE (%)
Diagnosed & treated	3 (0.7)	0 (0)	1 (0.2)	4 (1.0)
Suspected, but not diagnosed or treated	3 (0.7)	0 (0)	0 (0)	3 (0.7)
Unsuspected	14 (3.5)	2 (0.5)	36 (8.9)	52 (12.9)
Total	20 (5.0)	2 (0.5)	37 (9.2)	59 (14.6)

PE = pulmonary embolism
Reprinted with permission from Stein, PD, Henry JW. Prevalence of acute pulmonary embolism among patients in a general hospital and at autopsy. Chest 1995;108:978–981.

tions, contribute to death at autopsy, or cause death was estimated to have occurred in 0.6% of patients admitted to the hospital. In an estimated 0.4% of patients, pulmonary embolism was an incidental finding at autopsy.

Among 404 patients at autopsy, pulmonary embolism was observed in 14.6% (Table 1–2) (4). It was the likely cause of death in 5.0%, a contributing

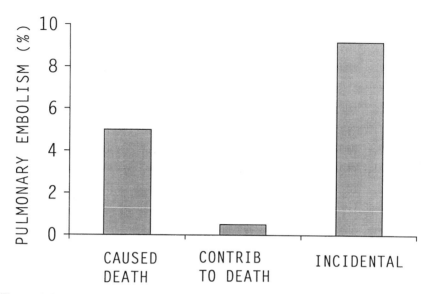

Figure 1–1. Percentage of 404 patients at autopsy in whom pulmonary embolism caused death, contrib. to death, or was incidental. (Data from Stein, PD, Henry JW. Prevalence of acute pulmonary embolism among patients in a general hospital and at autopsy. Chest 1995;108:978–981.)

cause of death in 0.5%, and an incidental finding in 9.2% (Fig. 1–1). The distribution of diagnosed and undiagnosed pulmonary embolism among these patients is shown in Table 1–2 and Figure 1–2.

Among 59 patients with pulmonary embolism at autopsy, pulmonary embolism was the likely cause of death in 33.9%, a contributing cause of death in 3.4%, and an incidental finding among 62.7% who died from other illnesses (Table 1–2 and Fig. 1–3) (4). Associated diagnoses in patients who showed incidental pulmonary embolism at autopsy are shown in Table 1–3.

Pulmonary embolism in patients at autopsy was unsuspected antemortem in 52 of 59 (88.1%) (4). Pulmonary embolism that caused death was unsuspected antemortem in 14 of 20 (70.0%)(Fig. 1–4). Most of these patients had advanced associated disease. Clinical diagnoses in these 14 patients who died from unsuspected pulmonary embolism are shown in Table 1–4. This experience is comparable to the experience of others (6). Among 92 patients at autopsy in whom pulmonary embolism was the cause of death, an antemortem diagnosis of pulmonary embolism was not considered in 51% (6). Testing for thromboembolic disease was not performed in 78%. Comorbid disease was present in most, and 54% had a guarded or poor prognosis independent of pulmonary embolism. Only 41% were short of breath and sudden hypotension was present in only 20%.

The prevalence of pulmonary embolism in a general hospital, based on clinical diagnoses, many of which were confirmed at autopsy, in an era prior to pulmonary angiography or ventilation-perfusion scans, was 0.2% (7). The prevalence of acute pulmonary embolism in patients in a clinic of digestive

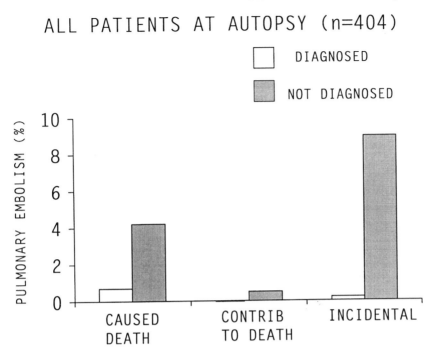

ALL PATIENTS AT AUTOPSY (n=404)

Figure 1-2. Percentage of 404 patients at autopsy in whom pulmonary embolism was diagnosed versus those in whom pulmonary embolism was not diagnosed. Patients are distributed according to whether pulmonary embolism caused death, contrib. to death, or was incidental. (Data from Stein, PD, Henry JW. Prevalence of acute pulmonary embolism among patients in a general hospital and at autopsy. Chest 1995;108:978–981.)

surgery, diagnosed by pulmonary angiography, high probability ventilation-perfusion scans or autopsy in patients with suspected pulmonary embolism, was 0.3% (8). Using comparable criteria, we found the same prevalence (0.3%) (4). The inclusion of patients estimated to have pulmonary embolism based on non-high probability interpretations of the ventilation-perfusion lung scans and the inclusion of patients with clinically undiagnosed pulmonary embolism at autopsy caused the estimated prevalence of pulmonary embolism to be higher, 1.0% (4). The prevalence of acute pulmonary embolism among general surgery patients calculated by meta-analysis of pooled data from randomized trials is 1.6% (9). There are, in addition, patients with silent pulmonary embolism, the frequency of which is undetermined (10).

The frequency of death from pulmonary embolism among patients admitted to the hospital that we estimated, 122 of 51,645 (0.2%), is the same order of magnitude as 212 of 287,370 (0.1%) reported by Hermann and associates in 1961 based on clinical diagnoses, often with autopsy confirmation (7).

The prevalence of acute pulmonary embolism at autopsy that we observed, 14.6%, was within the range reported by most others, 12.0% to 14.8% (11,12). Meticulous dissection and microscopical examination for minute and barely visible fragments has shown traces of fresh or old pulmonary embolism at autopsy in 52% and 64% of patients (1,13). The frequency of pulmonary embo-

PULMONARY EMBOLISM AT AUTOPSY (n=59)

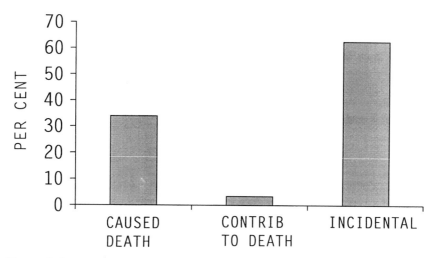

Figure 1–3. Distribution of 59 patients with pulmonary embolism at autopsy according to whether pulmonary embolism caused death, contrib. to death, or was incidental. (Data from Stein, PD, Henry JW. Prevalence of acute pulmonary embolism among patients in a general hospital and at autopsy. Chest 1995;108:978–981.)

lism as a cause or contributing cause of death at autopsy that we observed, 5.4%, was within the range of 3.4% to 8.9% reported by most others (9,11,14), but lower than reported by Morrell and Dunnill, 21.3% (1).

Among all patients who showed pulmonary embolism at autopsy, an antemortem diagnosis or suspicion of pulmonary embolism was present in only 11.9%. This was comparable with 7.9% to 9.3% of suspected or diagnosed pulmonary embolism reported by others (3,11,12,15). Most of the patients with pulmonary embolism at autopsy died from causes unrelated to pulmonary embolism. Even so, only 27.3% of patients in whom pulmonary embolism caused or contributed to death were suspected or diagnosed antemortem. Typically, these patients had advanced associated disease. Unsuspected fatal pulmonary embolism at autopsy was reported by others in 29.6% and 31.8% of patients (11,14).

In, conclusion, pulmonary embolism is common in a general hospital. The frequency of pulmonary embolism at autopsy has not changed over 3 decades. Unsuspected pulmonary embolism in patients at autopsy has not diminished, even among patients who die from acute pulmonary embolism. Such patients typically have advanced associated disease. Incidental pulmonary embolism among moribund patients is rarely diagnosed. Patients who suffer sudden and unexplained catastrophic events in the hospital are a group in whom the diagnosis might be suspected more frequently if physicians maintain a high index of suspicion.

Table 1–3. ASSOCIATED ILLNESSES OF PATIENTS WHO SHOWED
INCIDENTAL PULMONARY EMBOLISM AT AUTOPSY

MI, CHF, COPD, CABG
Pneumonia, decubitus ulcers, CVA
Metastatic carcinoma of bowel, pneumonia
Cirrhosis, UGI bleeding, esophageal varices
Malignant neoplasm with metastasis, renal failure
Pneumonia, cardiomyopathy
Adenocarcinoma with metastasis
Pneumonia, CVA with hemiplegia, diabetes mellitus
Cirrhosis, UGI bleeding, hepatic coma, bronchopneumonia
Cerebral hemorrhage, staph pneumonia
ARDS
Prosthetic valve endocarditis
MI complicating aorta-iliac bypass
Multiple lung abcesses, COPD
Subarachnoid hemorrhage
Diabetic ketoacidosis, ARDS, sepsis
COPD, old MI, pulmonary congestion
Cholecystectomy, abdominal aneurysm, brain stem infarct, hepatic failure
Cerebral hemorrhage
Old MI, CHF, pneumonia
Yeast enterocolitis, peritonitis
Adenocarcinoma lung
Subarachnoid hemorrhage
Hemorrhagic CVA, neurosurgical shunt, pneumonia
Hypertensive crisis, hypoxic encephalopathy
Metastatic CA lung
Ischemic cardiomyopathy, GI bleed
Carcinoma lung, pneumonia
Carcinomatosis, staphylococcal pneumonia
Diabetes mellitus, hypoglycemia
Mitral valve replacement, postop sepsis
Subarachnoid hemorrhage
Above knee amputation, septicemia, scleroderma
ASHD, CHF
CVA
MI, pulmonary edema, CA lung
COPD, CA larynx, CVA

MI, myocardial infarction
CHF, congestive heart failure
COPD, chronic obstructive pulmonary disease
CABG, coronary artery bypass graft
UGI, upper gastrointestinal
CVA, cerebral vascular accident
ARDS, adult respiratory distress syndrome
CA, carcinoma
ASHD, atherosclerotic heart disease

Reprinted with permission from Stein, PD, Henry JW. Prevalence of acute pulmonary embolism among patients in a general hospital and at autopsy. Chest 1995;108:978–981.

PULMONARY EMBOLISM AS CAUSE OF DEATH (n=20)

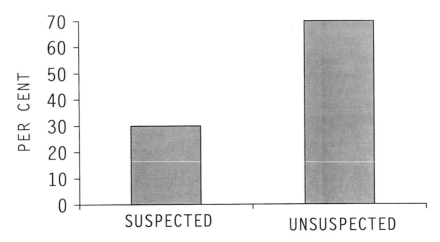

Figure 1–4. Among 20 patients who died from acute pulmonary embolism, the diagnosis was suspected in 30% and unsuspected in 70%. (Data from Stein, PD, Henry JW. Prevalence of acute pulmonary embolism among patients in a general hospital and at autopsy. Chest 1995;108:978–981.)

Table 1–4. ASSOCIATED DIAGNOSES IN PATIENTS WHO DIED FROM UNSUSPECTED PE

Postoperative radical neck dissection and laryngectomy for carcinoma of larynx complicated by postoperative CVA
Congestive heart failure (left- and right-sided)
CA breast
Diabetes mellitus, end-stage renal disease
CA prostrate, carcinomatosis, postorchiectomy
Hip fracture, dementia
Postprostatectomy
Atherosclerosis legs, postbelow-knee amputation
Carcinoma of tongue, duodenal ulcer
Pneumonia, left- and right-sided CHF, dementia
Bowel obstruction
Duodenal ulcer with bleeding, cardiomyopathy with CHF
CVA, sepsis, respiratory failure, mentally obtunded
Diabetes mellitus, end-stage renal disease

CA, carcinoma
CVA, cerebral vascular accident

Reprinted with permission from Stein, PD, Henry JW. Prevalence of acute pulmonary embolism among patients in a general hospital and at autopsy. Chest 1995;108:978–981.

REFERENCES

1. Morrell MT, Dunnill MS. The post-mortem incidence of pulmonary embolism in a hospital population. Br J Surg 1968; 55:347–352.
2. Dalen JE, Alpert JS. Natural history of pulmonary embolism. Prog Cardiovas Dis 1975;17:258–270.
3. Uhland H, Goldberg LM. Pulmonary embolism: a commonly missed clinical entity. Dis Chest 1964;45:533–536.
4. Stein PD, Henry JW. Prevalence of acute pulmonary embolism among patients in a general hospital and at autopsy. Chest 1995;108:978–981.
5. The PIOPED Investigators. Value of the ventilation/perfusion scan in acute pulmonary embolism: results of the Prospective Investigation of Pulmonary Embolism Diagnosis (PIOPED). J Amer Med Assoc 1990;263:2753–2759.
6. Morgenthaler TI, Ryu JH. Clinical characteristics of fatal pulmonary embolism in a referral hospital. Mayo Clin Proc 1995;70:417–424.
7. Hermann RE, Davis JH, Holden WD. Pulmonary embolism. Aclinical and pathologic study with emphasis on the effect of prophylactic therapy with anticoagulants. Am J Surg 1961;102:19–28.
8. Huber O, Bounameaux H, Borst F, Rohner A. Postoperative pulmonary embolism after hospital discharge: an underestimated risk. Arch Surg 1992;127:310–313.
9. Clagett GP, Reisch JS. Prevention of venous thromboembolism in general surgical patients. Ann Surg 1988;208:227–240.
10. Moser KM, Fedullo PF, LitteJohn JK, Crawford R. Frequent asymptomatic pulmonary embolism in patients with deep venous thrombosis. J Amer Med Assoc 1994;271:223–225.
11. Goldhaber SZ, Hennekens CH, Evans DA, Newton EC, Godleski JJ. Factors associated with correct antemortem diagnosis of major pulmonary embolism. Amer J Med 1982;73:822–826.
12. Coon WW, Coller FA. Clinicopathologic correlation in thromboembolism. Surg Gynecol Obstet 1959;109:259–269.
13. Freiman DG, Suyemoto J, Wessler S. Frequency of pulmonary thromboembolism in man. N Eng J Med 1965;272:1278–1280.
14. Rubenstein I, Murray D, Hoffstein V. Fatal pulmonary embolism in hospitalized patients: an autopsy study. Arch Int Med 1988;148:1425–1426.
15. Coon WW. The spectrum of pulmonary embolism: twenty years later. Arch Surg 1976;111:398–402. at autopsy. Chest 1995;108;978–981.

2

Changing Risks of Untreated Deep Venous Thrombosis and Acute Pulmonary Embolism

The frequency of fatal pulmonary embolism in patients with untreated deep venous thrombosis has diminished as diagnostic tests have made it possible to diagnose mild deep venous thrombosis (1). Before the use of venography and sensitive noninvasive tests for the early detection of deep venous thrombosis, the risk of fatal pulmonary embolism in untreated patients with clinically apparent deep venous thrombosis was 37% (2) (Fig. 2–1). In patients with untreated deep venous thrombosis diagnosed with radioactive fibrinogen scintiscans, the risk of fatal pulmonary embolism, most of which was subclinical, was approximately 5% (3). It is apparent that the risk of fatal pulmonary embolism was greater among patients with more severe deep venous thrombosis.

The percentage of patients with acute pulmonary embolism (pulmonary embolism) who have clinically detectable deep venous thrombosis has diminished as physicians have developed the ability to diagnose subtle pulmonary embolism (2). Among patients who died from acute pulmonary embolism, 53% had clinically identified deep venous thrombosis (4) (Fig. 2–2). In an investigation of patients with massive or submassive acute pulmonary embolism diagnosed by pulmonary angiography (the Urokinase Pulmonary Embolism Trial), 34% of patients had clinically identifiable deep venous thrombosis (5). Among patients with mild as well as severe acute pulmonary embolism (PIO-PED), only 15% of patients had clinically apparent deep venous thrombosis (Stein, PD. Unpublished data from Prospective Investigation of Pulmonary Embolism Diagnosis). Clinically apparent deep venous thrombosis, therefore, is more frequent in patients with more severe acute pulmonary embolism.

In the present era of early diagnosis of acute pulmonary embolism, the risk of fatal recurrent pulmonary embolism as well as the risk of death from the initial pulmonary embolism in untreated patients is lower than in patients with severe pulmonary embolism reported in prior years (1). Among untreated

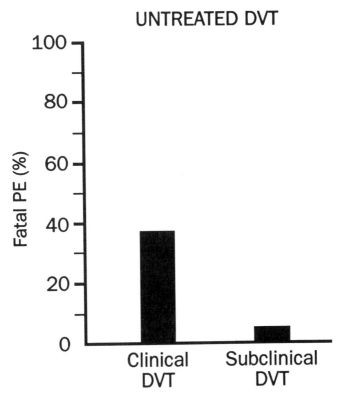

Figure 2–1. Frequency of fatal pulmonary embolism (PE) in untreated patients with clinically apparent deep venous thrombosis (DVT), and patients, most of whom had subclinical DVT diagnosed by radioactive fibrinogen scintiscans. (Data from Byrne JJ. Phlebitis: A study of 748 cases at the Boston City Hospital. New Engl J Med 1955;253:579–586. and Collins R, Scrimgeour A, Yusuf S, Peto R. Reduction in fatal pulmonary embolism and venous thrombosis by perioperative administration of subcutaneous heparin. New Engl J Med 1988;318:1162–1173. Reprinted with permission from Stein PD. Changing patterns of risk of untreated thromboembolic disease. Seminars of Respiratory and Critical Care Medicine 1996;17:3–6.)

patients with acute pulmonary embolism diagnosed on the basis of clinical features that included evidence of right ventricular failure, pulmonary infarction, or both, Barritt and Jordan reported a 26% mortality from the initial pulmonary embolism, although some of these patients, perhaps, died from recurrent pulmonary embolism (6). Information that Barritt and Jordan relied upon to diagnose pulmonary infarction included pleuritic pain, hemoptysis, pleural friction rub, loss of resonance at the lung base, rales, and the chest radiograph. Features that they relied upon to diagnose acute right ventricular failure were faintness, chest pain, fall of blood pressure, rise of jugular venous pressure, and the electrocardiogram.

In 1961, Hermann and associates calculated a 37% mortality from the initial pulmonary embolism (7). The diagnosis was based on clinical features, and autopsy among those who died. The treatment of these patients was not reported, although data were collected between 1943 and 1957, and anticoagulant

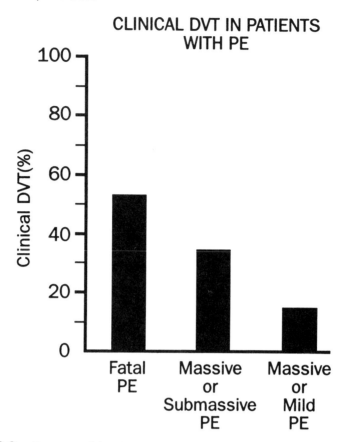

Figure 2–2.   Frequency of clinically apparent deep venous thrombosis (DVT) among patients with fatal acute pulmonary embolism (PE), massive or submassive pulmonary embolism, or massive or mild pulmonary embolism. (Data based on Byrne JJ, O'Neil EE. Fatal pulmonary emboli. A study of 130 autopsy-proven fatal emboli. Am J Surg 1952;83:47–54, A National Cooperative Study. Clinical and electrocardiographic observations. The Urokinase Pulmonary Embolism Trial. Circulation 1973;47/48(Suppl II):60–65, and Stein, PD. Unpublished data from the Prospective Investigation of Pulmonary Embolism Diagnosis. Reprinted with permission from Stein PD. Changing patterns of risk of untreated thromboembolic disease. Seminars of Respiratory and Critical Care Medicine 1996;17:3–6.)

therapy was not in general used before 1947 (7). Hermann and associates found a 36% frequency of fatal recurrent pulmonary embolism. The total estimated frequency of death that included the original pulmonary embolism and recurrent pulmonary embolism was 73% (7). There was, in addition, a 21% frequency of nonfatal recurrent pulmonary embolism among untreated patients with clinically diagnosed pulmonary embolism (7). Presumably, pulmonary embolism was severe among these patients with overt clinical features. A high mortality from the initial pulmonary embolism, therefore, was predictable.

In an investigation of the clinical course of acute pulmonary embolism, Carson and associates observed that in the Prospective Investigation of Pulmo-

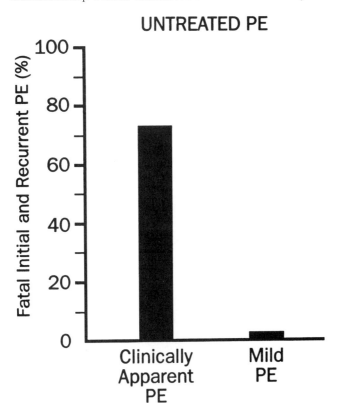

Figure 2–3. Fatal initial and fatal recurrent pulmonary embolism (PE) among untreated patients. Comparison is made between patients in whom the diagnosis was clinically apparent, and presumably pulmonary embolism was severe, and patients in whom pulmonary embolism was mild. (Data from Hermann RE, Davis JH, Holden WD. Pulmonary embolism: A clinical and pathologic study with emphasis on the effect of prophylactic therapy with anticoagulants. Am J Surg 1961;102:19–28. and Stein PD, Henry JW. Untreated patients with pulmonary embolism: Outcome, clinical and laboratory assessment. Chest 1995;107:931–935. Reprinted with permission from Stein PD. Changing patterns of risk of untreated thromboembolic disease. Seminars of Respiratory and Critical Care Medicine 1996;17:3–6.)

nary Embolism Diagnosis (PIOPED), 24 patients escaped treatment in the hospital (8). However, four patients started anticoagulant therapy during the first month after discharge. We evaluated the 20 patients who received no treatment for pulmonary embolism during the first 3 months of follow-up (9). Only one of these patients died of pulmonary embolism (8,9). In the present era of early diagnosis by ventilation-perfusion lungs scans and pulmonary angiography, mortality from the initial pulmonary embolism and from recurrent pulmonary embolism among patients with untreated mild pulmonary embolism was 1 of 20 (5%) (Fig. 2–3) (9).

The circumstances involving no therapy in these 20 patients from PIOPED are as follows: 19 had pulmonary angiograms interpreted as showing no pulmonary embolism by the local radiologist, but the interpretation of no pulmonary

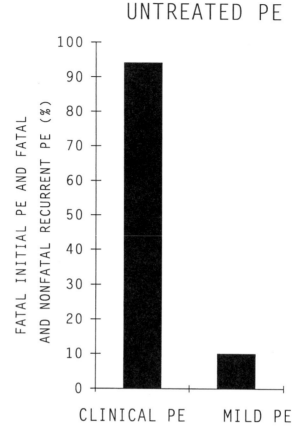

Figure 2–4. Fatal initial pulmonary embolism (PE), fatal recurrent PE, and nonfatal recurrent PE among patients with clinically apparent severe PE and patients with mild PE. (Data from Hermann RE, Davis JH, Holden WD. Pulmonary embolism: A clinical and pathologic study with emphasis on the effect of prophylactic therapy with anticoagulants. Am J Surg 1961;102:19–28. and Stein PD, Henry JW. Untreated patients with pulmonary embolism: Outcome, clinical and laboratory assessment. Chest 1995;107:931–935.)

embolism was reversed in 18 after re-evaluation by the central panel of angiogram readers (9). The diagnosis of no pulmonary embolism was reversed in one patient because pulmonary embolism was found at autopsy 6 days after the pulmonary angiogram. One patient had no pulmonary angiogram; that patient died of unrelated causes 4 days after a ventilation-perfusion lung scan, and autopsy showed small peripheral pulmonary embolism.

The untreated patient who died was a 33-year-old woman with underlying primary pulmonary hypertension with right ventricular failure (9). Organized and fresh pulmonary emboli were shown at autopsy 6 days after a pulmonary angiogram that failed to show pulmonary embolism. Whether this death resulted from the original pulmonary embolism or recurrent pulmonary embolism is uncertain.

In regard to the course of untreated mild pulmonary embolism over 1 year, there were no instances of fatal recurrent pulmonary embolism (9). This assumes that the cause of death in the only patient who died was the original pulmonary embolism. Fatal recurrent pulmonary embolism, therefore, was 0 of 19 (0%) among untreated survivors of mild pulmonary embolism during months 4 to 12 of observation (9).

One patient died of aspiration pneumonia after hysterectomy for endometrial carcinoma 4 days after an intermediate probability ventilation-perfusion lung scan was obtained (9). Multiple small thromboemboli in peripheral branches were observed at autopsy. These thromboemboli did not contribute to death. Based on clinical assessment, recurrent pulmonary embolism was thought to have occurred. The frequency of nonfatal recurrent pulmonary embolism among survivors of the first pulmonary embolism was 1 of 19 (5.3%).

The frequency of fatal initial pulmonary embolism, fatal recurrent pulmonary embolism, and nonfatal recurrent pulmonary embolism over the course of 1 year among untreated patients with acute pulmonary embolism was 2 of 20 (10%) (Fig. 2–4).

Untreated patients with pulmonary embolism had mild pulmonary embolism as suggested by the following data. Among patients who had measurements of the PaO_2 while breathing room air, the PaO_2 was lower in untreated patients compared with treated patients (39 ± 16 versus 55 ± 31 mm Hg) (P<.001) (9). The pulmonary artery mean pressure did not show a statistically significant difference between untreated and treated patients (23 ± 13 mm Hg versus 24 ± 10 mm Hg).

Ventilation-perfusion lung scans were interpreted as high probability in a smaller percent of untreated patients with pulmonary embolism than treated patients, 0 of 20 (0%) versus 160 of 376 (43%) (P<.001) (9). Low probability, nearly normal, or normal ventilation-perfusion scans were more frequent among untreated patients, 10 of 20 (50%) versus 58 of 376 (15%) (P<.001). Ventilation-perfusion lung scans among untreated patients more often showed no mismatched segmental equivalent perfusion defects than among treated patients, 14 of 20 (70%) versus 122 of 376 (32%) (P<.01) (9). All untreated patients, 20 of 20 (100%) showed fewer than 3 mismatched segmental equivalent perfusion defects compared with 227 of 376 (60%) among treated patients (P<.001).

Pulmonary angiograms at the time of PIOPED entry were obtained in 19 untreated patients and 362 treated patients (9). Thromboemboli involved only segmental pulmonary arteries or smaller branches in 16 of 19 (84%) untreated patients and 132 of 362 (36%) treated patients (P<.001). Only peripheral vessels were involved in 7 of 19 (37%) untreated patients and 13 of 362 (4%) treated patients (P<.001). Thromboemboli were not observed on the angiogram of one untreated patient, but were shown at autopsy 6 days later.

The frequency of fatal initial and fatal recurrent pulmonary embolism in untreated patients with mild pulmonary embolism (5.0%) is strikingly lower than the mortality from untreated pulmonary embolism reported in past decades among patients who presumably had severe pulmonary embolism (6,7). This lower mortality appears to relate to the milder severity of pulmonary embolism in these untreated patients. The mortality of untreated patients with mild pulmonary embolism is comparable to the mortality from fatal pulmonary embolism in untreated patients with subtle deep venous thrombosis, approximately 5% (3).

REFERENCES

1. Stein PD. Changing patterns of risk of untreated thromboembolic disease. Seminars of Respiratory and Critical Care Medicine 1996;17:3–6.
2. Byrne JJ. Phlebitis: a study of 748 cases at the Boston City Hospital. New Engl J Med 1955;253:579–586.
3. Collins R, Scrimgeour A, Yusuf S, Peto R. Reduction in fatal pulmonary embolism and venous thrombosis by perioperative administration of subcutaneous heparin. New Engl J Med 1988;318:1162–1173.
4. Byrne JJ, O'Neil EE. Fatal pulmonary emboli. A study of 130 autopsy-proven fatal emboli. Am J Surg 1952;83:47–54.
5. A National Cooperative Study. Clinical and electrocardiographic observations. The Urokinase Pulmonary Embolism Trial. Circulation 1973;47/48(Suppl II):60–65.
6. Barritt DW, Jordan SC. Anticoagulant drugs in the treatment of pulmonary embolism: a controlled trial. Lancet 1960;1:1309–1312.
7. Hermann RE, Davis JH, Holden WD. Pulmonary embolism: a clinical and pathologic study with emphasis on the effect of prophylactic therapy with anticoagulants. Am J Surg 1961;102:19–28.
8. Carson JL, Kelley MA, Duff A, et al. The clinical course of pulmonary embolism. New Engl J Med 1992;326:1240–1245.
9. Stein PD, Henry JW. Untreated patients with pulmonary embolism: outcome, clinical and laboratory assessment. Chest 1995;107:931–935.

CHAPTER 3

Pulmonary Embolism Among Patients with Negative Pulmonary Angiograms

The occurrence of pulmonary embolism on follow-up among patients with negative pulmonary angiograms is small. There is, however, a real and measurable rate of clinically important pulmonary embolism over the subsequent 12 months that is higher than reported in the general population of patients admitted to the hospital. Patients with suspected pulmonary embolism, therefore, even if their angiogram is negative, might benefit from definitive studies of the lower extremities to exclude deep venous thrombosis (1). The cost-benefit ratio of this, however, has not been evaluated.

Among patients with negative pulmonary angiograms who received no anticoagulant therapy, 6 of 380 (1.6%) suffered clinical pulmonary embolism during the year of follow-up (Table 3–1) (1). Pulmonary embolism may have contributed to death in 2 of 380 (0.5%). Both deaths were in the first month of follow-up. Among 291 patients with negative pulmonary angiograms who survived unrelated illnesses during the year of follow-up, nonfatal pulmonary embolism occurred in 4 (1.4%).

The symptoms among patients with negative angiograms who developed subsequent pulmonary embolism did not differ to a statistically significant extent from symptoms among patients who did not develop pulmonary embolism, nor did the signs or chest radiographic abnormalities (1). The partial pressure of oxygen in arterial blood (PaO_2) among patients with subsequent pulmonary embolism versus patients with no subsequent pulmonary embolism was 70 ± 20 mm Hg versus 69 ± 17 mm Hg (NS). The alveolar arterial oxygen difference among patients with subsequent pulmonary embolism versus patients with no subsequent pulmonary embolism was 51 ± 19 mm Hg versus 37 ± 17 mm Hg (NS). The pulmonary artery mean pressure, however, was higher in patients who had a subsequent pulmonary embolism compared with patients who did not, 34 ± 25 mm Hg versus 22 ± 10 mm Hg (P<0.01).

Among patients who had a history of thrombophlebitis, compared with those who had no history of thrombophlebitis, a trend suggested that future pulmonary embolism was more likely, 3 of 40 (7%) versus 3 of 340 (0.9%), but the difference was not statistically significant (1).

Pulmonary embolism was more frequent among patients with at least 1 leg test that showed deep venous thrombosis than among patients with normal leg studies, 2 of 3 (67%) compared with 0 of 26 (0%) (P<0.01) (1). Among patients who had a history of thrombophlebitis or at least 1 leg test that showed deep venous thrombosis, compared with those who had neither, pulmonary embolism on follow-up occurred in 2 of 5 (40%) versus 0 of 24 (0%) (P<0.05).

Among patients who showed pulmonary embolism on follow-up, 5 of 6 (83%) had a history of deep venous thrombosis or at least 1 objective test that showed deep venous thrombosis. This suggests that deep venous thrombosis may have been present in these patients.

Pulmonary embolism during the year of follow-up of patients who had a negative pulmonary angiogram was uncommon in our experience (1.6%), and it was uncommon in the experience of others (2–4). Cheely and associates followed patients with negative pulmonary angiograms an average of 13 months (2). Nonfatal pulmonary embolism occurred in 3 of 112 (2.7%) survivors of unrelated illnesses, and pulmonary embolism was observed in 3 of 11 autopsied patients. The total frequency of pulmonary embolism, therefore, was 6 of 144 (4.2%). Hull and associates, studying 44 patients with negative pulmonary angiograms, observed 1 fatal pulmonary embolism (2.3%) that occurred within 2 weeks of the pulmonary angiogram in a patient with untreated calf vein thrombosis (3). Novelline and associates followed 167 untreated patients with negative pulmonary angiograms a minimum of 6 months (4). They reported that 20 patients died of unrelated illnesses, and observed incidental pulmonary embolism in 3 of 10 patients at autopsy. There was no evidence of pulmonary embolism among 147 survivors. The frequency of any pulmonary embolism during follow-up was 3 of 167 (1.8%). The frequency of pulmonary embolism on follow-up that we observed in untreated patients with negative pulmonary angiograms (1) was comparable to the frequency of pulmonary embolism reported by Hull and associates among untreated patients with negative serial leg tests for deep venous thrombosis, 1.9% (5).

Whether pulmonary embolism after a negative pulmonary angiogram represents a recurrent pulmonary embolism in patients in whom the prior pulmo-

Table 3–1.   PATIENTS WITH NEGATIVE PULMONARY ANGIOGRAMS
(n = 380)

	Number (%)
Died, death perhaps related to PE	2 (0.5)
Nonfatal PE, in 1-year follow-up	4 (1.1)
Total PE	6 (1.6)

PE, pulmonary embolism
Data from Henry JW, Stein PD. Continuing risk of thromboemboli among patients with negative pulmonary angiograms. Chest 1995;107:1375–1378.

nary embolism could not be definitively diagnosed, or whether the pulmonary embolism was the first pulmonary embolism in a patient with a prior negative pulmonary angiogram is uncertain. Many of the patients who had negative pulmonary angiograms were at risk of pulmonary embolism, and had clinical findings that suggested deep venous thrombosis.

Even though the frequency of pulmonary embolism was low during 1 year of follow-up of patients with a negative pulmonary angiogram, the frequency of pulmonary embolism in this group was higher than in the general population of patients admitted to the hospital. In the general population of patients admitted to the hospital, using the same criteria as those used in the follow-up of PIOPED patients (a clinical suspicion confirmed by pulmonary angiography, a high probability interpretation of the ventilation-perfusion lung scan, or confirmed at autopsy), pulmonary embolism was diagnosed in 0.3% (6). Using the same criteria, Huber and associates reported an identical prevalence (7). These criteria for the prevalence of pulmonary embolism are more strict than we used for assessing the prevalence of pulmonary embolism in the general hospital population (6) (Chapter 1).

REFERENCES

1. Henry JW, Stein PD. Continuing risk of thromboemboli among patients with negative pulmonary angiograms. Chest 1995;107:1375–1378.
2. Cheely R, McCartney WH, Perry JR, et al. The role of noninvasive tests versus pulmonary angiography in the diagnosis of pulmonary embolism. Amer J Med 1981;70:17–22.
3. Hull RD, Hirsh J, Carter CJ, et al. Pulmonary angiography, ventilation lung scanning, and venography for clinically suspected pulmonary embolism with abnormal perfusion lung scan. Ann Intern Med 1983;98:891–899.
4. Novelline RA, Baltarowich OH, Athanasoulis CA, et al. The clinical course of patients with suspected pulmonary embolism and a negative pulmonary arteriogram. Radiology 1978;126:561–567.
5. Hull RD, Raskob GE, Ginsberg JS, et al. A noninvasive strategy for the treatment of patients with suspected pulmonary embolism. Arch Intern Med 1994;154:289–297.
6. Stein PD, Henry JW. Prevalence of acute pulmonary embolism in a general hospital. Chest 1995;108:978–981.
7. Huber O, Bounameaux H, Borst F, Rohner A. Postoperative pulmonary embolism after hospital discharge: an underestimated risk. Arch Surg 1992;127:310–313.

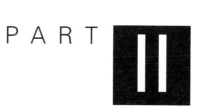

The History, Physical Examination, and Laboratory Tests

CHAPTER 4

Sensitivity and Specificity of Examination of the Lower Extremities for Deep Venous Thrombosis

Thrombosis of the veins of the lower extremities usually occurs without inflammation (1). Inflammation of the walls of the veins, when it occurs, is usually secondary to the thrombosis (1). No clear evidence indicates that inflammation of the veins prevents embolization, or that embolization is more frequent in those patients with thrombi not associated with venous inflammation.

In the past, patients who had thrombosed veins of the lower extremities accompanied by signs of inflammation were diagnosed as having thrombophlebitis, based on the presumption that the primary event was inflammation of the walls of the veins. Patients with no clinical signs in the lower extremities, who had thrombosis that resulted in pulmonary embolism, were said to have phlebothrombosis. Histological investigations have not supported a distinction between the clinical diagnoses of thrombophlebitis and phlebothrombosis. A thrombus can induce inflammation in the underlying wall of the vein, and this inflammation in some patients is extensive enough to produce pain, tenderness, swelling, and fever (2).

In an investigation of deep venous thrombosis at autopsy, all unsuspected, and therefore untreated, thrombi that we observed had fresh components, indicating that thrombosis was continuing (1) (Fig. 4–1). A patient with clinical signs and symptoms of deep venous thrombosis showed lymphocytic infiltration in the media of the veins (Fig. 4–2). The inflammation occurred not only at the sites of attachment of the thrombus, but also where the thrombus was apposed to the endothelium without being attached, suggesting that the thrombus induced the inflammation.

The valve pockets were a frequent site of origin of thrombi (Figs. 4–1, 4–3, 4–4). Thrombi located in valve pockets consisted of organized fibrous points of attachment capped by fresh fibrin and red cell clot (1).

Clinically unsuspected deep venous thrombosis at autopsy was often extensive, causing collateral circulation around occlusions and dilatation of collateral

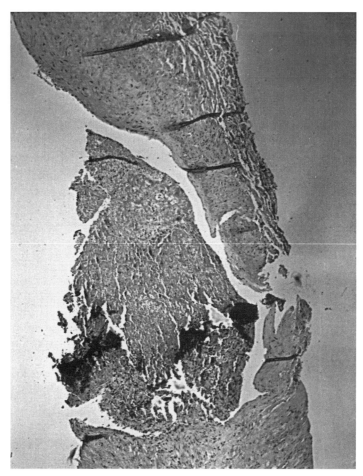

Figure 4–1.   Photomicrograph showing thrombus originating in valve pocket of a posterior tibial vein. The well-organized fibrous point of attachment is capped by a fresh red cell, platelet, and fibrin clot. There is no inflammation of the vein. Hematoxylin and eosin. (Previously unpublished figure from Stein PD, Evans H. An autopsy study of leg vein thrombosis. Circulation 1967;35:671–681.)

veins (1) (Figs. 4–5,4–6). Normal postmortem venograms are shown for comparison in Figures 4–7 and 4–8. Thrombi were found to originate both in veins of the thigh and in veins of the calf (1). Origin in the veins of the calf was more common, and in every case in which the veins of the thigh and the calf were thrombosed in continuity, the thrombi in the calf were older than those in the thigh. This supports the concept that forward thrombosis is more common than retrograde thrombosis.

Many say that the clinical diagnosis of deep venous thrombosis is inaccurate because of a low sensitivity and specificity (3) and low positive predictive value (4–7). The "dogma" that clinical assessment is of no use in the diagnostic assessment of deep venous thrombosis has been challenged by use of a clinical model that combines a pretest probability by a clinical model with ultrasonography, which can simplify and improve the diagnostic process (8). With this clinical model, patients with suspected deep venous thrombosis were stratified into groups with high, intermediate, or low clinical likelihood, based on a point grading system using specific risk factors, symptoms and signs that the investigators designated as major or minor. Major diagnostic items were active cancer, paralysis, paresis, recent plaster immobilization, major surgery, localized tenderness along the distribution of the deep venous system, thigh and calf swollen, calf swollen 3 cm or more, more than 2 first-degree relatives with deep venous thrombosis. A high clinical likelihood and an abnormal ultrasound in combination always indicated deep venous thrombosis based on venography. A concordantly low clinical likelihood of deep venous thrombosis based on a point grading system in combination with a negative ultrasound of the lower extremities was associated with deep venous thrombosis in only 2% of patients. Deep venous thrombosis was shown by venography in 32% of patients with a discordantly high clinical likelihood of deep venous thrombosis and negative ultrasound. Venograms indicated that the ultrasound was falsely positive in 37% of patients in whom there was a discordantly low likelihood clinical assessment for deep venous thrombosis and the ultrasound was abnormal.

Physical examination remains the initial diagnostic modality that calls attention to the potential diagnosis and upon which physicians must rely. It would be useful, therefore, to know the sensitivity and specificity of individual signs and combinations of signs of deep venous thrombosis.

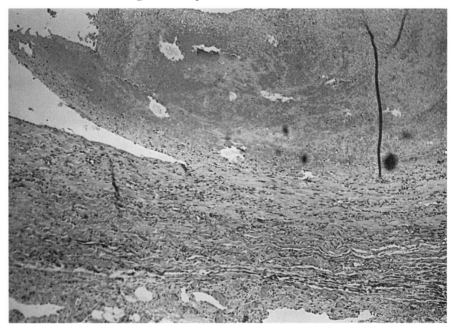

Figure 4–2. Thrombus attached to femoral vein. Lymphocytic infiltrate is shown throughout the wall of the vein. The patient had signs and symptoms of deep venous thrombosis. Hematoxylin and eosin. (Previously unpublished figure from Stein PD, Evans H. An autopsy study of leg vein thrombosis. Circulation 1967;35:671–681.)

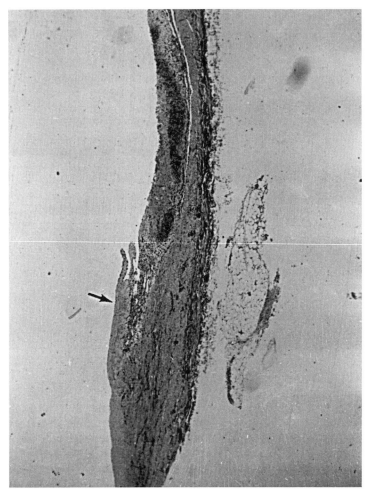

Figure 4–3. Thrombus attached to valve pocket in femoral vein and propagating along the vein. Venous valve is shown (arrow). Hematoxylin and eosin. (Previously unpublished figure from Stein PD, Evans H. An autopsy study of leg vein thrombosis. Circulation 1967;35:671–681.)

Regarding clinical manifestations in general, without specific information about individual signs, among patients who died of trauma or burns, 13 of 32 (41%) with autopsy-proven deep venous thrombosis were diagnosed antemortem (9). Among patients who died of pulmonary embolism, 63 of 118 (53%) with autopsy-proven deep venous thrombosis had antemortem clinical signs of deep venous thrombosis (10). Among 37 legs of patients screened by ^{125}I fibrinogen scans, the clinical signs showed a similar sensitivity (49%) (11). The specificity of clinical signs among 16 legs evaluated by venography was also low (56%), but these data are biased because patients were selected because of clinical findings (12).

Data on the sensitivity and specificity of individual clinical findings are even more sparse. In 12 extremities of patients with deep venous thrombosis shown by dissection at autopsy, the sensitivity of ankle asymmetry ≥ 1.27 cm was 83%, Homans' sign was 8%, and local tenderness was 41% (13). The specificity among 18 extremities of patients in whom deep venous thrombosis was excluded by dissection at autopsy for both ankle asymmetry and Homans' sign was 94% and the specificity of local tenderness was 89% (13). Among patients referred for venography because of clinical findings, however, the specificity was 59% or less (14).

To assess the sensitivity and specificity of signs of deep venous thrombosis, it would be ideal to survey a population of patients by performing tests on the

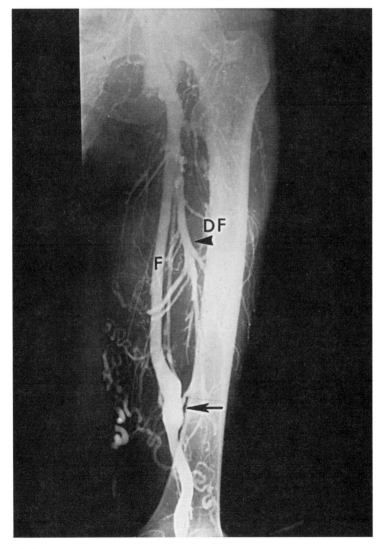

Figure 4–4.   Postmortem venogram showing dilated valve pocket in femoral (F) vein of left thigh (arrow). The deep femoral vein (DF) is also shown. (Reprinted with permission from Stein PD, Evans H. An autopsy study of leg vein thrombosis. Circulation 1967;35:671–681.)

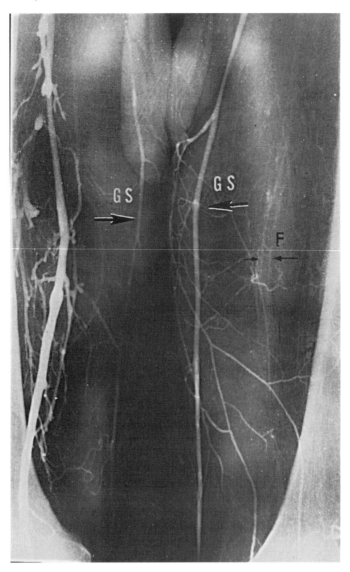

Figure 4–5.   Postmortem venogram of the veins of both thighs. Extensive thrombosis of the femoral, deep femoral, and popliteal veins was found by dissection of the left thigh. The venogram of the left thigh shows absence of filling of the popliteal and deep femoral veins and only a faint outline of the femoral vein (F). The left greater saphenous vein is dilated and joined by numerous collateral vessels. The veins of the right thigh were normal. (Reprinted with permission from Stein PD, Evans H. An autopsy study of leg vein thrombosis. Circulation 1967;35:671–681.)

entire group to determine if deep venous thrombosis were present, and evaluate the clinical findings among those with deep venous thrombosis and those in whom there was no deep venous thrombosis. Unfortunately, no database with this information exists. Patients referred for objective tests of the lower extremi-

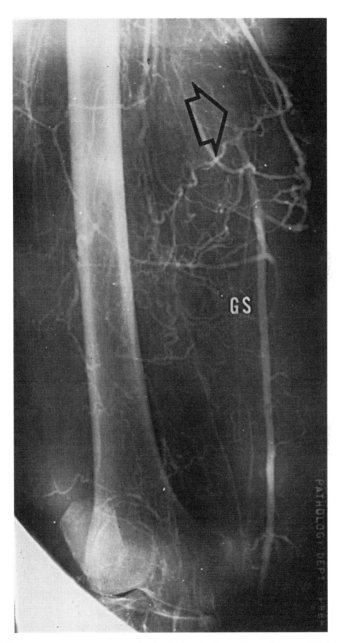

Figure 4–6.   Postmortem venogram of right thigh. The femoral vein has not filled with contrast material because of a completely occluding thrombus. The greater saphenous (GS) vein is distended. Collateral vessels formed at the site of an occluding thrombus in the greater saphenous vein (arrow). (Reprinted with permission from Stein PD, Evans H. An autopsy study of leg vein thrombosis. Circulation 1967;35:671–681.)

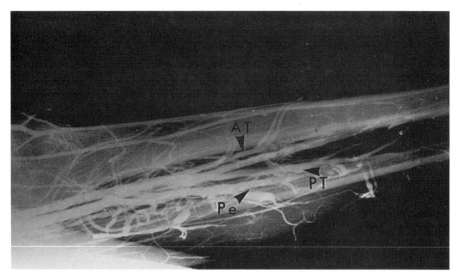

Figure 4–7. Normal postmortem venogram of calf (lateral projection) showing anterior tibial (AT), posterior tibial (PT), and peroneal (Pe) veins. The deep veins are paired. (Reprinted with permission from Stein PD, Evans H. An autopsy study of leg vein thrombosis. Circulation 1967;35:671–681.)

ties typically are referred because of clinical findings that suggest deep venous thrombosis. Patients with no clinical findings seldom are referred for diagnostic studies of the lower extremities. The sensitivity and specificity of clinical findings in the lower extremities, therefore, have been incompletely determined. Because of sparse data, we evaluated the sensitivity and specificity of individual signs of deep venous thrombosis (Stein PD, Henry JW, Relyea B. Unpublished data from the Prospective Investigation of Pulmonary Embolism Diagnosis), and these observations will be described. Sensitivity was defined as the proportion of patients with deep venous thrombosis who were correctly diagnosed by a particular sign, or combination of signs. Specificity was defined as the proportion of negative tests among patients in whom deep venous thrombosis was absent.

We assessed the sensitivity and specificity of signs of deep venous thrombosis in 2 diagnostic categories of patients, the results of which gave a range in which the sensitivity and specificity of clinical findings are included. The first diagnostic category was 350 patients from the Prospective Investigation of Pulmonary Embolism Diagnosis (PIOPED) (15) with pulmonary embolism proven by pulmonary angiography and in whom deep venous thrombosis was estimated to be present. The second diagnostic category was 30 patients from PIOPED in whom deep venous thrombosis was diagnosed by objective leg tests of the lower extremities. The first diagnostic category is advantageous for the investigation of the sensitivity of signs of deep venous thrombosis because these patients, in general, were identified on the basis of respiratory complaints associated with pulmonary embolism. Fewer than 1 percent of these patients were referred for ventilation-perfusion scans in PIOPED because of apparent deep venous thrombosis (16). There was little bias, therefore, in the selection of patients for the evaluation of signs of deep venous thrombosis in this diagnostic category. A disadvantage of using this category, however, is that some patients may have had thromboemboli from sources other than the lower extremities. Deep venous thrombosis of the lower extremities in patients with pulmonary embolism has been documented by dissection in 83% and 91% of patients who had pulmonary embolism at autopsy (10,17). The sensitivity of signs of deep venous thrombosis in these patients with pulmonary embolism who were estimated to have deep venous thrombosis would be lower than the actual value because 9 to 17% of these patients may not have had deep venous thrombosis (10,17).

The second diagnostic category in which the sensitivity of signs of deep venous thrombosis was evaluated consisted of 30 patients with suspected pulmonary embolism in whom deep venous thrombosis was diagnosed by objective tests of the lower extremities. The advantage of this diagnostic category is that the diagnosis of deep venous thrombosis was made with confidence. The disadvantage is that bias was present in the referral of many of these patients

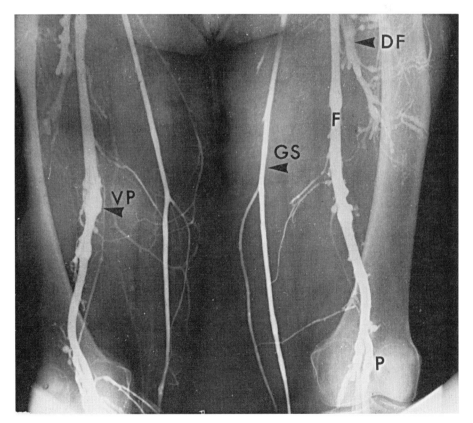

Figure 4–8. Normal postmortem venogram of the thighs (anteroposterior projection) showing the femoral (F), deep femoral (DF), greater saphenous (GS), and popliteal (P) veins. Valve pockets are shown. (Reprinted with permission from Stein PD, Evans H. An autopsy study of leg vein thrombosis. Circulation 1967;35:671–681.)

Table 4–1. SIGNS OF DEEP VENOUS THROMBOSIS

Sign	Positive Leg Test Sensitivity N/n (%)	PE+, Assumed DVT Sensitivity N/n (%)	Leg Test Neg Specificity N_1/n_1 (%)
Any Edema	14/30 (47)	79/350 (23)	40/47 (85)
Unilateral Edema	-	30/350 (9)	43/47 (91)
Bilateral Edema	-	49/350 (14)	44/47 (94)
Erythema	5/30 (17)	21/350 (6)	43/47 (91)
Calf Tender	5/30 (17)	47/350 (13)	39/47 (83)
Palpable Cord	0/30 (0)	8/350 (2)	46/47 (98)
Homans' Sign	1/30 (3)	9/350 (3)	44/47 (94)

PE = pulmonary embolism, DVT = deep venous thrombosis
N = number of patients with sign
n = number of patients with deep venous thrombosis
N_1 = number of patients with no sign
n_1 = number of patients with no deep venous thrombosis
Stein PD, Henry JW, Relyea B. Unpublished data from PIOPED.

for noninvasive leg tests. Many patients presumably had leg tests because of clinical manifestations that suggested deep venous thrombosis. This bias would increase the apparent sensitivity of clinical findings. However, among the entire group of patients in whom leg tests were performed (30 with deep venous thrombosis and 47 with no deep venous thrombosis), 48 of 77 (62%) had no qualitative signs of deep venous thrombosis, and 29 of 77 (38%) had no qualitative signs or measured asymmetry. Therefore, a significant number of patients were referred for objective leg tests only because they had a suspicion of pulmonary embolism.

The two methods of diagnosing deep venous thrombosis give an envelope of results within which the sensitivity of signs of deep venous thrombosis is likely to be accurate.

Patients with deep venous thrombosis diagnosed by objective tests had an impedance plethysmogram, Doppler ultrasound, or venogram of the lower extremities within 2 weeks of the physical clinical examination. Some patients had more than one test performed. Patients were excluded if one objective test showed deep venous thrombosis and another objective test of the same extremity showed no deep venous thrombosis.

Deep venous thrombosis was absent in 47 patients. In these patients, all objective tests of the lower extremities showed no evidence of deep venous thrombosis. In addition, these patients had no evidence of pulmonary embolism.

The individual qualitative signs of deep venous thrombosis (edema, erythema, calf tenderness, palpable cord, Homans' sign) showed a sensitivity of 47% or less, irrespective of whether deep venous thrombosis was diagnosed by objective tests of the lower extremities or whether it was assumed to be present in patients with pulmonary embolism (Table 4–1). Edema was the most sensitive sign. Unilateral edema was not statistically significantly more sensitive or specific than bilateral edema. All signs showed a specificity of 83% or higher (Table 4–1). The specificities of signs did not differ to a statistically significant extent. Calf asymmetry indicates a need for noninvasive diagnostic tests of the lower extremities to determine whether deep venous thrombosis is present (18). Asymmetry of the circumference of the ankle, calf or thigh ≥1 cm has been shown in 90% of patients with deep venous thrombosis, but such asymmetry was also shown in 92% of patients with suspected deep venous thrombosis in whom the diagnosis was excluded (14). A difference ≥3 cm of calf circumference, however, was associated with a high likelihood of having deep venous thrombosis (19,20).

We measured the circumference of the calves 10 cm below the tibial tuberosity. Asymmetry of the calves ≥1 cm was defined as a quantitative sign. A difference of circumference of the calves ≥1 cm is abnormal (18). As the difference of calf circumference increased from ≥1 cm to ≥4 cm, the sensitivity decreased from 43% or 53% to 4% or 10%, and the specificity increased from 57% to 98% (Table 4–2, Fig. 4–9).

Homans' sign is active and/or passive dorsiflexion of the foot associated with any of the following: (1) pain, (2) incomplete dorsiflexion (with equal pressure applied) to prevent pain, or (3) flexion of the knee to release tension in the posterior muscles with dorsiflexion (21). A Homans' sign was present in 44% of patients with deep venous thrombosis of the lower leg, and in 60% of patients with femoral venous thrombosis (22).

The elicitation of pain with inflation of a blood pressure cuff around the calf to 60 to 150 mm Hg has been recommended as a test for deep venous thrombosis (23). This test, however, was not shown to be more helpful than the assessment of direct tenderness or leg circumference (22).

The presence of any sign (edema, erythema, calf tenderness, palpable cord, or Homans' sign) or measured asymmetry of the calves increased the sensitivity for detection of deep venous thrombosis above the sensitivity of a physical sign alone or asymmetry alone (Table 4–3) The specificity varied inversely with the sensitivity.

The combination of a sign on physical examination (edema, erythema, calf tenderness, palpable cord, or Homans' sign) plus asymmetry was associated

Table 4–2. CALF ASYMMETRY WITH DEEP VENOUS THROMBOSIS

Circum Diff (cm)	Positive Leg Test Sensitivity N/n (%)	PE+, Assumed DVT Sensitivity N/n (%)	Leg Test Neg Specificity N_1/n_1 (%)
≥1	16/30 (53)	149/350 (43)	27/47 (57)
≥2	8/30 (27)	59/350 (17)	41/47 (87)
≥3	4/30 (13)	23/350 (7)	45/47 (96)
≥4	3/30 (10)	13/350 (4)	46/47 (98)

N = number of patients with sign
n = number of patients with deep venous thrombosis
N_1 = number of patients with no sign
n_1 = number of patients with no deep venous thrombosis
Circum Diff, circumference difference of calves, DVT = deep venous thrombosis, PE = pulmonary embolism
Stein PD, Henry JW, Relyea B. Unpublished data from PIOPED.

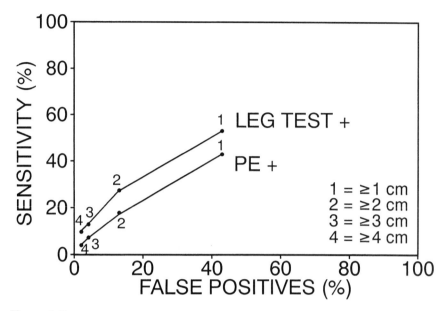

Figure 4–9.   Relation of sensitivity of measured calf asymmetry to the frequency of false positive findings. The upper curve (Leg Test +) shows data of patients in whom objective tests of the lower extremities showed deep venous thrombosis. The lower curve (PE+) shows data of patients in whom deep venous thrombosis was estimated to be present because of pulmonary embolism (PE). The numbers indicate the measured difference of calf circumference. (Stein PD, Henry JW, Relyea B. Unpublished data from PIOPED.)

Table 4–3.   SIGNS OF DEEP VENOUS THROMBOSIS AND/OR CALF ASYMMETRY

Sign +/Or Circum Diff (Cm)	Positive Leg Test Sensitivity N/n (%)	PE+, Assumed DVT Sensitivity N/n (%)	Leg Test Neg Specificity N_1/n_1 (%)
Any Sign +/or ≥1 Cm	24/30 (80)	192/350 (55)	23/47 (49)
Any Sign +/or ≥2 Cm	23/30 (67)	131/350 (37)	33/47 (70)
Any Sign +/or ≥3 Cm	19/30 (63)	111/350 (32)	35/47 (74)
Any Sign +/or ≥4 Cm	18/30 (60)	104/350 (30)	35/47 (74)

N = number of patients with sign
n = number of patients with deep venous thrombosis
N_1 = number of patients with no sign
n_1 = number of patients with no deep venous thrombosis
Circum Diff, circumference difference of calves, PE = pulmonary embolism, DVT = deep venous thrombosis
Stein PD, Henry JW, Relyea B. Unpublished data from PIOPED.

Table 4–4. IPSILATERAL SIGNS OF DEEP VENOUS THROMBOSIS AND CALF ASYMMETRY

Sign and Circum Diff (cm)	Positive Leg Test Sensitivity N/n (%)	PE+, Assumed DVT Sensitivity N/n (%)	Leg Test Neg Specificity N_1/n_1 (%)
Any sign and ≥1 cm	10/30 (33)	52/350 (15)	41/47 (87)
Any sign and ≥2 cm	5/30 (17)	27/350 (8)	43/47 (91)
Any sign and ≥3 cm	3/30 (10)	11/350 (3)	45/47 (96)
Any sign and ≥4 cm	2/30 (7)	8/350 (2)	46/47 (98)

N = number of patients with sign
n = number of patients with deep venous thrombosis
N_1 = number of patients with no sign
n_1 = number of patients with no deep venous thrombosis
Circum Diff, circumference difference of calves, PE = pulmonary embolism, DVT = deep venous thrombosis
Stein PD, Henry JW, Relyea B. Unpublished data from PIOPED.

with a sensitivity of 33% or lower, but the specificity was 87% or higher (Table 4–4). Among the 3 to 10% of patients who had one or more qualitative signs plus ≥3 cm calf asymmetry, the specificity for deep venous thrombosis was 96%. Among patients in whom deep venous thrombosis was diagnosed by objective leg tests, signs of deep venous thrombosis or measured asymmetry showed a higher sensitivity than in patients in whom deep venous thrombosis was estimated to be present because of pulmonary embolism (Fig. 4–10). If either a qualitative sign or measured asymmetry was present, the presence of one or both was more sensitive than a qualitative sign plus measured asymmetry. The former, however, showed more false positive values than qualitative signs and ipsilateral measured calf swelling. As the measured difference of calve circumferences increased from ≥1 cm to ≥4 cm in combination with qualitative signs, the sensitivity diminished, and the presence of false positive values also diminished.

The area under the receiver operating characteristic curve of patients with deep venous thrombosis diagnosed on the basis of objective leg tests was 0.7018. The area under the receiver operating characteristic curve of patients in whom deep venous thrombosis was estimated to be present because of pulmonary embolism was 0.5199. The probability, therefore, of correctly identifying a randomly selected pair of patients (one with deep venous thrombosis and another without deep venous thrombosis) was between 52% and 70% (24).

Among patients with deep venous thrombosis diagnosed by objective leg tests, 2 of 30 (7%) had leg pain, but no qualitative signs or asymmetry ≥1 cm. An additional 1 of 30 (3%) reported swelling in the leg or foot, but had no leg pain, qualitative signs, or asymmetry ≥1 cm. The sensitivity for the detection of deep venous thrombosis of one or more symptoms, qualitative signs, or asymmetry ≥1 cm was 27 of 30 (90%). Among patients with deep venous thrombosis estimated to be present on the basis of pulmonary embolism, the addition of symptoms of tenderness or swelling to the qualitative or quantitative signs increased the sensitivity for the detection of deep venous thrombosis to 229 of 350 (65%).

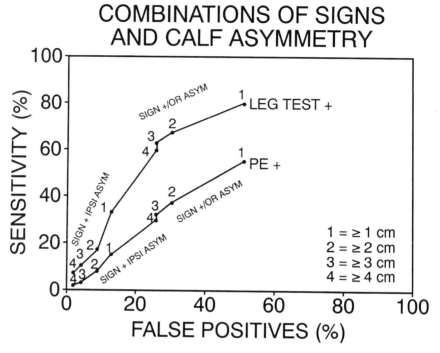

Figure 4–10. Relation of sensitivity of combinations of qualitative signs and measured calf asymmetry to the frequency of false positive findings. The upper curve (Leg Test +) shows data of patients in whom objective tests of the lower extremities showed deep venous thrombosis. The lower curve (PE+) shows data of patients in whom deep venous thrombosis was estimated to be present because of pulmonary embolism (PE). The numbers indicate the measured difference of calf circumference. Sign +/or asym indicates patients who had a qualitative sign and/or asymmetry. Sign + IPSI ASYM indicates patients who had a qualitative sign plus ipsilateral asymmetry. (Stein PD, Henry JW, Relyea B. Unpublished data from PIOPED.)

The addition of symptoms of tenderness or swelling to qualitative signs or measured asymmetry ≥1 cm decreased the specificity of one or more of any of these findings to 18 of 47 (38%).

Not all patients with pulmonary embolism have deep venous thrombosis. The heart has been reported as a source of pulmonary embolism in 8 to 17% (10,17). Thrombosis confined to the iliac vein, without involvement of the veins of the lower extremity, is uncommon (1 of 149 patients with deep venous thrombosis shown by dissection at autopsy) (25). Thrombosis confined to the inferior vena cava is equally uncommon (1 of 149) (25). Although autopsy showed deep venous thrombosis of the lower extremities in 83 to 91% of patients with pulmonary embolism (10,17), venography of the lower extremities showed deep venous thrombosis in only 71% of patients with pulmonary embolism diagnosed by pulmonary angiography (26). The identification of fewer patients with deep venous thrombosis by venography than by dissection suggests that the venogram itself may not be entirely sensitive. Regarding this possibility, dissection of the veins of the lower extremities accompanied by postmortem venograms showed that the detection of deep venous thrombosis of the veins of the calves was less reliable on postmortem venograms than deep venous thrombosis of the veins of the thighs (1).

Deep venous thrombosis of the upper extremities caused by the insertion of central venous catheters may be a source of pulmonary embolism. Among 86 patients with deep venous thrombosis of the upper extremities caused by central venous catheters, 13 (15%) developed pulmonary embolism (27). Two of these patients died of massive recurrent pulmonary embolism despite adequate therapy with heparin. In a series of 34 patients with long-term indwelling central venous catheters for parenteral nutrition, 10 patients suffered a pulmonary embolism (28).

In conclusion, regarding signs and symptoms of deep venous thrombosis of the lower extremity, combinations of qualitative signs and measured asymmetry of the calves do not reliably identify patients with deep venous thrombosis, nor does the absence of such signs exclude deep venous thrombosis. However, in occasional patients who have ≥3 cm asymmetry of the calves, the finding is 96% specific.

REFERENCES

1. Stein PD, Evans H. An autopsy study of leg vein thrombosis. Circulation 1967;35:671–681.
2. Allen EV, Barker NW, Hines EA Jr. Peripheral vascular diseases. Philadelphia: WB Saunders, 1962;559–569.
3. Hirsh J, Hull RD, Raskob GE. Clinical features and diagnosis of venous thrombosis. J Am Coll Cardiol 1986;8:114B–127B.
4. Vine HS, Hillman B, Hessel SJ. Deep venous thrombosis: predictive value of signs and symptoms. Am J Roentgenol 1981;136:167–171.
5. Barnes RW, Wu KK, Hoak JC. Fallibility of the clinical diagnosis of venous thrombosis. JAMA 1975;234:605–607.
6. Nicholas GG, Miller FJ Jr, Demuth WE Jr, et al. Clinical vascular laboratory diagnosis of deep venous thrombosis. Ann Surg 1977;186:213–215.
7. Sandler DA, Martin JF, Duncan JS, et al. Diagnosis of deep-vein thrombosis: comparison of clinical evaluation, ultrasound, plethysmography, and venoscan with x-ray venogram. Lancet 1984;2:716–719.
8. Wells PS, Hirsh J, Anderson DR, et al. Accuracy of clinical assessment of deep-vein thrombosis. Lancet 1995;345:1326–1330.
9. Sevitt S, Gallagher N. Venous thrombosis and pulmonary embolism: A clinicopathological study in injured and burned patients. Br J Surg 1961;48:475–489.
10. Byrne JJ, O'Neil EE. Fatal pulmonary emboli. A study of 130 autopsy-proven fatal emboli. Am J Surg 1952;83:47–54.
11. Milne RM, Gunn AA, Griffiths JMT, et al. Postoperative deep venous thrombosis: a comparison of diagnostic techniques. Lancet 1971;2:445–447.
12. Johnson WC. Evaluation of newer techniques for the diagnosis of venous thrombosis. J Surg Res 1974;16:473–481.
13. McLachlin J, Richards T, Paterson JC. An evaluation of clinical signs in the diagnosis of venous thrombosis. Arch Surg 1962;85:738–744.
14. Cranley JJ, Canos AJ, Sull WJ. The diagnosis of deep venous thrombosis: fallibility of clinical signs and symptoms. Arch Surg 1976;111:34–36.
15. A Collaborative Study by the PIOPED Investigators. Value of the ventilation/perfusion scan in acute pulmonary embolism: results of the Prospective Investigation of Pulmonary Embolism Diagnosis (PIOPED). JAMA 1990;263:2753–2759.
16. Stein PD, Saltzman HA, Weg JG. Clinical characteristics of patients with acute pulmonary embolism. Am J Cardiol 1991;68:1723–1724.

17. Short DS. A survey of pulmonary embolism in a general hospital. Brit Med J 1952;1:790–796.
18. Stein PD, Henry JW, Gopalakrishnan D, et al. Asymmetry of the calves in the assessment of patients with suspected acute pulmonary embolism. Chest 1995;107:936–939.
19. Lambie JM, Mahaffy RG, Barber DC, et al. Diagnostic accuracy in venous thrombosis. Brit Med J 1970;2:142–143.
20. Nypaver TJ, Shepard AD, Kiell CS, et al. Outpatient duplex scanning for deep vein thrombosis: parameters predictive of a negative study result. J Vasc Surg 1993;18:821–826.
21. Homans J. Disease of the veins. New Engl J Med 1944;231:51–60.
22. DeWeese JA, Rogoff SM. Phlebographic patterns of acute deep venous thrombosis of the leg. Surgery 1963;53:99–108.
23. Lowenberg RI. Early diagnosis of phlebothrombosis with aid of a new clinical test. JAMA 1954;155:1566.
24. Hanley JA, McNeil BJ. The meaning and use of the area under a receiver operating characteristic (ROC) curve. Radiology 1982;143:29–36.
25. Gibbs NM. Venous thrombosis of the lower limbs with particular reference to bed-rest. Brit J Surg 1957;45:209–236.
26. Hull RD, Hirsh J, Carter CJ, et al. Pulmonary angiography, ventilation lung scanning, and venography for clinically suspected pulmonary embolism with abnormal perfusion lung scan. Ann Intern Med 1983;98:891–899.
27. Monreal M, Raventos A, Lerma R, et al. Pulmonary embolism in patients with upper extremity DVT associated to venous central lines—a prospective study. Thromb Haemost 1994;72:548–550.
28. Dollery CM, Sullivan ID, Bauraind O, et al. Thrombosis and embolism in long-term central venous access for parenteral nutrition. Lancet 1994;344:1043–1045.

CHAPTER 5

The History and Physical Examination in Patients with No Prior Cardiopulmonary Disease

The clinical manifestations of pulmonary embolism are recognized to be nonspecific. When considered together, however, they can strongly suggest the need for further diagnostic evaluation (1,2).

To characterize the diagnostic features of the history and physical examination in patients with acute pulmonary embolism, it is useful to evaluate patients in whom the diagnosis is not confused by pre-existing cardiac or pulmonary disease. In such patients, the features of acute pulmonary embolism become clear, and manifestations related to coexistent disease are excluded.

We evaluated patients who had no history or evidence of pre-existing cardiac or pulmonary disease and who participated in the national collaborative Prospective Investigation of Pulmonary Embolism Diagnosis (PIOPED) (3). There were 117 patients with pulmonary embolism diagnosed by pulmonary angiography or autopsy. Pulmonary embolism was excluded in 248 patients. Pulmonary embolism was excluded by a normal pulmonary angiogram in 176 patients and by the absence of adverse events over the course of 1 year in 72 patients who did not receive anticoagulant therapy (4).

Patients with pulmonary embolism were 54 ± 17 years of age (mean ± standard deviation). Patients in whom pulmonary embolism was excluded were younger, 48 ± 17 years of age (P<.01). Among the patients with pulmonary embolism, 57 of 117 (49%) were males. Among those in whom pulmonary embolism was excluded, 80 of 248 (32%) were males.

Patients were considered to have no pre-existing cardiac or pulmonary disease if they had no history or evidence of valvular heart disease, coronary artery disease, myocardial infarction, "other heart disease," or if before this acute episode they had not suffered left or right-sided congestive heart failure. Such patients had no history of asthma, chronic obstructive pulmonary disease, interstitial lung disease, or "other lung disease" and no recognized acute pneu-

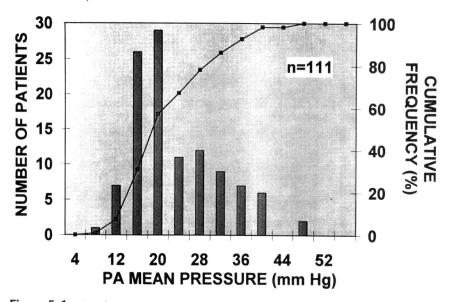

Figure 5–1. Distribution and cumulative frequency of pulmonary artery (PA) mean pressure among randomized patients with pulmonary embolism and no prior cardiopulmonary disease. (Data are from Stein PD, Relyea B, and previously unpublished from PIOPED.)

monia or acute respiratory distress syndrome at the time of the evaluation for suspected pulmonary embolism. These patients also had no previous history of pulmonary embolism.

The pulmonary artery mean pressure exceeded the upper limits of normal (20 mm Hg) in only 42% of 111 randomized patients with no prior cardiopulmonary disease in whom measurements were obtained (Fig. 5–1) (Stein PD, Relyea B. Unpublished data from PIOPED). Pulmonary artery mean pressure was 30 mm Hg or higher in only 15% of these patients. Right atrial mean pressure was less than the upper limits of normal (8 mm Hg) in 75% of 109 patients with pulmonary embolism and no prior cardiopulmonary disease (Fig. 5–2). Right atrial mean pressure was rarely elevated in patients in whom the pulmonary artery mean pressure was normal. Even among patients in whom pulmonary artery mean pressure exceeded 20 mm Hg, a poor correlation existed with right atrial mean pressure (r = 0.11).

Predisposing Factors

Immobilization, irrespective of cause, was the most prevalent predisposing factor. Data from PIOPED (3) indicate, as others have shown (5), that immobilization of even 1 or 2 days may predispose to pulmonary embolism. Among 117 patients with pulmonary embolism who had no pre-existing cardiac or pulmonary disease, immobilization usually from surgery occurred in 56% of patients (Table 5–1) (3). Among the 66 patients in whom immobilization was a predisposing factor, 43 (65%) were immobilized ≥ 2 weeks. Immobilization of 2 days or less preceded pulmonary embolism in 8 of 117 (7%). A history of

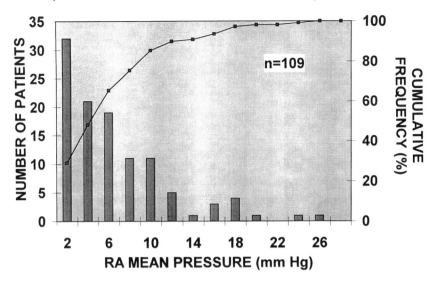

Figure 5–2. Distribution and cumulative frequency of right atrial (RA) mean pressure among randomized patients with pulmonary embolism and no prior cardiopulmonary disease. (Data are from Stein PD, Relyea B, and previously unpublished from PIOPED.)

Table 5–1. PREDISPOSING FACTORS IN PATIENTS WITH PULMONARY EMBOLISM AND NO PREVIOUS CARDIAC OR PULMONARY DISEASE

	Number	(%)
Immobilization	66	(56)
Surgery	63	(54)
Malignancy	27	(23)
Thrombophlebitis, ever	16	(14)
Trauma—lower extremities	12	(10)
Estrogen	10	(9)
Stroke	8	(7)
Postpartum ≤3 mo.	5	(4)

Modified and reprinted with permission from Stein PD, Terrin ML, Hales CA, et al. Clinical, laboratory, roentgenographic and electrocardiographic findings in patients with acute pulmonary embolism and no pre-existing cardiac or pulmonary disease. Chest 1991;100:598–603.

neoplasia occurred in 23% and a history of thrombophlebitis occurred in 14% of patients with pulmonary embolism and no prior cardiac or pulmonary disease. Stroke, estrogen therapy, or trauma of the leg occurred in 7 to 10% of patients with pulmonary embolism. Only 4% were ≤ 3 months postpartum (Table 5–1).

PULMONARY EMBOLISM AND NO PRIOR CARDIOPULMONARY DISEASE (n=117)

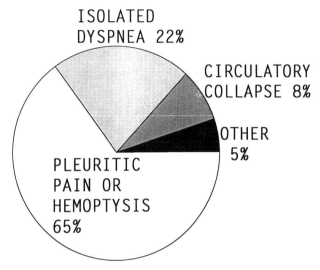

Figure 5–3.   Presenting syndromes of acute pulmonary embolism among patients with no prior cardiopulmonary disease.

One or more of these predisposing factors were present in 96 of 117 (82%) of patients with pulmonary embolism and in 162 of 248 (65%) with no pulmonary embolism (P=.001).

Syndromes of Acute Pulmonary Embolism

Consideration of the diagnosis of pulmonary embolism in terms of its presenting syndrome may focus one's thinking about the diverse manifestations of pulmonary embolism. The syndrome of pleuritic pain or hemoptysis, in the absence of circulatory collapse, was the most prevalent mode of presentation of patients with acute pulmonary embolism and no pre-existing cardiac or pulmonary disease (3). It occurred in 76 of 117 (65%) (Fig. 5–3). A syndrome of dyspnea in the absence of hemoptysis or pleuritic pain or circulatory collapse occurred in 26 of 117 (22%). Circulatory collapse (systolic blood pressure < 80 mm Hg or loss of consciousness) was an uncommon mode of presentation (9 of 117) (8%).

The syndrome of pleuritic pain or hemoptysis was the most prevalent syndrome (or perhaps the most readily diagnosed). This syndrome occurred in 65% of PIOPED patients with no pre-existing cardiac or pulmonary disease,

Table 5–2. SYMPTOMS IN PATIENTS WITH PULMONARY EMBOLISM
AND NO PRE-EXISTING CARDIAC OR PULMONARY DISEASE

	Number	(%)
Dyspnea	85	(73)
Pleuritic pain	77	(66)
Cough	43	(37)
Leg swelling	33	(28)
Leg pain	30	(26)
Hemoptysis	15	(13)
Palpitations	12	(10)
Wheezing	10	(9)
Angina-like pain	5	(4)

Modified and reprinted with permission from Stein PD, Terrin ML, Hales CA, et al. Clinical, laboratory, roentgeno-graphic and electrocardiographic findings in patients with acute pulmonary embolism and no pre-existing cardiac or pulmonary disease. Chest 1991;100:598–603.

and it occurred in 66% of patients enrolled in the Urokinase Pulmonary Embolism Trial (UPET) (6). The syndrome of uncomplicated dyspnea perhaps was overlooked in some patients because of its nonspecificity. In PIOPED, circulatory collapse was less frequent than reported among UPET patients with no pre-existing cardiac or pulmonary disease (8% versus 19%). This may reflect the selection of more severe patients for UPET. In UPET, patients were selected only if the pulmonary embolism was large enough to involve at least one segmental artery, which was defined as submassive pulmonary embolism (6).

Symptoms of Acute Pulmonary Embolism

Among 117 patients with pulmonary embolism and no prior cardiac or pulmonary disease, dyspnea was the most common symptom, occurring in 73% (Table 5–2) (3). Pleuritic chest pain (66% of patients with pulmonary embolism) occurred much more often than hemoptysis (13% of patients with pulmonary embolism).

Cough was common (37%) among patients with pulmonary embolism. The cough, when present, was nonspecific. It may have been nonproductive, or productive of purulent or bloody sputum. When hemoptysis occurred, the sputum typically was blood-streaked, but can be pure blood or blood-tinged. Hemoptysis occurred in 13% of patients with pulmonary embolism. Purulent sputum was present in 7% with pulmonary embolism.

The relation of the sensitivity of individual symptoms (percent of patients with pulmonary embolism who had the particular symptoms) to the percent of false positives among patients who did not have pulmonary embolism is shown in Figure 5–4.

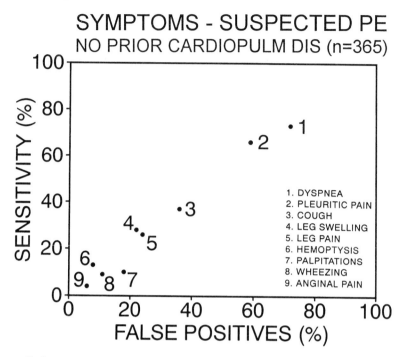

Figure 5–4. Sensitivity and frequency of false positive symptoms in patients with suspected acute pulmonary embolism (PE) who had no prior cardiopulmonary disease (cardiopulm dis). The numbers refer to the individual symptoms shown in the insert.

Dyspnea was somewhat less frequent among PIOPED patients (73%) than among UPET patients with no prior cardiopulmonary disease (84%). This may relate to the greater severity of pulmonary embolism in UPET (6).

The angina-like pain that occurred in patients with pulmonary embolism did not radiate to either arm or to the jaw, and this may help distinguish it from true angina. Angina-like chest pain occurred in only 5 of 117 patients (4%) with pulmonary embolism and no prior cardiac or pulmonary disease. It was usually located in the anterior chest (4 of 5). The angina-like pain was described as heavy in 4 of these patients.

Signs of Acute Pulmonary Embolism

Tachypnea (respiratory rate ≥ 20/min) was the most common sign of acute pulmonary embolism among patients with no prior cardiac or pulmonary disease (70% of patients) (Table 5–3) (3). Tachycardia (heart rate > 100/min) occurred in 30% of patients with pulmonary embolism. The pulmonary component of the second sound was accentuated in 23% of patients with pulmonary embolism. Deep venous thrombosis was clinically apparent in 11%. A right ventricular lift, third heart sound, or pleural friction rub were uncommon, each occurring ≤ 4% of patients with pulmonary embolism. The relation of the sensitivity of

Table 5–3.   SIGNS OF ACUTE PULMONARY EMBOLISM IN PATIENTS
WITH NO PRE-EXISTING CARDIAC OR PULMONARY DISEASE
(n = 117)

	Number	(%)
Tachypnea (≥20/min)	82	(70)
Rales (crackles)	60	(51)
Tachycardia (>100/min)	35	(30)
Fourth heart sound	28	(24)
Increased pulmonary component of second sound	27	(23)
Deep venous thrombosis	13	(11)
Diaphoresis	13	(11)
Temperature >38.5°C	8	(7)
Wheezes	6	(5)
Homans' sign	5	(4)
Right ventricular lift	5	(4)
Pleural friction rub	3	(3)
Third heart sound	3	(3)
Cyanosis	1	(1)

Modified and reprinted with permission from Stein PD, Terrin ML, Hales CA, et al. Clinical, laboratory, roentgeno-graphic and electrocardiographic findings in patients with acute pulmonary embolism and no pre-existing cardiac or pulmonary disease. Chest 1991;100:598–603.

individual signs (percent of patients with pulmonary embolism who had the particular signs) to the percent of false positives among patients who did not have pulmonary embolism is shown in Figure 5–5.

Rales (crackles) were heard in 60 of 117 patients with pulmonary embolism (51%). Most patients with pulmonary embolism who had rales (53 of 60) (88%) had pulmonary parenchymal abnormalities, atelectasis or a pleural effusion on the chest radiograph. Rales, therefore, appeared to relate to the effects of pulmonary infarction or atelectasis.

A larger percent of patients (85%) with no prior cardiopulmonary disease were tachypneic in the Urokinase Pulmonary Trial (UPET) (6) than were observed in PIOPED (3). This may relate to the greater severity of pulmonary embolism in UPET. The UPET included only patients with massive or submassive pulmonary embolism (6). Among patients in UPET with no prior cardiopulmonary disease, the most severe pulmonary embolism, as assessed by pulmonary arteriography, occurred in patients with shock or syncope (1). In patients with uncomplicated dyspnea, the severity of pulmonary embolism was almost as great. Patients with the pulmonary hemorrhage/infarction syndrome had the least severe pulmonary embolism (1).

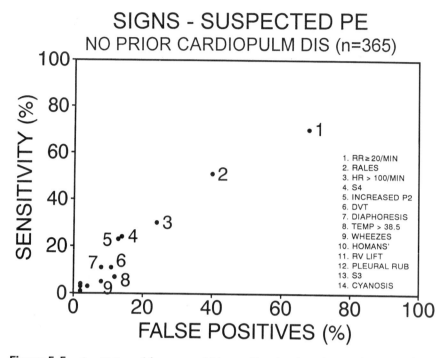

SIGNS - SUSPECTED PE
NO PRIOR CARDIOPULM DIS (n=365)

1. RR ≥ 20/MIN
2. RALES
3. HR > 100/MIN
4. S4
5. INCREASED P2
6. DVT
7. DIAPHORESIS
8. TEMP > 38.5
9. WHEEZES
10. HOMANS'
11. RV LIFT
12. PLEURAL RUB
13. S3
14. CYANOSIS

Figure 5–5.   Sensitivity and frequency of false positive signs in patients with suspected acute pulmonary embolism (PE) who had no prior cardiopulmonary disease (cardiopulm dis). The numbers refer to the individual signs shown in the insert.

Syncope was more frequent in patients with massive pulmonary embolism than submassive pulmonary embolism (17% versus 4%) (1). Strikingly, among patients in shock from pulmonary embolism, only 71% were dyspneic and only 38% had pleuritic pain. Apprehension, diaphoresis, and tachypnea were more frequent with massive pulmonary embolism than with submassive pulmonary embolism. However, patients with submassive pulmonary embolism, compared with patients with massive pulmonary embolism, more often had pleuritic pain (85% versus 67%) or a pleural friction rub (26% versus 14%).

Combinations of Signs and Symptoms

Dyspnea or tachypnea (respiratory rate ≥ 20/min) was present in 105 of 117 patients (90%) with pulmonary embolism (Fig. 5–6) (3). Dyspnea, tachypnea, or signs of deep venous thrombosis were present in 107 of 117 (91%). Dyspnea, tachypnea, or pleuritic pain was present in 113 of 117 (97%). Dyspnea, tachypnea, pleuritic pain, radiographic evidence of atelectasis, or a parenchymal abnormality was present in 115 of 117 (98%). The remaining 2% had either deep venous thrombosis or an unexplained low PaO_2. The prevalence of various

PATIENTS WITH PULMONARY EMBOLISM AND NO PRIOR CARDIOPULMONARY DISEASE
(n=117)

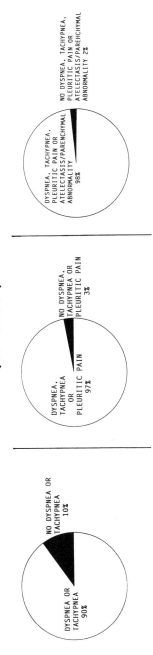

Figure 5–6. Combinations of signs and symptoms in patients with acute pulmonary embolism and no prior cardiopulmonary disease.

Table 5–4.   CLINICAL ASSESSMENT PATIENTS WITH NO PREVIOUS
CARDIAC OR PULMONARY DISEASE

Clinical Assessment	Pulmonary Embolism (Assessment by Fellow) PE/n (%)	Pulmonary Embolism (Assessment by Staff) PE/n (%)
High Probability	26/41 (63)	15/17 (88)
Intermediate Probability	47/99 (47)	74/200 (37)
Low Probability	8/74 (11)	14/103 (14)

PE = pulmonary embolism
n = number of patients
Differences between assessments by fellows and staff were not significant
Data are from Stein PD, Terrin ML, Hales CA, et al. Clinical, laboratory, roentgenographic and electrocardiographic findings in patients with acute pulmonary embolism and no preexisting cardiac or pulmonary disease. Chest 1991;100:598–603.

signs and symptoms and their combinations was comparable among patients with and without pulmonary embolism. Conversely, in the absence of some manifestations, particularly dyspnea, tachypnea or pleuritic pain, pulmonary embolism was rarely diagnosed by angiography (3).

Comparable observations among patients with no prior cardiopulmonary disease were also made in the Urokinase Pulmonary Embolism Trial (6). Either dyspnea or tachypnea (respiratory rate ≥ 20/min) occurred in 90% of patients in PIOPED (3), but this combination was observed in 96% of patients with no pre-existing cardiac or pulmonary disease in UPET (6). These observations may relate to the greater severity of pulmonary embolism among patients in UPET. Dyspnea, hemoptysis, or pleuritic pain occurred in 97% of PIOPED patients and in 94% UPET patients. Either dyspnea, tachypnea, or signs of deep venous thrombosis in the present PIOPED were observed in 91% of patients; this combination was nearly universal in patients with no pre-existing cardiac or pulmonary disease in UPET, occurring in 99%.

Clinical Assessment

Based on clinical assessment, physicians were more consistent in their ability to exclude pulmonary embolism than they were in their ability to make the diagnosis of pulmonary embolism. In the majority of patients, however, physicians were suspicious of the diagnosis of pulmonary embolism, but were not confident in their assessment. Senior staff correctly diagnosed pulmonary embolism in 15 of 17 patients (88%) in whom their clinical assessment indicated a high probability of pulmonary embolism, and fellows correctly diagnosed pulmonary embolism in 26 of 41 (63%) (Table 5–4) (3). This difference in the ability to diagnose pulmonary embolism did not differ significantly between staff and fellows. Fellows were able to correctly exclude pulmonary embolism in 66 of 74 patients (89%), and staff were able to correctly exclude pulmonary embolism in 89 of 103 (86%) of patients in whom their clinical assessment indicated a low probability of pulmonary embolism. The fellows were more

Table 5–5. RELATION BETWEEN SIGNS, SYMPTOMS, RIGHT-SIDED PRESSURES AND PaO$_2$

	PA Mean (mm Hg)	RA Mean (mm Hg)	P$_a$O$_2$ (mm Hg)
Dyspnea	23 ± 9 (n = 121)	6 ± 5 (n = 114)	69 ± 14 (n = 98)
Pleuritic pain	21 ± 8 (n = 115)	5 ± 4 (n = 114)	73 ± 14 (n = 97)
Cough	24 ± 9 (n = 68)	6 ± 5 (n = 63)	71 ± 13 (n = 54)
Hemoptysis	22 ± 8 (n = 24)	5 ± 5 (n = 24)	74 ± 14 (n = 23)
Palpitations	27 ± 10 (n = 18)	6 ± 6 (n = 15)	64 ± 15 (n = 15)
Wheezing	21 ± 7 (n = 16)	4 ± 3 (n = 14)	70 ± 15 (n = 13)
Angina-like pain	25 ± 14 (n = 9)	3 ± 3 (n = 6)	62 ± 9 (n = 8)
Tachypnea	22 ± 9 (n = 118)	6 ± 5 (n = 112)	69 ± 15 (n = 95)
Rales	22 ± 8 (n = 81)	6 ± 4 (n = 78)	68 ± 14 (n = 68)
Tachycardia	24 ± 9 (n = 59)	7 ± 5 (n = 53)	69 ± 17 (n = 42)
Increased P2	23 ± 9 (n = 42)	6 ± 5 (n = 40)	67 ± 14 (n = 33)
Diaphoresis	26 ± 11 (n = 16)	8 ± 7 (n = 14)	61 ± 15 (n = 12)
RV Lift	28 ± 12 (n = 3)	8 ± 9 (n = 3)	67 ± 23 (n = 4)
Friction Rub	21 ± 8 (n = 6)	9 ± 6 (n = 6)	67 ± 4 (n = 5)
Third Sound	39 ± 2 (n = 3)	12 ± 8 (n = 4)	72 ± 9 (n = 3)

values are mean ± standard deviation
PA, pulmonary artery
RA, right atrium
RV, right ventricle
PaO$_2$, partial pressure of oxygen in arterial blood in patients breathing room air
P$_2$ = pulmonary component of second sound
Stein PD, Relyea B. Unpublished from PIOPED.

accurate in their ability to exclude pulmonary embolism than in their ability to diagnose pulmonary embolism (P<.001). Senior staff were uncertain of the diagnosis in more than half the patients they evaluated (200 of 320); and fellows were uncertain in almost half the patients they evaluated (99 of 214). The clinical assessment of the likelihood of acute pulmonary embolism was based upon all available noninvasive data with the exception of the ventilation-perfusion scan. The basis for arriving at the clinical likelihood estimate was individual clinical judgment, and not any specific predetermined criteria.

The initial identification of these patients by their attending physicians was based upon informed clinical judgment. Symptoms and signs of pulmonary embolism, therefore, would be expected among those in whom the diagnosis was suspected but subsequently excluded. Also, unusual presentations, not known to be suggestive of pulmonary embolism, may have been overlooked.

The relation of signs and symptoms to pulmonary artery mean pressure, right atrial mean pressure, and the partial pressure of oxygen in arterial blood (PaO$_2$) while breathing room air is shown in Table 5–5 (Stein PD, Relyea B. Unpublished data from PIOPED). In order to expand the database, we included both randomized and referred patients among the group with no prior cardiopulmonary disease. The pulmonary artery mean pressure was lowest in patients with pleuritic chest pain, and highest in those with a third heart sound, right ventricular lift, diaphoresis, and palpitations. A few statistically significant differences were shown at the P<0.01 level. The pulmonary artery mean pressure was higher in patients with a third heart sound than in patients with the following signs and symptoms who did not have a third heart sound: pleural friction rub, accentuated pulmonary component of the second sound, tachycardia, tachypnea, wheezing, hemoptysis, cough, pleuritic pain, and dyspnea. Patients with pleuritic pain had a lower pulmonary artery mean pressure than patients with palpitations and patients with tachypnea who did not have pleuritic pain. A poor correlation existed between pulmonary artery mean pressure and the PaO$_2$ (Fig. 5–7).

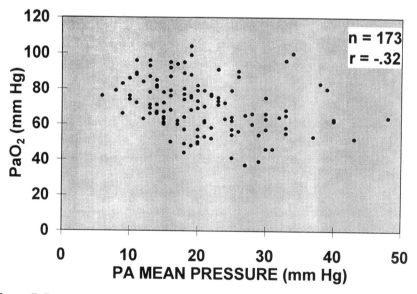

Figure 5–7. Relation of the partial pressure of oxygen in arterial blood (PaO$_2$) while breathing room air to the pulmonary artery (PA) mean pressure in patients with no prior cardiopulmonary disease. Both randomized and referred patients are included. (Data are from Stein PD, Relyea B, and previously unpublished from PIOPED.)

In conclusion, it is critical to recognize that important clues to the identification of acute pulmonary embolism are based upon nonspecific characteristics of the patient's history and physical examination. Among the patients in whom pulmonary embolism was identified, only a small percent did not have a number of important manifestations or combinations of manifestations. Clinical assessment is useful for the identification of patients for whom ventilation-perfusion scans are required and for whom angiography may be necessary.

REFERENCES

1. Stein PD, Willis PW III, DeMets DL. History and physical examination in acute pulmonary embolism in patients without pre-existing cardiac or pulmonary disease. Am J Cardiol 1981;47:218–223.
2. Wenger NK, Stein PD, Willis PW III. Massive acute pulmonary embolism: the deceivingly nonspecific manifestations. JAMA 1972;220:843–844.
3. Stein PD, Terrin ML, Hales CA, et al. Clinical, laboratory, roentgenographic and electrocardiographic findings in patients with acute pulmonary embolism and no pre-existing cardiac or pulmonary disease. Chest 1991;100:598–603.
4. The PIOPED Investigators. Value of the ventilation- perfusion scan in acute pulmonary embolism: results of the Prospective Investigation of Pulmonary Embolism Diagnosis (PIOPED). JAMA 1990;263:2753–2759.
5. Coon WW, Coller FA. Some epidemiologic considerations of thromboembolism. Surg Gynecol Obstet 1959;109:487–501.
6. National Cooperative Study. The Urokinase Pulmonary Embolism Trial. Circulation 1973;47/48(Suppl II):II-18–II-24, II-81–II-85.

CHAPTER 6

The History and Physical Examination in All Patients Irrespective of Prior Cardiopulmonary Disease

Evaluation of the clinical characteristics of acute pulmonary embolism in patients with no prior cardiopulmonary disease is particularly useful because it eliminates patients whose clinical findings may be caused by underlying disease as well as acute pulmonary embolism. Such an evaluation of the history and physical examination was made in Chapter 5. In this chapter, the characteristics of the history and physical examination in all patients with suspected acute pulmonary embolism are evaluated to know the clinical findings in the entire population of patients with suspected pulmonary embolism.

Data are from the Prospective Investigation of Pulmonary Embolism Diagnosis (PIOPED) (1), and include patients who were randomized for pulmonary angiography as described in the primary PIOPED report and patients who were referred for angiography. Referred patients were not described in the original PIOPED report. The patients with acute pulmonary embolism were 58 ± 17 years of age (mean ± standard deviation) and 54% were men (2).

Predisposing Factors

Predisposing factors are shown in Table 6–1. Immobilization was the most frequent predisposing factor, and surgery was the usual cause of immobilization. Although smoking was not included in Table 6–1 of predisposing factors, 54% of patients with pulmonary embolism had smoked at one time or continued to smoke at the time of their pulmonary embolism.

Syndromes of Acute Pulmonary Embolism

The syndrome of pleuritic pain or hemoptysis, in the absence of circulatory collapse, was the most frequent mode of presentation of patients with acute

Table 6–1. PREDISPOSING FACTORS ALL PATIENTS WITH PULMONARY EMBOLISM IRRESPECTIVE OF PREVIOUS CARDIAC OR PULMONARY DISEASE (n = 383)

	Number	(%)
Immobilization	206	(54)
Surgery	160	(42)
Lung disease	104	(27)
Malignancy	69	(18)
Coronary heart disease	76	(20)
Thrombophlebitis, ever	71	(19)
Myocardial infarction	48	(13)
Trauma—lower extremities	47	(12)
Heart failure	45	(12)
COPD	37	(10)
Stroke	37	(10)
Asthma	27	(7)
Pneumonia, acute	27	(7)
Prior pulmonary embolism	23	(6)
Estrogen	22	(6)
Collagen vascular disease	15	(4)
Postpartum ≤3 mos.	9	(2)
Interstitial lung disease	6	(2)

Unpublished data from PIOPED. COPD = chronic obstructive pulmonary disease

pulmonary embolism (2). It occurred in 60% of patients with acute pulmonary embolism (Fig. 6–1). The syndrome of dyspnea in the absence of hemoptysis, pleuritic pain or circulatory collapse occurred in 25% of patients with acute pulmonary embolism. Circulatory collapse (systolic blood pressure < 80 mm Hg or loss of consciousness) was an uncommon mode of presentation.

Symptoms of Acute Pulmonary Embolism

Among 383 patients with acute pulmonary embolism, dyspnea was the most common symptom, occurring in 78% (Table 6–2) (2). Pleuritic chest pain was observed in 59% of patients with pulmonary embolism. Cough was common and occurred in 43% of patients with pulmonary embolism.

Signs of Acute Pulmonary Embolism

Tachypnea (respiratory rate ≥ 20/min) was the most common sign of acute pulmonary embolism and was observed in 73% (Table 6–3) (2). Rales were

ALL PATIENTS WITH PULMONARY EMBOLISM (n=383)

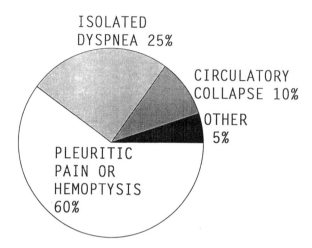

Figure 6–1. Presenting syndromes of acute pulmonary embolism among patients with all patients, irrespective of prior cardiopulmonary disease.

Table 6–2. SYMPTOMS ALL PATIENTS WITH PULMONARY EMBOLISM IRRESPECTIVE OF PRIOR CARDIOPULMONARY DISEASE

	Pulmonary Embolism (n = 383)	Number (%)
Dyspnea	299	(78)
Pleuritic pain	225	(59)
Cough	166	(43)
Leg swelling	118	(31)
Leg pain	103	(27)
Hemoptysis	62	(16)
Wheezing	54	(14)
Palpitations	48	(13)
Angina-like pain	23	(6)

Unpublished data from PIOPED and data from Stein and associates (2).

detected in 55% of patients with acute pulmonary embolism. Tachycardia (heart rate > 100/min) occurred in 30% of patients with pulmonary embolism.

In all patients in the Urokinase Pulmonary Embolism Trial, irrespective of the presence or absence of prior cardiopulmonary disease, syncope, accentu-

Table 6–3.   SIGNS OF ACUTE PULMONARY EMBOLISM IN ALL PATIENTS IRRESPECTIVE OF PRIOR CARDIOPULMONARY DISEASE

	Pulmonary Embolism (n = 383)	Number (%)
Tachypnea (20/min)	278	(73)
Rales (crackles)	210	(55)
Tachycardia (100/min)	115	(30)
Increased pulmonary component of second sound	87	(23)
Deep venous thrombosis	56	(15)
Wheezes	44	(11)
Diaphoresis	38	(10)
Temperature 38.5°C	27	(7)
Pleural friction rub	17	(4)
Third heart sound	21	(5)
Cyanosis	13	(3)
Homans' sign	10	(3)

Unpublished data from PIOPED and data from Stein and associates (2).

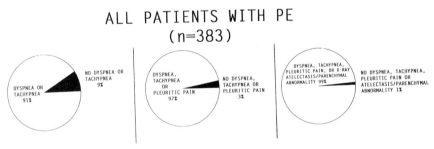

ALL PATIENTS WITH PE
(n=383)

Figure 6–2.   Combinations of signs and symptoms in patients with acute pulmonary embolism in all patients, irrespective of prior cardiopulmonary disease.

ated pulmonary component of the second sound, third or fourth heart sound (S_3 or S_4), and cyanosis, were more frequent among patients with massive PE than submassive PE (3). Pleuritic pain, however, was less frequent among patients with massive PE than submassive PE.

Combinations of Signs and Symptoms

Among 383 patients with acute pulmonary embolism, dyspnea or tachypnea (respiratory rate ≥ 20/min) was present in 91% (Fig. 6–2)(2). Dyspnea, tachypnea, or pleuritic pain were present in 97%. Dyspnea, tachypnea, pleuritic pain, unexplained radiographic evidence of atelectasis, or a parenchymal abnormality was observed in 99% of patients with pulmonary embolism. All patients with acute pulmonary embolism had dyspnea, tachypnea, pleuritic pain, unexplained radiographic evidence of atelectasis, a parenchymal abnormality, or an unexplained low PaO_2.

The characteristics of the history and physical examination were not specific for pulmonary embolism. The frequency of individual signs and symptoms in patients with pulmonary embolism did not differ to a statistically significant extent from signs and symptoms in patients in whom pulmonary embolism was suspected, but excluded. This is expected, because patients with suspected pulmonary embolism were identified for further diagnostic studies on the basis of signs and symptoms that suggested acute pulmonary embolism. As in patients with no prior cardiopulmonary disease (4), important nonspecific features of the history, physical examination, chest radiograph, and electrocardiogram, particularly in a patient who has been immobilized, combined with a high level of awareness of the possibility of pulmonary embolism, may lead to further diagnostic tests and a correct diagnosis.

REFERENCES

1. The PIOPED Investigators. Value of the ventilation-perfusion scan in acute pulmonary embolism: results of the Prospective Investigation of Pulmonary Embolism Diagnosis (PIOPED). JAMA 1990;263:2753–2759.
2. Stein PD, Saltzman HA, Weg JG. Clinical characteristics of patients with acute pulmonary embolism. Am J Cardiol 1991;68:1723–1724.
3. National Cooperative Study. The Urokinase Pulmonary Embolism Trial. Associated laboratory and clinical findings. Circulation 1973;47/48(Suppl II):II-81–II-85.
4. Stein PD, Terrin ML, Hales CA, et al. Clinical, laboratory, roentgenographic and electrocardiographic findings in patients with acute pulmonary embolism and no pre-existing cardiac or pulmonary disease. Chest 1991;100:598–603.

CHAPTER 7

The Electrocardiogram

In 1935, McGinn and White described the electrocardiograms of seven patients with acute cor pulmonale secondary to pulmonary embolism (1). They described the presence of a Q wave and late inversion of the T wave in lead III and a low origin of the T wave with a gradual staircase ascent of the ST segment in lead II. They also noted an S wave in lead I. Their description of the $S_1Q_3T_3$ complex became a traditional electrocardiographic manifestation of acute cor pulmonale. This observation was expanded by Murnaghan and associates (2) in 1943 with the report of 10 additional patients with acute cor pulmonale and no prior heart disease. An $S_1Q_3T_3$ pattern was again observed, sometimes associated with right axis deviation. Some of the patients showed a depressed ST segment; others showed ST segment elevation (2). However, even in the presence of pre-existent cardiac disease, these electrocardiographic indications of acute cor pulmonale were present in only about one-third of patients. Based upon studies of patients, and of dogs, Love and associates, in 1938, concluded that the typical electrocardiogram of pulmonary embolism was ST segment depression and T wave inversion (3).

Transient right bundle branch block in pulmonary embolism was reported in 1939 (4). Wood (5), and subsequently others (6–9), reported sharp T wave inversion in the precordial leads facing the right ventricle. Clockwise rotation was described by Wilson and associates in 1947 (10) and was later confirmed (9). A shift of the transitional zone to the left and evidence of incomplete right bundle branch block helped to distinguish the prominent Q waves of pulmonary embolism from those of myocardial infarction (7–11). P pulmonale in acute pulmonary embolism was described by Katz in 1946 (12).

By 1940, Sokolow and associates stated that no single electrocardiographic abnormality is consistently present in pulmonary embolism (13). Sokolow and associates, in a study of 50 patients, found that a large percentage had either normal electrocardiograms or nonspecific changes (13). The distinctive pattern described by McGinn and White occurred only in 10% of patients (1).

The prevalence of various electrocardiographic abnormalities in 90 patients with massive or submassive pulmonary embolism and in 89 patients with mild

Table 7–1. ELECTROCARDIOGRAPHIC MANIFESTATIONS: PATIENTS WITHOUT PRIOR CARDIAC OR PULMONARY DISEASE

Electrocardiogram	Pulmonary Embolism (%)	
	Mild to Massive (n = 89)*	Submassive to Massive (n = 90)**
Normal electrocardiogram	30	13
Rhythm disturbances		
Atrial flutter	1	0
Atrial fibrillation	4	0
Atrial premature contractions	4	2
Ventricular premature contractions	4	3
P Wave		
P pulmonale	2	6
QRS abnormalities		
Right axis deviation	2	7
Left axis deviation	13	7
Clockwise rotation (V5)	—	7
$S_1S_2S_3$	—	7
$S_1Q_3T_3$	—	12
Incomplete right bundle branch block	4	6
Complete right bundle branch block	6	9
Right ventricular hypertrophy	2	6
Pseudoinfarction	3	11
Low voltage (frontal plane)	3	6
ST segment and T wave		
Nonspecific T wave	—	42
ST segment depression	—	26
ST segment elevation	—	16
Nonspecific ST segment or T wave	49	—

Some patients had more than one abnormality.
* Data from Stein et al (15). **Data from Stein et al (14).

to massive pulmonary embolism, all of whom had no prior cardiopulmonary disease, is shown in Table 7–1 (14,15). Definitions of the various electrocardiographic abnormalities are shown in Table 7–2 (14). The electrocardiographic abnormalities observed in the patients with no prior cardiopulmonary disease who had submassive or massive pulmonary embolism were comparable to the electrocardiographic changes observed in patients with no prior cardiopulmonary disease in whom the severity of the pulmonary embolism ranged from mild to severe (Table 7–1)(15).

A normal electrocardiogram was shown in only 6% of patients with massive acute pulmonary embolism, whereas in those with submassive acute pulmonary embolism, it was normal in 23%. Although this would appear to suggest a trend, the difference was not statistically significant. In patients with mild to massive

Table 7–2.

Abnormalities of the P Wave
  Right atrial enlargement. The P wave was considered to be suggestive of right atrial enlargement if it was 0.25 mV (2.5 mm) in the extremity leads or over 0.15 mV in lead V_1 (31,32).
Abnormalities of the QRS Complex
  Right axis deviation. Right axis deviation was defined as a mean frontal plane QRS electrical axis greater than 90° (32).
  Left axis deviation. This was defined as a mean frontal plane QRS axis equal to or leftward of –30°. The A QRS was measured by the simplified method of Grant (33). Many patients with marked left axis deviation undoubtedly had left anterior fascicular block; but this was not indicated as a separate interpretation.
  $S_1S_2S_3$ pattern. This was defined as the occurrence of S waves in leads I, II, and III of at least 0.15 mV (1.5 mm) amplitude in each lead.
  Clockwise rotation. This was defined as a shift in the transition zone (R = S) in the precordial leads. Usually a shift to the V_4 position or further leftward is considered as clockwise rotation (16,20). For purposes of this study, a shift in the transition zone to V_5 was analyzed to avoid problems of interpretation that may occur with minor errors of precordial electrode position.
  Right bundle branch block (16,20). Incomplete right bundle branch block was diagnosed when the QRS duration was 0.10–0.11 sec and when the terminal QRS forces were directed rightward and anteriorly, causing the production of S waves in leads I and R waves in lead V_1.
  Complete right bundle branch block was considered to be present in those patients with a QRS duration of 0.12 sec or greater and with terminal QRS forces directed as previously described.
  $S_1Q_3T_3$ pattern (1,16,20). The presence of S waves in lead I and Q waves in lead III, each of amplitude exceeding 0.15 mV (1.5 mm), associated with inversion of the T wave in lead III constitutes the $S_1Q_3T_3$ pattern.
  Right ventricular hypertrophy (32,34). Right ventricular hypertrophy was considered to be present if the R wave in lead V_1 exceeded 0.5 mV (5 mm) or the R/S ratio in lead V_1 was greater than one. In this study, right axis deviation was not required to make this diagnosis nor was the presence of right axis deviation alone considered adequate for the diagnosis of the right ventricular hypertrophy.
  Low voltage QRS complexes. The QRS complexes were considered to be low voltage if the greatest overall deflection of the QRS was 0.5 mV (5 mm) or less in all of the limb leads (32).
  Pseudoinfarction pattern. This was defined as ST segment or T wave abnormalities associated with prominent Q waves which simulated a recent myocardial infarction.
  ST segment depression. This was considered present if the ST segment was depressed 0.05 mV (0.5 mm) or greater in any lead except aVR. No distinction was made between junctional or ischemic ST segment depression. Changes were considered primary in the absence of complete bundle branch block or ventricular hypertrophy.
  ST segment elevation. This was recorded as present when found in any lead except aVR if the ST segment was elevated at least 0.1 mV (1 mm) in the absence of ST depression in any other lead.
  T wave inversion. This was considered to be present if it occurred in any lead except aVL, III, aVR, or V_1. Changes were considered primary in the absence of complete bundle branch block or ventricular hypertrophy.

Reprinted with permission from Stein PD, Dalen JE, McIntyre KM, et al. The electrocardiogram in acute pulmonary embolism. Prog Cardiovasc Dis 1975;17:247–257.

pulmonary embolism, a normal electrocardiogram was shown in 30% (15). Cutforth and Oram reported 50 patients with pulmonary embolism, 49 of whom had patent coronary arteries, and 24% of these patients had normal electrocardiograms (16).

None of the patients who had massive or submassive pulmonary embolism with no prior cardiopulmonary disease had atrial flutter or atrial fibrillation (14), and only 5% of the patients with no prior cardiopulmonary disease in whom the severity of the pulmonary embolism ranged from mild to severe had atrial fibrillation or atrial flutter (15). None had second- or third-degree atrioventricular block (14,15). Only one patient had first-degree atrioventricular block (14,15). Among 23 patients with acute pulmonary embolism and no heart disease reported by Szucs and associates, only 4% (1 of 23) had atrial flutter or atrial fibrillation (17). This observation led Dalen to conclude that atrial flutter or atrial fibrillation in patients with pulmonary embolism is nearly always limited to individuals with prior heart disease (18).

Right axis deviation in pulmonary embolism has been observed for many years (1,11). Electrocardiographic manifestations of acute cor pulmonale ($S_1Q_3T_3$, complete right bundle branch block, P pulmonale, or right axis deviation) were less common than ST segment or T wave changes (Table 7–1)(14). One or more of these abnormalities occurred in 26% of patients with submassive or massive acute pulmonary embolism not associated with cardiac or pulmonary disease and occurred in 32% of such patients who suffered massive pulmonary embolism. Cutforth and Oram reported 14% of patients with pulmonary embolism had right bundle branch block and 28% had an $S_1Q_3T_3$ (16).

A pseudoinfarction pattern was seen in 11% of patients with submassive or massive pulmonary embolism who had no prior cardiopulmonary disease (14). A pseudoinfarction pattern, however, was seen in only 3% patients with no prior cardiopulmonary disease who had pulmonary embolism that ranged in severity from mild to massive (15). It is difficult to distinguish the prominent Q waves known to occur with pulmonary embolism from those of myocardial infarction (7,9). The electrocardiogram may simulate an inferior infarction with Q waves and T wave inversion in leads II, III, and aVF (7,19) or anteroseptal infarction characterized by QS or QR waves in V_1 and T wave inversion in the right precordial leads (16,20). The development of Q waves and extensive T wave inversion in the anterior and lateral leads was also observed in one patient after pulmonary embolism (21).

Leftward shifts of the frontal plane axis in pulmonary embolism are frequent (22,23). Karlen and Wolff noted a shift of the frontal plane axis toward the horizontal position in four patients with pulmonary embolism (19). An example of a patient with a previously normal frontal plane QRS axis that showed a shift to −25° after an acute pulmonary embolism, and subsequently reverted to normal is shown in Figure 7–1 (22). In a review of 115 patients with acute pulmonary embolism, a leftward shift of the frontal plane QRS axis was observed more frequently than a rightward shift, and left axis deviation was present more often than right axis deviation (23). In patients with submassive or massive pulmonary embolism and no prior cardiopulmonary disease, left axis deviation was recorded as frequently as right axis deviation (Table 7–1)(14). Among PIOPED patients with pulmonary embolism who had no prior cardiopulmonary disease, left axis deviation was more frequent than right axis deviation (Table 7–1)(15). Emphysema is also a cause of left axis deviation (24). Since the electrocardiogram of emphysema is usually easily recognized, the term pseudo left axis deviation has been used for such individuals to distinguish the electrocardiogram from that of left ventricular conduction abnormalities. Abnormal conduction through the emphysematous lungs has been postulated as a possible cause of the left axis deviation in these patients (24).

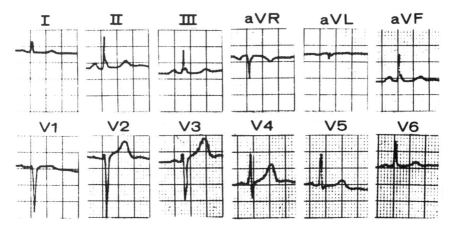

Figure 7–1A. Electrocardiogram 1 week prior to acute pulmonary embolism. Maximal frontal plane QRS axis, +70°, is within normal limits.

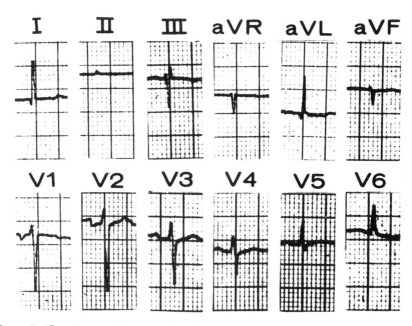

Figure 7–1B. Electrocardiogram on day of hospitalization for acute pulmonary embolism. The frontal plane QRS axis has shifted leftward to −25°. Nonspecific STsegment and T wave changes are also present.

Low voltage frontal plane QRS complexes in pulmonary embolism were first observed by Stein and associates (14). Six percent of patients with massive or submassive pulmonary embolism who did not have prior cardiopulmonary disease had low voltage QRS complexes (Table 7–1)(14). Among patients in PIOPED with mild to massive pulmonary embolism who had no prior cardiopul-

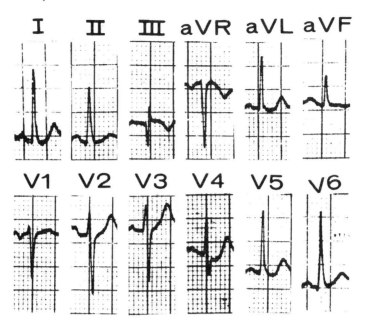

Figure 7–1C. Electrocardiogram 5 days after transvenous embolectomy shows return of frontal plane QRS axis toward control value. Frontal plane QRS axis is now +15°. (Reprinted with permission from Stein PD, Bruce TA. Left axis deviation as an electrocardiographic manifestation of acute pulmonary embolism. J Electrocardiol 1971;4:67–69.)

monary disease, 3% had low voltage QRS complexes (15). An electrocardiogram showing low voltage frontal plane QRS complexes that subsequently resolved is shown in Figure 7–2. Right ventricular endocardial potential is reduced in massive pulmonary embolism, possibly reflecting acute myocardial stress (25).

In 1938, Love and associates considered changes of the ST segment and T wave to be "the significant electrocardiographic changes noted" in acute pulmonary embolism (3). Abnormalities of the ST segment and T wave are by far the most frequent electrocardiographic manifestation of pulmonary embolism (14,15). Nonspecific T wave changes occurred in 42% of patients with massive or submassive embolization (14). A similar number of patients (41%) showed either depression or elevation of the ST segment (14). Nonspecific ST segment or T wave changes were observed in 49% of patients who had no prior cardiopulmonary disease and in whom the severity of pulmonary embolism ranged from mild to severe (15). Inversion of the T wave was also the most common electrocardiographic abnormality reported by Cutforth and Oram (46%) (16). They observed depression of the ST segment in 18% of patients with pulmonary embolism (16).

As early as 1935, the electrocardiographic abnormalities in acute pulmonary embolism were known to be transient and in some instances lasted only 48 hours (1). Among patients with submassive or massive pulmonary embolism and no prior cardiopulmonary disease, inversion of the T waves was the most persistent electrocardiographic abnormality (14). Abnormalities of the QRS complex appeared to be more transient (15).

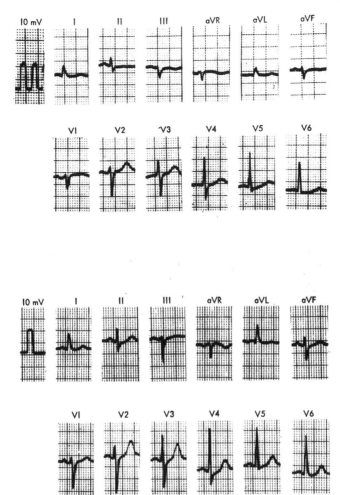

Figure 7–2. Top. Electrocardiogram on day of diagnostic pulmonary angiogram showing low voltage QRS complexes in frontal plane. Bottom. Electrocardiogram 13 days later. Amplitude of QRS complexes is normal. (Reprinted with permission from Stein PD, Dalen JE, McIntyre KM, et al. The electrocardiogram in acute pulmonary embolism. Prog Cardiovasc Dis 1975;17:247–257.)

The duration of electrocardiographic abnormalities after acute pulmonary embolism is shown in Table 7–3 (14). (The day of diagnostic arteriography and baseline electrocardiogram is considered as day 0). The acute pulmonary embolism, by history, may have occurred as many as 5 days previously. Abnormalities of repolarization tended to persist. Inversion of the T wave disappeared in only 22% of patients 5 or 6 days after the pulmonary embolism was diagnosed by arteriography, although it resolved in 49% by 2 weeks (14). Depression of the ST segment tended to resolve somewhat faster. In contradistinction to repolarization, many of the abnormalities of depolarization disappeared faster. In well over half of the patients with pseudoinfarction, $S_1S_2S_3$, $S_1Q_3T_3$, right

Table 7–3. DISAPPEARANCE OF ELECTROCARDIOGRAPHIC
ABNORMALITIES FOLLOWING ACUTE MASSIVE OR
SUBMASSIVE PULMONARY EMBOLISM

Electrocardiographic Abnormality*	Days after Diagnostic Pulmonary Angiography	
	5 or 6	**14**
P wave abnormality* P pulmonale	80% (4 of 5)	80% (4 of 5)
QRS abnormalities	60% (3 of 5)	60% (3 of 5)
Right axis deviation		
Left axis deviation	50% (3 of 6)	50% (3 of 6)
Clockwise rotation (V_5)	67% (4 of 6)	67% (4 of 6)
Incomplete right bundle branch block	80% (4 of 5)	100% (5 of 5)
Complete right bundle branch block	75% (6 of 8)	75% (6 of 8)
Right ventricular hypertrophy	60% (3 of 5)	80% (4 of 5)
$S_1S_2S_3$	67% (4 of 6)	80% (4 of 5)
$S_1Q_3T_3$	100% (11 of 11)	100% (11 of 11)
Pseudoinfarction	67% (6 of 9)	67% (6 of 9)
Low voltage (frontal plane)	0% (0 of 4)	67% (2 of 3)
Primary RST segment and T wave abnormalities	48% (11 of 23)	74% (17 of 23)
RST segment depression (not reciprocal)		
RST segment elevation (not reciprocal)	31% (4 of 13)	14% (2 of 14)[+]
T wave inversion	22% (8 of 37)	49% (18 of 37)

* Some patients had more than one abnormality.
[+] Recurrence noted in two patients.
Reprinted with permission from Stein PD, Dalen JE, McIntyre KM et al. The electrocardiogram in acute pulmonary embolism and no pre-existing cardiac or pulmonary disease. Chest 1991;100:598–603.

ventricular hypertrophy, or right bundle branch block, these abnormalities were no longer apparent on the electrocardiograms 5 or 6 days after the angiographic diagnosis. Examples of the occurrence and disappearance of a leftward axis shift are shown in Figure 7–1. Low voltage QRS complexes in the frontal plane occurring with acute pulmonary embolism are shown in Figure 7–2, and pseudoinfarction is shown in Figure 7–3.

Electrocardiographic abnormalities of acute massive or submassive pulmonary embolization were frequently related to the severity of the embolization as indicated by lung scans or pulmonary arteriography (14). Patients with ST segment abnormalities, T wave inversion, pseudoinfarction patterns, $S_1Q_3T_3$ patterns, incomplete right bundle branch block, right axis deviation, right ventricular hypertrophy, or ventricular premature beats had statistically significantly larger perfusion defects on the lung scan or larger defects on the pulmonary arteriogram than those with normal electrocardiograms (14).

Elevation of the pulmonary arterial mean pressure or right ventricular end-diastolic pressure was often associated with electrocardiographic abnormalities. In patients with right axis deviation, incomplete right bundle branch block, $S_1S_2S_3$ pattern, pseudoinfarction pattern, ST segment depression, or T wave

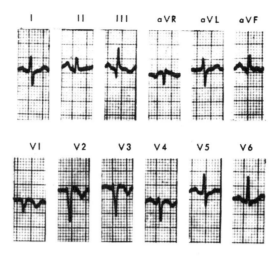

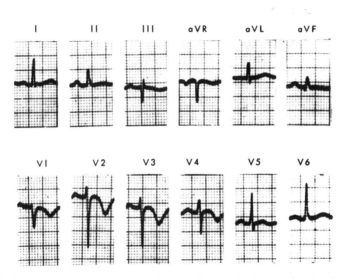

Figure 7–3. Top. Electrocardiogram on day of pulmonary angiogram showing Q waves in II, II, aVF and V_1 simulatingrecent inferior and anteroseptal myocardial infarction. Pulmonary artery pressure was 63/24 mm Hg and PaO$_2$ was 63 mm Hg. Bottom. Electrocardiogram next day shows no significant Q waves. Inversion of T waves persists. Pulmonary artery pressure decreased to 32/12 mm Hg and PaO$_2$ increased to 89 mm Hg. (Reprinted with permission from Stein PD, Dalen JE, McIntyre KM, et al. The electrocardiogram in acute pulmonary embolism. Prog Cardiovasc Dis 1975;17:247–257.)

inversion, either the pulmonary arterial mean pressure, right ventricular end-diastolic pressure, or both were significantly higher than in patients who had normal electrocardiograms (14).

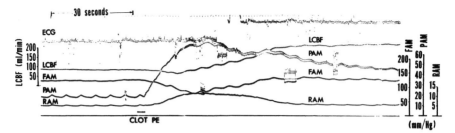

Figure 7–4. Simultaneous mean left circumflex coronary artery blood flow (LCBF), femoral artery mean pressure (FAM), pulmonary artery mean pressure (PAM), right atrial mean pressure (RAM), and electrocardiogram (ECG) in a dog during the administration of clot pulmonary embolism (PE). The LCBF was measured with an electromagnetic flow transducer placed around the artery. The LCBF increased from a control value of 88 cm^3/min to 210 cm^3/min 1 minute after PE. The PAM increased to 72 mm Hg by 25 seconds after PE, and decreased to 53 mm Hg 1 minute after PE. There was a transient reduction of FAM and a transient elevation of RAM. (Reprinted with permission from Stein PD, Alshabkhoun S, Hatem C, et al. Coronary artery blood flow in acute pulmonary embolism. Am J Cardiol 1968;21:32–37.)

The partial pressure of oxygen in arterial blood (PaO$_2$) of patients with various electrocardiographic abnormalities, with the exception of patients with right axis deviation, did not differ significantly from the depressed levels found in patients who had normal electrocardiograms (14). Even so, a contribution of hypoxemia to the electrocardiographic changes cannot be excluded. Neither right ventricular work nor the total pulmonary resistance of patients with abnormal electrocardiograms differed significantly from values measured in patients with normal electrocardiograms. The product of heart rate and pulmonary arterial peak pressure also showed no difference between groups. Peak brachial arterial pressure was 90 mm Hg or higher in all but three patients (96%).

The magnitude of the T wave inversion was not related to any of the measured hemodynamic abnormalities or to the severity of pulmonary embolism (14). Patients in whom the T wave was inverted 0.05 to 0.1 mV had hemodynamic, angiographic, and perfusion abnormalities comparable to patients in whom the T waves were inverted more than 0.3 mV in the frontal plane.

The electrocardiographic changes in pulmonary embolism are thought to be related to several etiologic mechanisms. Since some of the electrocardiographic abnormalities simulate myocardial ischemia, and even infarction, myocardial underoxygenation may be the cause (26). The right ventricle would be especially embarrassed by myocardial ischemia because of the load placed upon it by obstruction of the pulmonary circulation. The main cardiac effects of pulmonary embolism are: (1) strain upon the right ventricle, and (2) myocardial ischemia (26). The latter has been postulated to be caused by shock, hypoxemia, or vagal reflexes from the lung to the coronary arteries (26).

Myocardial necrosis, usually involving the left ventricle, has been observed at autopsies of patients who died of pulmonary embolism and had normal coronary arteries (26,27). Because left coronary flow (28) and right coronary blood flow (29) after induced acute pulmonary embolism in dogs and pigs showed an increased coronary flow (Fig. 7–4), rather than a reduction, reflex spasm of the coronary arteries appears unlikely. Shock also appears to be an unlikely cause, because electrocardiographic changes frequently occur in the absence of shock (14). An effect of hypoxemia upon the myocardium cannot be excluded. Such an effect, however, would be secondary, because the partial pressure of oxygen in arterial blood (PaO_2) in patients with abnormal electrocardiograms in general did not differ from that of patients with normal electrocardiograms (14). The possibility also exists that some patients may have had asymptomatic coronary heart disease. In the presence of acute pulmonary embolism and hypoxemia, such individuals would not be able to increase coronary flow adequately to compensate for the underoxygenation of arterial blood.

Love and associates concluded that dilatation of the right ventricle produced the electrocardiographic changes in pulmonary embolism (3). Mechanical obstruction of the pulmonary artery produced electrocardiographic changes similar to those produced by pulmonary embolism. The electrocardiographic abnormalities were preceded by visible and marked dilatation of the right ventricle (3). Section of the vagi or cervical sympathetic cords had no effect upon the production of the electrocardiographic changes (3). Wood also concluded that the essential factor in the production of electrocardiographic abnormalities in pulmonary embolism was right ventricular stress (5). Electrocardiographic changes appeared to depend on the size of the pulmonary embolism (5). Occlusion of the pulmonary artery of human beings during thoracic surgery produced some of the electrocardiographic changes observed in pulmonary embolism, thereby supporting this contention (30).

Occasional patients with a PaO_2 as low as 51 mm Hg and mean pulmonary arterial pressures as high as 31 mm Hg had normal electrocardiograms (14). Even so, most of the patients with electrocardiographic abnormalities had more severe evidence of pulmonary embolism as indicated by the lung scan or pulmonary angiogram than patients with normal electrocardiograms. The frequent association of electrocardiographic abnormalities with an elevated pulmonary arterial mean pressure or elevated right ventricular end-diastolic pressure supports the hypothesis that ventricular dilatation represents the major cause of the electrocardiographic changes. Arterial hypoxemia did not correlate with the electrocardiographic changes, although the PaO_2 was low in many patients and may have contributed to the observed abnormalities (14).

REFERENCES

1. McGinn S, White PD. Acute cor pulmonale resulting from pulmonary embolism. JAMA 1935;104:1473–1480.
2. Murnaghan D, McGinn S, White PD. Pulmonary embolism with and without acute cor pulmonale, with special reference to the electrocardiogram. Am Heart J 1943;25:573–597.
3. Love WS Jr, Brugler GW, Winslow N. Electrocardiographic studies in clinical and experimental pulmonary embolization. Ann Intern Med 1938;11:2109–2123.
4. Durant TM, Ginsburg IW, Roesler H. Transient bundle branch block and other electrocardiographic changes in pulmonary embolism. Am Heart J 1939;17:423–430.
5. Wood P. Pulmonary embolism: diagnosis by chest lead electrocardiography. Br Heart J 1941;3:21–29.
6. Myers GB, Klein HA, Stoffer BE. The electrocardiographic diagnosis of right ventricular hypertrophy. Am Heart J 1948;35:1–40.
7. Phillips E, Levine HD. A critical evaluation of extremity and precordial electrocardiography in acute cor pulmonale. Am Heart J 1950;39:205–216.

8. Wood P. Electrocardiographic appearances in acute and chronic pulmonary heart disease. Br Heart J 1948;10:87.
9. Eliaser M Jr, Giansiracusa F. The electrocardiographic diagnosis of acute cor pulmonale. Am Heart J 1952;43:533–545.
10. Wilson FN, Rosenbaum FF, Johnston FD. Interpretation of the ventricular complex of the electrocardiogram. Adv Intern Med 1947;2:1–63.
11. Kuo PT, Vander Veer JB. Electrocardiographic changes in pulmonary embolism with special reference to an early and transient shift of the electrical axis of the heart. Am Heart J 1950;40:825–838.
12. Katz LN. Electrocardiography. 2nd ed. Philadelphia: Lea & Febiger, 1946:401–406.
13. Sokolow M, Katz LN, Muscovitz AN. The electrocardiogram in pulmonary embolism. Am Heart J 1940;19:166–184.
14. Stein PD, Dalen JE, McIntyre KM, et al. The electrocardiogram in acute pulmonary embolism. Prog Cardiovasc Dis 1975;17:247–257.
15. Stein PD, Terrin ML, Hales CA, et al. Clinical, laboratory, roentgenographic and electrocardiographic findings in patients with acute pulmonary embolism and no pre-existing cardiac or pulmonary disease. Chest 1991;100:598–603.
16. Cutforth RH, Oram S. The electrocardiogram in pulmonary embolism. Br Heart J 1958;20:41–54.
17. Szucs MM Jr., Brooks HL, Grossman W, et al. Diagnostic sensitivity of laboratory findings in acute pulmonary embolism. Ann Intern Med 1971;74:161–166.
18. Dalen JE. Diagnosis of acute pulmonary embolism. In: Dalen JE, ed. Pulmonary embolism. New York: Medcom, 1972:28–39.
19. Karlen WS, Wolff L. The vectorcardiogram in pulmonary embolism. II. Am Heart J 1956;51:839–860.
20. Weber DM, Phillips JH Jr. A re-evaluation of electrocardiographic changes accompanying acute pulmonary embolism. Am J Med Sci 1966;251:381–398.
21. Romhilt D, Susilavorn B, Chou T. Unusual electrocardiographic manifestation of pulmonary embolism. Am Heart J 1970;80:237–241.
22. Stein PD, Bruce TA. Left axis deviation as an electrocardiographic manifestation of acute pulmonary embolism. J Electrocardiol 1971;4:67–69.
23. Lynch RE, Stein PD, Bruce TA. Leftward shift of frontal plane QRS axis as a frequent manifestation of acute pulmonary embolism. Chest 1972;61:443–446.
24. Pryor R, Blount SG Jr. The clinical significance of true left axis deviation: left intraventricular blocks. Am Heart J 1966;72:391–413.
25. Chatterjee K, Sutton GC, Miller GAH. Right ventricular endocardial potential in acute massive pulmonary embolism. Br Heart J 1972;34:271–273.
26. Horn H, Dack S, Friedberg CK. Cardiac sequelae of embolism of the pulmonary artery. Arch Intern Med 1939;64:296–321.
27. Dack S, Master AM, Horn H, et al. Acute coronary insufficiency due to pulmonary embolism. Am J Med 1949;7:464–477.
28. Stein PD, Alshabkhoun S, Hatem C, et al. Coronary artery blood flow in acute pulmonary embolism. Am J Cardiol 1968;21:32–37.
29. Stein, PD, Alshabkhoun S, Hawkins HF, et al. Right coronary blood flow in acute pulmonary embolism. Am Heart J 1969;77:356–362.
30. Semisch CW III, Merves L. Electrocardiographic studies on artificially produced pulmonary artery occlusion in human beings. Arch Intern Med 1942;69:417–428.
31. Thomas P, Dejong D. The P wave in the electrocardiogram in the diagnosis of heart disease. Br Heart J 1954;16:241–254.
32. Friedberg CK. Diseases of the Heart. 3rd ed. Philadelphia: WB Saunders, 1966:38,171,188.
33. Grant RP. Clinical electrocardiography. New York: McGraw-Hill, 1957:13.
34. Milnor WR. Electrocardiogram and vectorcardiogram in right ventricular hypertrophy and right bundle branch block. Circulation. 1957;16:348–367.

CHAPTER 8

The Plain Chest Radiograph

Some of the classic abnormalities on the plain chest radiograph of patients with pulmonary embolism were described in the late 1930s and early 1940s (1–3). The radiographic signs of acute pulmonary embolism include oligemia, pleonemia of the obstructed lung, dilated hilar arteries, elevated hemidiaphragm, dilated pulmonary artery trunk, pleural effusion, atelectasis, and infiltrate (4, 5). Occasionally, cavity formation may occur with pulmonary infarction (5). Dilatation of the azygos vein and superior vena cava has been described (4). Pulmonary edema has also been described (4). It was thought by some to reflect underlying heart disease (5), although pulmonary edema has been observed in patients with no prior cardiopulmonary disease (6).

Clearly, the plain chest radiograph cannot be considered a definitive examination (7). Still, the chest radiograph may provide an additional data point in the evaluation of patients with suspected acute pulmonary embolism. Among 108 patients with pulmonary embolism and 44 who did not have pulmonary embolism, the chest radiograph showed an average sensitivity of 33% and an average specificity of 59% (7). Greenspan and associates concluded that the major clinical importance of the plain chest radiograph (other than for use with interpretation of the ventilation-perfusion lung scan) may lie in the exclusion of disease processes, such as pneumothorax or rib fracture, which may simulate pulmonary embolism (7).

The frequency of abnormalities on the plain chest radiograph in 383 patients in the Prospective Investigation of Pulmonary Embolism Diagnosis (PIOPED) who had acute pulmonary embolism, the severity of which ranged from mild to massive, is shown in Table 8–1 (8). Many of these patients had prior cardiopulmonary disease. The frequency of abnormalities on the plain chest radiograph in 128 patients in the Urokinase Pulmonary Embolism Trial (UPET) who had submassive to massive pulmonary embolism is also shown in Table 8–1 (9). Approximately one-third of these patients had prior cardiopulmonary disease (10).

The first extensive investigation of the plain chest radiograph in patients with proven acute pulmonary embolism and no prior cardiopulmonary disease was based on combined data from the UPET and the Urokinase-Streptokinase

Table 8–1. PLAIN CHEST RADIOGRAPH IN PATIENTS WITH ACUTE
PULMONARY EMBOLISM, IRRESPECTIVE OF PRIOR
CARDIOPULMONARY DISEASE

	Mild to Massive PE (n = 383)* Percent	Submassive to Massive PE (n = 128)** Percent
Atelectasis or pulmonary parenchymal abnormality	69	—
Atelectasis	—	20
Consolidation		41
Pleural effusion	47	28
Pleural based opacity	34	—
Elevated hemidiaphragm	28	41
Decreased pulmonary vascularity	20	15
Prominent central pulmonary artery	20	23
Cardiomegaly	16	—
Westermark's sign***	6	—
Pulmonary edema	10	—
Pulm venous hypertension pattern	—	3
Pulm arterial hypertension pattern	—	3

Data are from Stein and associates (8)* based on data from PIOPED and The Urokinase Pulmonary Embolism Trial (9)**.
*** Prominent central pulmonary artery and decreased pulmonary vascularity
Pulm = pulmonary

Embolism Trial (11). Among 169 patients with submassive or massive acute pulmonary embolism and no prior cardiopulmonary disease, the various signs of the plain chest radiograph are shown in Table 8–2 (11). None of the signs on the plain chest radiograph was specific (11). Subsequently, based on data from PIOPED, findings on the plain chest radiograph in 117 patients with pulmonary embolism of severity that ranged from mild to massive and who had no prior cardiopulmonary disease were reported (6). The radiographic signs in these 117 with acute pulmonary embolism are shown in Table 8–2 (6). The sensitivity in relation to the frequency of false positive radiographic signs among 364 patients with no prior cardiopulmonary disease in whom pulmonary emboism was suspected is shown in Figure 8–1 (6). As in the investigation of signs on the plain chest radiograph of patients with submassive or massive pulmonary embolism, none of the signs was specific (Fig. 8–1).

Among the 169 patients with submassive or massive acute pulmonary embolism and no prior cardiopulmonary disease, a normal chest radiograph was observed in 34% (11). The frequency of a normal plain chest radiograph was similar among patients with submassive pulmonary embolism (25%) and submassive pulmonary embolism (24%). Among 117 patients with pulmonary embolism that ranged in severity from mild to massive, and who had no prior cardiopulmonary disease, the plain chest radiograph was normal in 16% (6). The chest radiograph, when normal in a patient who is dyspneic, may hint that pulmonary embolism is a diagnostic possibility (12).

Among the 169 patients with submassive or massive acute pulmonary embolism and no prior cardiopulmonary disease, one or more parenchymal signs (elevated hemidiaphragm, consolidation, pleural effusion, or atelectasis)

Table 8–2. PLAIN CHEST RADIOGRAPH IN PATIENTS WITH ACUTE PULMONARY EMBOLISM AND NO PRIOR CARDIOPULMONARY DISEASE

	Mild to Massive PE (n = 117)* Percent	Submassive to Massive PE (n = 169)** Percent
Atelectasis or pulmonary parenchymal abnormality	68	—
Atelectasis	—	28
Consolidation		39
Pleural effusion	48#	30
Pleural based opacity	35	—
Elevated hemidiaphragm	24	46
Decreased pulmonary vascularity	21	22
Prominent central pulmonary artery	15	21
Cardiomegaly	12	—
Westermark's sign***	7	—
Pulmonary edema	4	—
Pulm venous hypertension pattern	—	4
Pulm arterial hypertension pattern	—	2

Data are from Stein and associates (6)* and (11)** and are reproduced with permission.
*** Prominent central pulmonary artery and decreased pulmonary vascularity
# Among patients with a pleural effusion, 86% had only blunting of the costophrenic angle. None had a pleural effusion that occupied more than one-third of a hemithorax.
Pulm = pulmonary

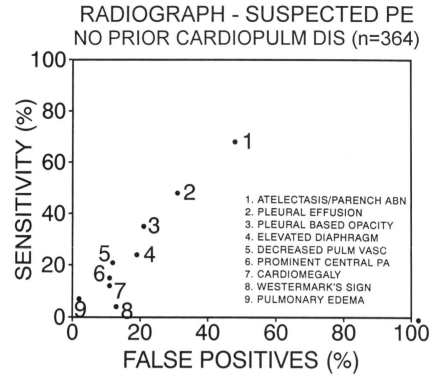

Figure 8-1. Sensitivity and frequency of false positive values of various abnormalities on the plain chest radiograph. (Data are from Stein PD, Terrin ML, Hales CA, et al. Clinical, laboratory, roentgenographic and electrocardiographic findings in patients with acute pulmonary embolism and no pre-existing cardiac or pulmonary disease. Chest 1991;100:598–603, in 364 patients with suspected acute pulmonary embolism and no prior cardiopulmonary disease. The numbers refer to the individual radiographic abnormalities, which are listed in the insert.)

occurred in 67% (11). Parenchymal signs occurred with comparable frequency among patients with submassive pulmonary embolism (71%) and massive pulmonary embolism (65%). Either consolidation, atelectasis, or pleural effusion occurred in 62% with submassive pulmonary embolism and 50% with massive pulmonary embolism (11). Atelectasis and a pulmonary parenchymal abnormality were the most frequent abnormalities on the plain chest radiograph in patients with no prior cardiopulmonary disease who had mild to massive pulmonary embolism (Table 8–2) (6). Among these patients, a pleural effusion occurred in 48% (6). Only blunting of the costophrenic angle was shown in 86% of patients with pulmonary embolism who had a pleural effusion. No patients with pulmonary embolism and no prior cardiopulmonary disease had a pleural effusion that occupied more than one-third of a hemithorax (6).

Among patients with no prior cardiopulmonary disease, one or more vascular signs (focal oligemia, distension of the proximal pulmonary artery, pulmonary artery hypertension pattern, or pulmonary venous hypertension pattern) occurred in 37%. Vascular signs on the plain chest radiograph were more frequent among patients with massive pulmonary embolism than with submassive pulmonary embolism (43% versus 28%) (11). Either focal oligemia or distension of the proximal portion of the pulmonary artery, or both, occurred more frequently among patients with massive pulmonary embolism than submassive pulmonary embolism (42% versus 26%) (11). Pulmonary edema occurred in 4% of patients with pulmonary embolism and no prior cardiopulmonary disease (6). Alveolar pulmonary edema occurred in only 1% and interstitial edema occurred in 3%.

Literature on the plain chest radiograph before the data from the Urokinase Pulmonary Embolism Trial is sparse. Among 25 patients with massive acute pulmonary embolism that involved 50% or more of the pulmonary arterial tree, 96% of whom had no prior cardiopulmonary disease, Kerr and associates identified zones of focal oligemia in all patients (13). Other findings were hyperemic zones (40%), pulmonary infarction (56%), hilar enlargement (56%), elevated hemidiaphragm (32%) and enlarged pulmonary trunk (12%). They concluded that changes in vascularity were the important diagnostic changes seen on the plain chest radiograph and that the extent of these changes may aid in the assessment of the severity of pulmonary embolism. The other signs, including changes of hilar shape, infarct shadows, and elevated hemidiaphragm, were considered supplementary (13).

Among 41 patients (the number with prior cardiopulmonary disease was unstated), Moses and associates observed that the most common signs on the plain chest radiograph were infiltrate (54%), pleural effusion (51%), and atelectasis (27%) (14). An elevated hemidiaphragm was observed only in 17%. Focal oligemia was uncommon (2%) as was a pattern of pulmonary hypertension (5%). A normal plain chest radiograph was uncommon (7%).

Among 126 patients who had pulmonary embolism (the number with prior cardiopulmonary disease was unstated), Laur (15) reported an elevated hemidiaphragm in 74% of severe cases and 50% of mild cases of pulmonary embolism. Dilatation of the hilar vessels was shown in 77% of severe cases and 48% of the mild cases of pulmonary embolism. Dilatation of the pulmonary artery was noted in 57% of severe cases and 22% of mild cases of pulmonary embolism. An inverse relation between the radiographic signs of pleural effusion and the severity of pulmonary embolism was noted. An inverse relation between the radiographic signs of pulmonary infarction and the severity of pulmonary embolism was also noted (15).

Among 38 patients with pulmonary embolism, 5 of whom had heart failure, Wiener and associates (16) observed an elevated hemidiaphragm in 32% and changes that suggested pleuritis in 45%. A negative plain chest radiograph was observed in 21%.

Among 22 patients with pulmonary hypertension from unresolved pulmonary embolism, Woodruff and associates (17) reported oligemia in 68%, enlargement of the right descending pulmonary artery in 55%, azygos vein enlargement in 27%, atelectasis or pleural effusion in 23%, and pleural thickening in 14%.

Among 29 patients with pulmonary embolism, Follath and associates (18) reported dilatation of the right pulmonary artery in 59% and dilatation of the left pulmonary artery in 45%. Dilatation of the main pulmonary artery was observed in fewer, 27%. Infiltrates occurred in 45% and oligemia in 17%.

Table 8–3.   PULMONARY ARTERY MEAN PRESSURE AND CHEST
RADIOGRAPHIC ABNORMALITIES AMONG 123 PATIENTS
WITH ACUTE PULMONARY EMBOLISM AND NO PRIOR
CARDIOPULMONARY DISEASE

	Number (%)	PA Mean Pressure (mm Hg)
Normal	10 (8)	16 ± 5
Atelectasis or pulmonary parenchymal abnormality	94 (72)	21 ± 9
Pleural effusion	71 (55)	21 ± 10
Pleural based opacity	45 (35)	23 ± 10
Elevated diaphragm	33 (25)	23 ± 8
Decreased pulmonary vascularity	26 (20)	24 ± 11
Prominent central pulmonary artery	20 (15)	30 ± 14
Cardiomegaly	15 (12)	34 ± 13
Westermark's sign	7 (5)	31 ± 11
Pulmonary edema	5 (4)	25 ± 10

Westermark's sign = prominent central pulmonary artery and decreased pulmonary vascularity
PA = Pulmonary artery
Values are mean ± standard deviation
Reprinted with permission from Stein PD, Athanasoulis C, Greenspan RH, et al. Relation of plain chest radiographic findings to pulmonary arterial pressure and arterial blood oxygen levels in patients with acute pulmonary embolism. Am J Cardiol 1992;69:394–396.

Radiographic Abnormalities Related to Pulmonary Artery Mean Pressure

Patients with no prior cardiopulmonary disease and pulmonary embolism who had normal plain chest radiograph had the lowest pulmonary artery mean pressures (Table 8–3) (19). Patients with a normal plain chest radiograph had a lower pulmonary artery mean pressure than patients with an elevated diaphragm, pleural based opacity, decreased pulmonary vascularity, prominent central pulmonary artery, Westermark's sign, or cardiomegaly. Patients with normal chest radiographs also had pulmonary artery mean pressures lower than patients with atelectasis or patients with a pleural effusion, but these differences may not have been statistically significant because of multiple comparisons.

The highest pulmonary artery mean pressures were in patients with no prior cardiopulmonary disease who had pulmonary embolism that ranged in severity from mild to massive and a prominent central pulmonary artery or cardiomegaly (Table 8–3) (19). Patients with a prominent central pulmonary artery had pulmonary artery mean pressures higher than patients with atelectasis, a pulmonary parenchymal abnormality, or pleural effusion. Patients with cardiomegaly had pulmonary artery mean pressures higher than in patients with atelectasis, a pulmonary parenchymal abnormality, or pleural effusion. Patients with cardiomegaly also had higher pulmonary artery mean pressures than patients with a pleural based opacity, elevated diaphragm, or decreased pulmonary vascularity. Patients with cardiomegaly and a dilated central pulmonary artery had a higher pulmonary artery mean pressure than patients with a prominent central pulmonary artery not accompanied by cardiomegaly.

Radiographic Abnormalities Related to the Partial Pressure of Oxygen in Arterial Blood (PaO₂) and the Alveolar-Arterial Oxygen Gradient

Among patients with pulmonary embolism that ranged in severity from mild to massive and who had no prior cardiopulmonary disease, the PaO_2 among patients with a normal chest radiograph was higher than among patients with pulmonary edema (Table 8–4) (19). The PaO_2 among patients with various

Table 8–4. PARTIAL PRESSURE OF OXYGEN IN ARTERIAL BLOOD ALVEOLAR-ARTERIAL OXYGEN GRADIENT, AND CHEST RADIOGRAPHIC ABNORMALITIES AMONG 93 PATIENTS WITH ACUTE PULMONARY EMBOLISM AND NO PRIOR CARDIOPULMONARY DISEASE

	Number (%)	PaO₂ (mm Hg)	A-a Gradient (mm Hg)
Normal	10 (11)	75 ± 14	30 ± 16
Atelectasis or pulmonary parenchymal abnormality	71 (76)	70 ± 13	36 ± 15
Pleural effusion	53 (57)	72 ± 15	35 ± 17
Pleural based opacity	31 (33)	70 ± 15	37 ± 14
Elevated diaphragm	25 (27)	67 ± 12	39 ± 14
Decreased pulmonary vascularity	16 (17)	69 ± 15	39 ± 17
Prominent central pulmonary artery	11 (12)	61 ± 11	44 ± 16
Cardiomegaly	9 (10)	61 ± 16	48 ± 22
Westermark's sign	4 (4)	60 ± 14	41 ± 18
Pulmonary edema	2 (2)	55 ± 4	58 ± 2

Westermark's sign = prominent central pulmonary artery and decreased pulmonary vascularity
values are mean ± standard deviation
PaO₂ = partial pressure of oxygen in arterial blood
A-a = Alveolar–arterial
Reprinted with permission from Stein PD, Athanasoulis C, Greenspan RH, et al. Relation of plain chest radiographic findings to pulmonary arterial pressure and arterial blood oxygen levels in patients with acute pulmonary embolism. Am J Cardiol 1992;69:394–396.

other abnormalities on the chest radiograph did not differ significantly. The alveolar-arterial oxygen difference was higher among patients with pulmonary edema than among patients with a normal chest radiograph, elevated diaphragm, or decreased pulmonary vascularity. The plain chest radiograph, therefore, assists in assessment of the severity of pulmonary hypertension in acute pulmonary embolism.

The observation that atelectasis, a pulmonary parenchymal abnormality, or pleural effusion was associated with lower pressures than cardiomegaly or a prominent pulmonary artery is compatible with the previous observation of others that pulmonary infarction or pulmonary hemorrhage (defined as the abrupt onset of pleuritic pain with or without hemoptysis and infiltrate on the chest radiograph) was uncommon when emboli obstructed the central pulmonary artery (20). However, pulmonary infarction was frequent when distal arteries were occluded (20). Presumably, those with central pulmonary artery occlusion had higher pulmonary artery pressures.

In summary the findings on the plain chest radiograph are not specific, but when used together with the history, physical examination, electrocardiogram, and simple laboratory tests, the findings on the plain chest radiograph assist in identifying a syndrome of pulmonary embolism. The chest radiograph, when normal in a patient who is dyspneic, may hint that pulmonary embolism is a diagnostic possibility. When various abnormalities are present on the plain chest radiograph, these may suggest a need for further diagnostic evaluation.

REFERENCES

1. Westermark N. On the Roentgen diagnosis of lung embolism. Acta Radiol 1938;19:357–372.
2. Hampton AO, Castleman B. Correlation of postmortem chest teleroentgenograms with autopsy findings: with special reference to pulmonary embolism and infarction. Am J Roentgen 1940;43:305–326.
3. Fleischner F. Hampton AO, Castleman B. Linear shadows in the lung (interlobar pleuritis, atelectasis and healed infarction). Am J Roentgen 1941;46:610–618.
4. Fleischner FG. Pulmonary embolism. Clin Rad 1962;13:169–182.
5. Kelly MJ, Elliot LP. The radiologic evaluation of the patient with suspected pulmonary thromboembolic disease. Med Clin North Am 1974;59:3–36.
6. Stein PD, Terrin ML, Hales CA, et al. Clinical, laboratory, roentgenographic and electrocardiographic findings in patients with acute pulmonary embolism and no pre-existing cardiac or pulmonary disease. Chest 1991;100:598–603.
7. Greenspan RH, Ravin CE, Polansky SM, et al. Accuracy of the chest radiograph in diagnosis of pulmonary embolism. Invest Radiol 1982;17:539–543.
8. Stein PD, Saltzman HA, Weg JG. Clinical characteristics of patients with acute pulmonary embolism. Am J Cardiol 1991;68:1723–1724.
9. National Cooperative Study. The Urokinase Pulmonary Embolism Trial: associated clinical and laboratory findings. Circulation 1973;(Suppl II);47/48:81–85.
10. National Cooperative Study. The Urokinase Pulmonary Embolism Trial: clinical and electrocardiographic observations. Circulation 1973;(Suppl II);47/48:60–65.
11. Stein PD, Willis PW III, DeMets DL, et al. Plain chest roentgenogram in patients with acute pulmonary embolism and no pre-existing cardiac or pulmonary disease. Am J Noninvas Cardiol 1987;1:171–176.
12. Stein PD, Alavi A, Gottschalk A, et al. Usefulness of non-invasive diagnostic tools for diagnosis of acute pulmonary embolism in patients with a normal chest radiograph. Am J Cardiol 1991;67:1117–1120.

13. Kerr IH, Simon G, Sutton GC. The value of the plain radiograph in acute massive pulmonary embolism. Brit J Radiol 1971;44:751–757.
14. Moses DC, Silver TM, Bookstein JJ. The complementary roles of chest radiography in the diagnosis of pulmonary embolism. Circulation 1974;49:179–188.
15. Laur A. Roentgen diagnosis of pulmonary embolism and its differential from myocardial infarction. Am J Roentgen 1963; 90:632–637.
16. Wiener SN, Edelstein J, Charms BL. Observations on pulmonary embolism and the pulmonary angiogram. Am J Roentgen 1966;98:859–873.
17. Woodruff WW III, Hoeck BE, Chitwood WR, et al. Radiologic findings in pulmonary hypertension in unresolved embolism. Am J Roentgen 144:681–686.
18. Follath F, Burkart F, Fridrich R. Zur Beurteilung des Thoraxbildes bei akuter Lungenembolie. Schweiz med Wschr 1968;41:1589–1592.
19. Stein PD, Athanasoulis C, Greenspan RH, et al. Relation of plain chest radiographic findings to pulmonary arterial pressure and arterial blood oxygen levels in patients with acute pulmonary embolism. Am J Cardiol 1992;69:394–396.
20. Dalen JE, Haffajee CI, Alpert JS, et al. Pulmonary embolism, pulmonary hemorrhage and pulmonary infarction. New Eng J Med 1977;296;1431–1435.

CHAPTER 9

Arterial Blood Gases and the Alveolar-Arterial Oxygen Difference

Arterial Blood Gases

The partial pressure of oxygen in arterial blood (PaO_2), when low in patients with suspected acute pulmonary embolism, is a helpful adjunct in the diagnostic assessment (1). Patients with acute pulmonary embolism, however, may have a normal PaO_2 (2–4). Among 132 patients with acute pulmonary embolism and no prior cardiopulmonary disease who had measurements of the PaO_2 while breathing room air, 24% had a PaO_2 of 80 mm Hg or higher (Fig. 9–1) (Stein PD, Relyea B. Unpublished data from PIOPED.). These data were obtained from patients in the randomized arm and the referred arm of the Prospective Investigation of Pulmonary Diagnosis (PIOPED) (5).

Even among patients with submassive or massive acute pulmonary embolism, 12% had a PaO_2 of 80 mm Hg or higher (2). The distribution of levels of the PaO_2 among 88 randomized patients with PE who had no prior cardiopulmonary disease was comparable to the distribution of the PaO_2 among 202 such patients in whom PE was suspected, but excluded (3). Among 277 patients with acute pulmonary embolism, 53% of whom had prior cardiopulmonary disease, the PaO_2 was 80 mm Hg or higher in 19% (6). Clearly, acute pulmonary embolism cannot be excluded on the basis of a normal PaO_2. Typically, however, among patients with acute pulmonary embolism, the PaO_2 is low.

The distribution of the partial pressure of carbon dioxide in arterial blood ($PaCO_2$) among 132 patients with acute pulmonary embolism and no prior cardiopulmonary disease who had measurements while breathing room air is shown in Figure 9–2. The $PaCO_2$ was less than 35 mm Hg in 49% of these patients, and it was greater than 45 mm Hg in 2% of patients (Stein PD, Relyea B. Unpublished data from PIOPED). The pH of arterial blood was greater than 7.44 in 53% of these patients and less than 7.38 in 4% patients (Fig. 9–3) (Stein PD, Relyea B. Unpublished data from PIOPED).

Alveolar-Arterial Oxygen Difference

A normal alveolar-arterial oxygen difference (alveolar-arterial oxygen gradient) does not exclude acute pulmonary embolism (3,6,7). Among 88 patients

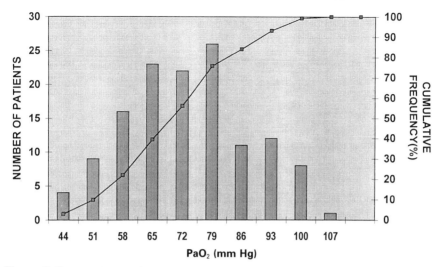

Figure 9–1.   Distribution of partial pressure of oxygen in arterial blood (PaO_2) and cumulative frequency while breathing room air, among 132 patients with angiographically proven pulmonary embolism (PE) and no pre-existing cardiac or pulmonary disease. The number of patients with indicated values of the PaO_2 is shown on the left and the cumulative percent of patients with the indicated values of the PaO_2 is shown of the right. (Stein PD, Relyea B. Unpublished data from PIOPED.)

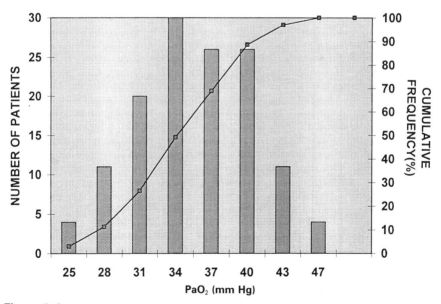

Figure 9–2.   Distribution of partial pressure of carbon dioxide in arterial blood ($PaCO_2$) and cumulative frequency while breathing room air, among 132 patients with angiographically proven pulmonary embolism (PE) and no prior cardiopulmonary disease. (Stein PD, Relyea B. Unpublished data from PIOPED.)

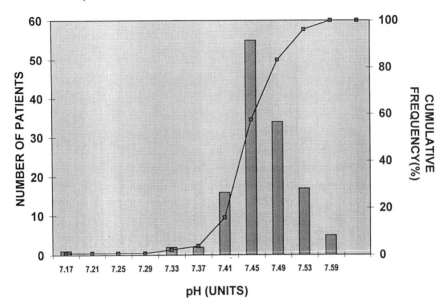

Figure 9–3. Distribution of pH of arterial blood and cumulative frequency while breathing room air, among 132 patients with angiographically proven pulmonary embolism (PE) and no prior cardiopulmonary disease. (Stein PD, Relyea B. Unpublished data from PIOPED.)

with acute pulmonary embolism who had no prior cardiopulmonary disease and in whom the alveolar-arterial oxygen difference was measured while breathing room air, the alveolar-arterial oxygen difference was ≤20 mm Hg in 14% of patients with pulmonary embolism (3). The distribution of values of the alveolar-arterial oxygen differences in patients with acute pulmonary embolism and in patients in whom acute pulmonary embolism was excluded is shown in Figure 9–4 (3). No value of the alveolar-arterial oxygen difference was diagnostic of pulmonary embolism, and no value excluded pulmonary embolism.

After the publication of our observations on the alveolar-arterial oxygen difference in patients with no prior cardiopulmonary disease, interest was rekindled in the ability of a normal alveolar-arterial oxygen difference to exclude pulmonary embolism. McFarlane and Imperiale indicated that only 1.9% of patients with a normal alveolar-arterial oxygen difference and no history of prior pulmonary embolism or prior deep venous thrombosis had pulmonary embolism (8). They concluded, therefore, that a normal alveolar-arterial oxygen difference among patients with no prior pulmonary embolism or prior deep venous thrombosis makes the diagnosis of pulmonary embolism so unlikely that further diagnostic evaluation may be unnecessary in this subgroup. Because the alveolar-arterial oxygen difference seemed to be more useful in the experience of these investigators than our data showed, we evaluated further the value of the alveolar-arterial oxygen difference among patients in PIOPED (6). We used more than one definition of a normal alveolar-arterial oxygen difference. We stratified according to categories of patients in whom a normal alveolar-arterial oxygen difference is thought by some to assist in excluding the diagnosis of pulmonary embolism. We used an expanded database from PIO-PED that included patients randomized for obligatory pulmonary angiography and patients referred for pulmonary angiography by their physicians.

The alveolar-arterial oxygen difference was calculated according to the following equation (9):

Alveolar-arterial oxygen difference = $150 - 1.25PaCO_2 - PaO_2$

where $PaCO_2$ equals partial pressure of carbon dioxide in arterial blood (mm Hg), and PaO_2 equals partial pressure of oxygen in arterial blood (mm Hg). Measurements of arterial blood gases were obtained with the patient breathing room air. All measurements were obtained within 24 hours before the diagnostic pulmonary angiogram. This may have been as long as 48 hours after the onset of symptoms, although usually it was less than 36 hours after the onset of symptoms (5).

The normal alveolar-arterial oxygen difference increases with age. Most patients have an alveolar-arterial oxygen difference ≤20 mm Hg (10–13). Normal age-related values obtained from data reported by Mellemgaard (10) are as follows. Patients 15 to 19 years of age had an alveolar-arterial oxygen difference ≤14 mm Hg. Patients 20 to 29 years of age had an alveolar-arterial oxygen difference ≈20 mm Hg. Patients ≥30 years of age (with one exception) had an

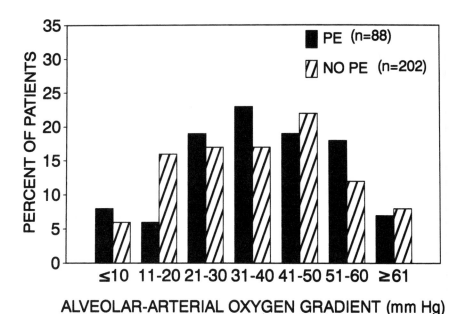

Figure 9–4.   Distribution of alveolar-arterial oxygen gradient among 88 patients with angiographically proven PE and no pre-existing cardiac or pulmonary disease (solid bars) and 202 such patients in whom PE was excluded (striped bars). (Reprinted with permission from Stein PD, Terrin ML, Hales CA, et al. Clinical, laboratory, roentgenographic, and electrocardiographic findings in patients with acute pulmonary embolism and no pre-existing cardiac or pulmonary disease. Chest 1991;100:598–603.)

alveolar-arterial oxygen difference ≤27 mm Hg (10). These values correspond closely with normal age-related values of the alveolar-arterial oxygen difference reported by Harris and associates (11), and Kanber and associates (13). Others reported somewhat lower normal values of the alveolar-arterial oxygen difference, which did not exceed 20 mm Hg in subjects 23 to 60 years of age (12). Normal values of the alveolar-arterial oxygen difference also were approximated by the equation: age/4 + 4 (8,14). This equation is restrictive, however. It would have excluded 28% of normal patients reported by Mellemgaard (10), 20% reported by Kanber and associates (13), 27% reported by Harris and associates (11), and 16% reported by Filley and associates (12). Averaging these data, the age-corrected equation would incorrectly define as abnormal 19% of patients (6).

Irrespective of how a normal alveolar-arterial oxygen difference was defined, comparable percentages of patients with normal alveolar-arterial oxygen differences had pulmonary embolism or no pulmonary embolism (6). This applied to all patients with pulmonary embolism, including patients with prior cardiopulmonary disease. It applied to patients stratified according to the absence of prior cardiopulmonary disease, and it applied to patients stratified according to the absence of prior pulmonary embolism or prior deep venous thrombosis.

All Patients

Among 280 patients with acute pulmonary embolism, including patients with prior cardiopulmonary disease as well as patients with prior pulmonary embolism and/or prior deep venous thrombosis), 12% had an alveolar-arterial oxygen difference ≤20 mm Hg versus 16% among patients who did not have pulmonary embolism (Table 9–1) (6). Among patients with a normal alveolar-arterial oxygen difference based on reported age-related values, 20% with pulmonary embolism had a normal alveolar-arterial oxygen difference versus 25% among patients who did not have pulmonary embolism. If a normal alveolar-arterial oxygen difference was defined on the basis of the equation age/4 + 4, then 8% had a normal alveolar-arterial oxygen difference versus 12% who did not have pulmonary embolism. None of these comparisons of patients with pulmonary embolism to those without pulmonary embolism showed statistically significant differences.

Patients with No Prior Cardiopulmonary Disease

Among 130 patients with no prior cardiopulmonary disease, 14% with an alveolar-arterial oxygen difference ≤20 mm Hg had acute pulmonary embolism versus 20% among patients who did not have pulmonary embolism (Table 9–1)(6). Among patients with a normal alveolar-arterial oxygen based on reported age-related values, 23% with pulmonary embolism had a normal alveolar-arterial oxygen difference versus 27% with no pulmonary embolism. Using the age/4 + 4 equation to define normal values of the alveolar-arterial oxygen difference, 10% with pulmonary embolism had normal values of the alveolar-arterial oxygen difference versus 12% among patients who did not have pulmonary

Table 9–1. FREQUENCY OF NORMAL A-a GRADIENTS AMONG PATIENTS WITH PE AND PATIENTS WITH NO PE[a]

| | A-a Gradient Normal ≤ 20 mm Hg | | | | A-a Gradient Normal ≤ Age/4 + 4 | | | | A-a Gradient Normal = Age-Related Data | | | |
| | PE | | No PE | | PE | | No PE | | PE | | No PE | |
	A-a ≤ NI # of Pts	(%)	A-a ≤ NI # of Pts	(%)	A-a ≤ NI # of Pts	(%)	A-a ≤ NI # of Pts	(%)	A-a ≤ NI # of Pts	(%)	A-a ≤ NI # of Pts	(%)
All patients	33/280	(12)	82/499	(16)	23/280	(8)	59/499	(12)	57/280	(20)	123/499	(25)
No prior CPD	18/130	(14)	40/200	(20)	13/130	(10)	24/200	(12)	30/130	(23)	54/200	(27)
No prior PE or DVT	21/190	(11)	55/365	(15)	15/190	(8)	40/365	(11)	38/190	(20)	86/365	(24)

[a] CPD, cardiopulmonary disease, PE = pulmonary embolism, A-a = Alveolar-arterial
DVT, deep venous thrombosis
NI, normal
Pts, patients
All differences (PE versus no PE), not significant
Reprinted with permission from Stein PD, Goldhaber SZ, Henry JW. Alveolar-arterial oxygen gradient in the assessment of acute pulmonary embolism. Chest 1995;107;139–143.

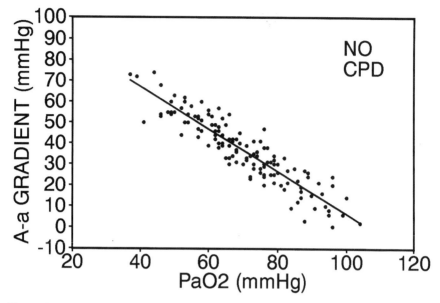

Figure 9–5. Alveolar-arterial (A-a) oxygen difference shown as a function of the partial pressure of oxygen in arterial blood (PaO_2) among patients with no prior cardiopulmonary disease (no CPD). Correlation coefficient (r) = -0.917 (P<0.005). (Reprinted with permission from Stein PD, Goldhaber SZ, Henry JW. Alveolar-arterial oxygen gradient in the assessment of acute pulmonary embolism. Chest 1995;107:139–143.)

embolism. None of these comparisons of patients with pulmonary embolism to those without pulmonary embolism showed statistically significant differences.

Patients with No Prior Pulmonary Embolism or Prior Deep Venous Thrombosis

Among 190 patients with no prior pulmonary embolism or prior deep venous thrombosis, 11% with acute pulmonary embolism had an alveolar-arterial oxygen difference ≤20 mm Hg versus 15% who did not have pulmonary embolism (Table 9–1) (6). Among patients with a normal alveolar-arterial oxygen difference based on reported age-related values, 20% had pulmonary embolism and 24% did not have pulmonary embolism. Based on the equation for age-corrected values of the alveolar-arterial oxygen difference, 8% with pulmonary embolism had a normal alveolar-arterial oxygen difference versus 11% with no pulmonary embolism. None of these comparisons of patients with pulmonary embolism to those without pulmonary embolism showed statistically significant differences.

Relation of Alveolar-Arterial Oxygen Difference to the PaO_2

The alveolar-arterial oxygen difference showed a strong inverse linear correlation with the PaO_2 among patients with pulmonary embolism and no prior cardiopulmonary disease (Fig. 9–5) (6). The alveolar-arterial oxygen difference also showed a strong inverse linear correlation with the PaO_2 and patients with pulmonary embolism who had prior cardiopulmonary disease (Fig. 9–6). This indicates that the value of both tests for screening for acute pulmonary embolism is similar. Neither values of the alveolar-arterial oxygen difference nor values of the PaO_2 can be used to exclude pulmonary embolism.

Relation of Alveolar-Arterial Oxygen Difference to Pulmonary Pressure and to the Ventilation/Perfusion Lung Scan

Patients with less severe pulmonary embolism were more likely to have a normal alveolar-arterial oxygen difference than those with more severe pulmonary embolism.

The alveolar-arterial oxygen difference showed a loose linear correlation with the pulmonary artery mean pressure among patients with pulmonary embolism and no prior cardiopulmonary disease (r=0.32, P<.005) and among patients with pulmonary embolism who had prior cardiopulmonary disease (r= 0.34, P<.005) (6).

The alveolar-arterial oxygen difference showed a loose linear correlation with the number of mismatched perfusion defects on the ventilation-perfusion lung scan among patients with pulmonary embolism and no prior cardiopulmonary disease (r=0.04, P<.005) (6). The alveolar-arterial oxygen difference also

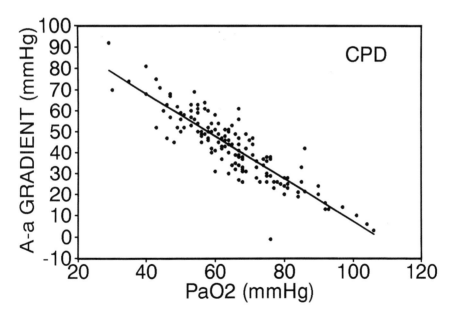

Figure 9–6. Alveolar-arterial (A-a) oxygen difference shown as a function of the partial pressure of oxygen in arterial blood (PaO_2) among patients with any prior cardiopulmonary disease (CPD). Correlation coefficient (r) = -0.842 (P<0.005). (Reprinted with permission from Stein PD, Goldhaber SZ, Henry JW. Alveolar-arterial oxygen gradient in the assessment of acute pulmonary embolism. Chest 1995;107:139–143.)

Table 9–2.   NEGATIVE PREDICTIVE VALUE OF BLOOD GASES AND
ALVEOLAR-ARTERIAL OXYGEN GRADIENT, ALONE OR IN
COMBINATION

	No Prior CPD No PE/Test Neg (%)	Prior CPD No PE/Test Neg (%)	All Patients No PE/Test Neg (%)
$PaCO_2 \geq 35$	105/171 (61)	142/211 (67)	247/382 (65)
$PaO_2 \geq 80$	55/87 (63)	62/84 (74)	117/171 (68)
A-a $\leq$ 20	40/58 (69)	38/50 (76)	78/108 (72)
$PaCO_2 \geq 35$ and $PaO_2 \geq 80$	30/49 (61)	28/36 (78)	58/85 (68)
$PaCO_2 \geq 35$ and A-a $\leq$ 20	30/46 (65)	28/33 (85)	58/79 (73)
$PaO_2 \geq 80$ and A-a $\leq$ 20	36/54 (67)	34/45 (76)	70/99 (71)
$PaCO_2 \geq 35$ and $PaO_2 \geq 80$ and A-a $\leq$ 20	26/42 (62)	24/28 (86)	50/70 (71)

Blood gases and alveolar-arterial (A-a) oxygen differences are in mm Hg
PE = pulmonary embolism, CPD = cardiopulmonary disease
NEG = negative
Reprinted with permission from Stein PD, Goldhaber SZ, Henry JW, et al. Arterial blood gas analysis in the
assessment of suspected acute pulmonary embolism. Chest 1996;109:178–81.

showed a loose linear correlation with the number of mismatched perfusion
defects on the ventilation-perfusion lung scan among patients with pulmonary
embolism who had prior cardiopulmonary disease (r=0.39, P<.005).

Blood Gases in Combination with the Alveolar-Arterial Oxygen Difference

Some suggest that if both the $PaCO_2$ and the alveolar-arterial oxygen difference are normal, this can be used as evidence against the presence of pulmonary
embolism (15). This is based on the observation among patients with essentially
no prior cardiac or pulmonary disease who had pulmonary embolism, that
93% had hypoxemia or hypocapnia and 98% had an increased alveolar-arterial
oxygen difference or hypocapnia (15). We tested this among patients in PIOPED
to determine if normal values of one or more blood gases, alone or in combination, could be used to exclude the diagnosis of acute pulmonary embolism (16).

Based on data from PIOPED, we were not able to exclude pulmonary
embolism based on an absence of abnormal values of the PaO_2, $PaCO_2$ or
alveolar-arterial oxygen difference (16). In patients who did not have prior
cardiopulmonary disease, pulmonary embolism was present 38% when the
PaO_2 and $PaCO_2$ were not low and the alveolar-arterial oxygen difference was
normal (Table 9–2).

Among patients with prior cardiopulmonary disease, the highest negative predictive value was shown with the combination PaO_2 ≥80 mm Hg, $PaCO_2$ ≥35 mm Hg and alveolar-arterial oxygen difference ≤20 mm Hg (Table 9–2) (16). With this combination, pulmonary embolism was absent in 86% of patients who had prior cardiopulmonary disease. Conversely, in patients with prior cardiopulmonary disease, pulmonary embolism was present 14% when the PaO_2 and $PaCO_2$ were not low and the alveolar-arterial oxygen difference was normal.

We observed, as have others, that arterial blood gases are abnormal in most patients with pulmonary embolism. Among patients with pulmonary embolism and no prior cardiopulmonary disease, 88% had either a low $PaCO_2$ or a high alveolar-arterial oxygen difference (16). We also observed that 97% of patients with prior cardiopulmonary disease who had pulmonary embolism had a low $PaCO_2$ or a high alveolar-arterial oxygen difference. Pulmonary embolism, however, could not be excluded on the basis of such blood gases (16). No combinations of blood gases were identified that reliably excluded pulmonary embolism. The PaO_2 and the alveolar-arterial oxygen difference may be included among laboratory and clinical findings that typically are abnormal in patients with pulmonary embolism, but may be normal in some patients with pulmonary embolism.

REFERENCES

1. Szucs MM, Brooks HL, Grossman W, et al. Diagnostic sensitivity of laboratory findings in acute pulmonary embolism. Ann Intern Med 1971;74:161–166.
2. National Cooperative Study. The Urokinase Pulmonary Embolism Trial. Circulation 1973;47/48(Suppl II):II-18–II-21,II-81–II-85.
3. Stein PD, Terrin ML, Hales CA, et al. Clinical, laboratory, roentgenographic, and electrocardiographic findings in patients with acute pulmonary embolism and no pre-existing cardiac or pulmonary disease. Chest 1991;100:598–603.
4. Menzoian JO, Williams LF. Is pulmonary angiography essential for the diagnosis of acute pulmonary embolism? Am J Surg 1979;137:543–548.
5. A collaborative study by the PIOPED investigators. Value of the ventilation-perfusion scan in acute pulmonary embolism: results of the Prospective Investigation of Pulmonary Embolism Diagnosis (PIOPED). JAMA 1990;263:2753–2759.
6. Stein PD, Goldhaber SZ, Henry JW. Alveolar-arterial oxygen gradient in the assessment of acute pulmonary embolism. Chest 1995;107:139–143.
7. Overton DT, Bocka JJ. The alveolar-arterial oxygen gradient in patients with documented pulmonary embolism. Arch Int Med 1988;148:1617–1619.
8. McFarlane MJ, Imperiale TF. Use of the alveolar-arterial oxygen gradient in the diagnosis of pulmonary embolism. Amer J Med 1994;96:57–62.
9. Guenter CA, Welch MH, eds. Pulmonary medicine. 2nd ed. Philadelphia: Lippincott, 1982:168.
10. Mellemgaard K. The alveolar-arterial oxygen difference: its size and components in normal man. Acta Physiol Scand 1966; 67:10–20.
11. Harris EA, Kenyon AM, Nisbet HD, et al. The normal alveolar-arterial oxygen-tension gradient in man. Clin Sci Mol Med 1974;46:89–104.
12. Filley GF, Gregoire F, Wright GW. Alveolar and arterial oxygen tensions and the significance of the alveolar-arterial oxygen tension difference in normal men. J Clin Invest 1954;33:517–529.
13. Kanber GJ, King FW, Eshchar YR, et al. The alveolar-arterial oxygen gradient in young and elderly men during air and oxygen breathing. Amer R Respir Dis 1968;97:376–381.

14. Skorodin MS. Respiratory diseases and A-a gradient measurement. JAMA 1984;252:1344.
15. Cvitanic O, Marino PL. Improved use of arterial blood gas analysis in suspected pulmonary embolism. Chest 1989;95:48–51.
16. Stein PD, Goldhaber SZ, Henry JW, et al. Arterial blood gas analysis in the assessment of suspected acute pulmonary embolism. Chest 1996;109:178–81.

CHAPTER 10

D-dimer in Diagnosis

D-dimer is a specific degradation product released into the circulation by endogenous fibrinolysis of a cross-linked fibrin clot (1). The use of D-dimer to exclude acute deep venous thrombosis was reviewed by Bounameaux and associates (2). A D-dimer measured by the an enzyme-linked immunosorbent assay (ELISA) below a cutoff of 300 ng/ml to 540 ng/ml (the values differed slightly from one study to another) made the diagnosis of deep venous thrombosis unlikely (2–13). Because of a large number of false positive values, a concentration of D-dimer above the cutoff level was not useful for a positive diagnosis (2).

To exclude acute pulmonary embolism, Bounameaux and associates analyzed pooled data from 908 patients with suspected acute pulmonary embolism, among whom 342 had pulmonary embolism (1). The average weighted sensitivity for acute pulmonary embolism was 97% and the average specificity was 45% when using the ELISA method(1, 14–22).

A diagnostic strategy that combines the use of ventilation-perfusion lung scans with measurement of quantitative plasma D-dimer levels may be useful in evaluating patients with suspected pulmonary embolism (23). Patients who had the rare combination of a low probability lung scan and a normal plasma D-dimer level had a negative predictive value for acute pulmonary embolism of 100% (14). The sample size was small, however, and the patient population was selected. The usefulness of this combination, therefore, needs further evaluation.

Low plasma D-dimer values in surgical patients, although helpful, are rare (14). Because surgical patients tend to have elevated D-dimer levels, it appears that the assay is likely to be less useful in this population than in medical patients (14). In contrast, 28% of medical patients had D-dimer levels less that 500 ng/ml.

The ELISA technique is not appropriate for emergency use. To overcome this shortcoming, several investigators used latex agglutination tests for plasma D-dimer levels in patients suspected of deep venous thrombosis. The pooled weighted sensitivity and specificity of these tests were approximately 83% and 68% for deep venous thrombosis (2). This was insufficient for either ruling in or out the presence of deep venous thrombosis (2). For pulmonary embolism, the sensitivity of latex agglutination tests was higher, 92% (1). However, these figures were derived from a relatively small sample (167 patients with acute pulmonary embolism) (2).

Bounaneaux and associates found poor agreement of levels of D-dimer measured with latex agglutination compared with ELISA (2). Different latex agglutination assays also have poor agreement with each other (24). Some say a normal latex agglutination D-dimer is unreliable for excluding pulmonary embolism (25,26), and should not be used.

A whole blood assay for D-dimer that can be performed and interpreted at the bedside within 5 minutes showed good preliminary results (27). In patients with suspected pulmonary embolism, the test showed a sensitivity of 94%. The technique uses a bispecific antibody whose epitopes are portions of D-dimer and red cells. In the presence of elevated levels of D-dimer, the antibody causes agglutination of the patient's red blood cells. More extensive evaluation is needed.

Although investigations of the use of the D-dimer to exclude acute pulmonary embolism have shown optimistic results, most members of the American College of Chest Physicians Consensus Committee on Pulmonary Embolism believe that if there is a high clinical suspicion of acute pulmonary embolism, diagnostic tests should proceed in spite of a normal plasma D-dimer (28). At the present time, data on the use of the D-dimer are insufficient to allow complete reliance on this test (28).Some recommend that if there is only a low level of clinical suspicion, a normal plasma D-dimer may strengthen the likelihood that no thromboembolic disease is present (28). Extreme caution was recommended by several panel members of the American College of Chest Physicians Consensus Committee on Pulmonary Embolism because of limited data in the use of the D-dimer tests (29).

REFERENCES

1. Bounameaux H, Perrier A. Role of D-dimers in the exclusion of pulmonary embolism. Semin in Resp and Crit Care Med 1996;17:31–37.
2. Bounameaux H, de Moerloose P, Perrier A, et al. Plasma measurement of D-dimer as diagnostic aid in suspected venous thromboembolism. Thromb Haemost 1994;71:1–6.
3. Heaton DC, Billings JD, Hickton CM. Assessment of D-dimer assays for the diagnosis of deep vein thrombosis. J Lab Clin Med 1987;110:588–591.
4. Rowbotham BJ, Carroll P, Whitaker AN, et al. Measurement of crosslinked fibrin derivatives—use in the diagnosis of venous thrombosis. Thromb Haemost 1987;57:59–61.
5. Ott P, Astrum L, Hartving Jensen R, et al. Assessment of D-dimer in plasma: diagnostic value in suspected deep venous thrombosis of the leg. Acta Med Scand 1988;224:263–7.
6. Bounameaux H, Schneider PA, Reber G, et al. Measurement of plasma D-dimer for diagnosis of deep venous thrombosis. Am Clin Pathol 1989;82–85.
7. Chapman CS, Akhtar N, Campbell S, et al. The use of D-dimer assay by enzyme immunoassay and latex agglutination techniques in the diagnosis of deep vein thrombosis. Clin Lab Haemat 1990;12:37–42.
8. Mossaz A, Grandrille S, Vitoux JF, et al. Valeur des D-dimeres dans le diagnostic en urgence des thromboses veineuses. Presse med 1990;19:1055.
9. van Bergen PFMM, Knot EAR, Jonker JJC, et al. Is quantitative determination of fibrin(ogen) degradation products and thrombin-antithrombin III complexes useful

to diagnose deep venous thrombosis in outpatients? Thromb Haemost 1989;62:1043–1045.

10. Elias A, Aillaud MF, Roul C, et al. Assessment of D-dimer measurement by ELISA or latex methods in deep vein thrombosis diagnosed by ultrasonic duplex scanning. Fibrinolysis 1990;4:237–40.

11. Boneu B, Bes G, Pelzer H, et al. D-dimers, thrombin-antithrombin III complexes and prothrombin fragments 1+2: diagnostic value in clinically suspected deep vein thrombosis. Thromb Haemost 1991;65:28–32.

12. Chang-Liem GS, Lustermans FAT, van Wersch JWJ. Comparison of the appropriateness of the latex and Elisa D-dimer determination for the diagnosis of deep venous thrombosis. Haemostasis 1991;21:106–10.

13. Heijboer H, Ginsberg JS, Buller HR, et al. The use of the D-dimer test in combination with non-invasive testing alone for the diagnosis of deep-vein. Thromb Haemost 1992;67:510–513.

14. Goldhaber SZ, Simons GR, Elliott CG, et al. Quantitative D-dimer levels among patients undergoing pulmonary angiography for suspected pulmonary embolism. JAMA 1993;270:2819–2822.

15. Bounameaux H, Cirafici P, de Moerloose P, et al. Measurement of D-dimer in plasma as diagnostic aid in suspected pulmonary embolism. Lancet 1991;196–200.

16. Bounameaux H, Schneider PA, Slosman D, et al. Plasma D-dimer in suspected pulmonary embolism: a comparison with pulmonary angiography and ventilation-perfusion scintigraphy. Blood Coag Fibrinol 1990;1:557–559.

17. Rowbotham RJ, Egerton-Vernon J, Whitaker AN, et al. Plasma cross-linked fibrin degradation products in pulmonary embolism. Thorax 1990;45:684–687.

18. Goldhaber SZ, Vaughn DE, Tumeh SS, et al. Utility of cross-linked fibrin degradation products in the diagnosis of pulmonary embolism. Am Heart J 1989;116:505–508.

19. Lichey J, Reschofski I, Dissmann T, et al. Fibrin degradation product D-dimer in the diagnosis of pulmonary embolism. Klin Wschr 1991;69:522–526.

20. Demers C, Ginsberg JS, Gohnston M, et al. D-dimer and thrombin-antithrombin III complexes in patients with clinically suspected pulmonary embolism. Thromb Haemost 1992:67:408–412.

21. van Beek EJR, van den Ende B, Berckmans RJ, et al. A comparative analysis of D-dimer assays in patients with clinically suspected pulmonary embolism. Thromb Haemost 1993;70:408–413.

22. Bounameaux H, Slosman D, de Moerloose P, et al. Diagnostic value of plasma D-dimer in suspected pulmonary embolism. Lancet 1988;2:628–629.

23. Perrier A, Bounameaux H, Morabia A, et al. Contribution of plasma D-dimer and lower limb venous ultrasound to the diagnosis of pulmonary embolism: a decision analysis model. Am Heart J 1994;127:624–635.

24. de Boer WA, de Haan MA, Huisman JW, et al. D-dimer latex assay as screening method in suspected deep venous thrombosis of the leg. A clinical study and review of the literature. Neth J Med 1991;38:65–69.

25. Ginsberg JS, Brill-Edwards PA, Demers C, et al. D-dimer in patients with clinically suspected pulmonary embolism. Chest 1993;104:1679–1684.

26. de Meerloose P, Minazio P, Reber G, et al. D-dimer determination to exclude pulmonary embolism: a two-step approach using latex assay as a screening tool. Thromb Haemost 1994;72:89–91.

27. Ginsberg JS, Wells PS, Brill-Edwards P, et al. Application of a novel and rapid whole blood assay for D-dimer in patients with clinically suspected pulmonary embolism. Thromb Haemost 1995;73:35–38.

28. ACCP Consensus Committee on Pulmonary Embolism. Opinions regarding the diagnosis and management of venous thromboembolism. Chest 1996;109:233–237.

29. Moser KM. Diagnosing pulmonary embolism. D-dimer needs rigorous evaluation. Brit Med J 1994;309:1525–1526.

CHAPTER 11

Neural Network Computer Assisted Diagnosis

All patients in the Prospective Investigation of Pulmonary Embolism Diagnosis (PIOPED) were studied because of a clinical suspicion of pulmonary embolism. (1) Primary physicians, aware of the signs and symptoms of pulmonary embolism, were suspicious if patients had well-known clinical manifestations. Because of this method of selection, patients with pulmonary embolism had signs, symptoms, chest radiographs, electrocardiograms, and blood gases similar to those in patients who did not have pulmonary embolism (2,3). Even so, physicians in PIOPED who were experienced with pulmonary embolism were often able to correctly estimate the likelihood of pulmonary embolism, based on undefined clinical judgment (1). This suggests that there were details of the clinical characteristics not recorded in the PIOPED database. It also suggests that there may be recorded combinations of observations that were weighted by physicians in reaching a correct clinical assessment. We attempted to determine if objective clinical characteristics that could be readily identified by physicians without special knowledge of pulmonary embolism could be evaluated by computer to achieve a correct estimate of the likelihood of pulmonary embolism (4). To accomplish this, we used a neural network (4).

A neural network is an artificial intelligence paradigm that integrates multiple clinical variables to arrive at a correct diagnosis. It has been used for clinical problems such as myocardial infarction and low back disorders (5,6). Neural network paradigms also have been applied to the evaluation of ventilation-perfusion lung scans, with good results (7,8). Neural network paradigms have been reported that perform computerized interpretations of scintillation data on thallium scans of the heart (9).

Data were from PIOPED. Characteristics of the history and objective data from the physical examination, chest radiograph, electrocardiogram, and blood gases were tabulated for each patient. A clinical assessment by physicians in PIOPED of the likelihood of acute pulmonary embolism was based on all available noninvasive data with the exception of the ventilation-perfusion scan.

Table 11–1. VARIABLES PRESENTED TO THE NEURAL NETWORK

Alveolar-arterial gradient	Stroke, ever
PaO_2	Postpartum ($\leq$3 mo)
Ilypoxia (PaO_2 < 60)	Cough ($\leq$3 d)
QRS axis > 120 and < −30	$PaCO_2$
ST segment and/or T-wave changes	Cyanosis
Recent surgery ($\leq$3 mo)	Prominent pulmonary artery (radiograph)
Lower extremity trauma ($\leq$3 mo)	Pulmonary edema (radiography)
Angina-like pain ($\leq$3 d)	Right ventricular hypertrophy (ECG)
Palpitations ($\leq$3 d)	Asthma, ever
History of chronic obstructive pulmonary disease	Estrogen use (at onset of symptoms)
A-a gradient > twice age-corrected	Pleuritic chest pain ($\leq$3 d)
History of immobilization ($\leq$3 mo)	Wheezing
T-wave changes alone	Pleural friction rub
Incomplete right bundle branch block	Cardiomegaly (radiograph)
Loss of consciousness ($\leq$1 wk)	ST segment depression alone
Calf tenderness	P-pulmonale
Thrombophlebitis (ever)	Respiratory alkalosis ($PaCO_2 \leq$ 30 mm Hg)
Leg or foot swelling, not joints	Palpable venous cord
Any leg pain, not arthritic	Left ventricular hypertrophy (ECG)
Leg erythema	Atrial fibrillation
Homan's sign	Diaphoresis
Low voltage QRS complexes	Premature atrial contractions
Premature ventricular contractions	Malignancy ($\leq$3 mo)
Complaints of dyspnea	Complete right bundle branch block
Hemoptysis ($\leq$1 mo)	

mo = months, d = days, wk = weeks
Reprinted with permission from Patil S, Henry JW, Rubenfire M, et al. Neural network in the clinical diagnosis of acute pulmonary embolism. Chest 1993;104:1685–1689.

The basis for arriving at the estimate of clinical likelihood was individual clinical judgment, and not any specific predetermined criteria.

Artificial neural network models were developed by presenting clinical data to the neural network in the form of numeric input variables (4). Fifty characteristics of the history, physical examination, chest radiograph, electrocardiogram, and arterial blood gases were presented to the computer algorithm (Table 11–1). The interpretations of the ventilation-perfusion scans were not included in the data presented to the neural network. Variables were coded as either binary variables (present or absent) or continuous variables.

The neural network models were developed using specific software (Neuroshell, Ward Systems, Frederick, Md). This software used a feed-forward single hidden-layer back propagation training algorithm with a sigmoidal transfer function.

The percentage of patients with pulmonary embolism was determined for deciles of risk estimated on the basis of clinical assessment by physicians in PIOPED (4). This was compared with deciles of risk estimated by neural network clinical assessment (Fig. 11–1). In general, there was good agreement between the likelihood of pulmonary embolism estimated by physicians in PIOPED and estimated by the neural network.

A receiver operating characteristic (ROC) curve is a useful method of evaluating tests that have more than two categories of classification and differing

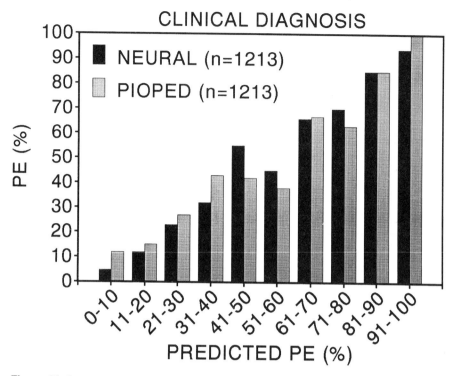

Figure 11–1. The percentage of patients with pulmonary embolism (PE) for deciles of predicted risk based on PIOPED clinical assessment and on neural network clinical assessment. (Reprinted with permission from Patil S, Henry JW, Rubenfire M, et al. Neural network in the clinical diagnosis of acute pulmonary embolism. Chest 1993;104:1685–1689.)

sensitivities and specificities at each classification level (10). The area under the ROC curve is a measure of performance of the test (10). The area under the ROC curve relating sensitivity to the frequency of false positive values was calculated for clinical assessment by PIOPED physicians (4). The area under the ROC curve relating sensitivity to the frequency of false positive values was also calculated for clinical assessment estimated by the neural network. The areas under the ROC curves did not differ significantly, indicating that the neural networks performed as well in achieving a clinical diagnosis as physicians knowledgeable and experienced in the diagnosis of acute pulmonary embolism.

Data that were of particular value to the neural network in making or rejecting the diagnosis of pulmonary embolism were identified (4). Among these were a high alveolar-arterial gradient, a low PaO_2 on room air, atrial flutter, marked right-axis or left-axis deviation, ST segment depression, T-wave inversion, and surgery within the last 3 months. It is important to keep in mind that all the patients evaluated were selected on the basis of important clinical characteristics that suggested acute pulmonary embolism. The fundamental and well-known features of acute pulmonary embolism, therefore, were not useful to the neural network in distinguishing between patients with pulmonary embolism and those without pulmonary embolism.

It may be that the neural network would perform better if more detailed clinical information were available. For example, a clinician may assess the suddenness of onset of shortness of breath, its severity, whether a patient is in acute distress, and whether the patient is using accessory muscles of respiration. Data from the PIOPED database that were supplied to the neural network had available only the presence or absence of shortness of breath and respiratory rate.

In summary, a neural network computer assisted diagnosis, based on readily obtained characteristics of the history, physical examination, chest radiograph, and electrocardiogram, performed as well as experienced physicians in making and excluding the diagnosis of acute pulmonary embolism.

REFERENCES

1. A Collaborative Study by the PIOPED Investigators. Value of the ventilation/perfusion scan in acute pulmonary embolism: results of the Prospective Investigation of Pulmonary Embolism Diagnosis (PIOPED). JAMA 1990;263:2753–2759.
2. Stein PD, Terrin ML, Hales CA, et al. Clinical, laboratory, roentgenographic, and electrocardiographic findings in patients with acute pulmonary embolism and no pre-existing cardiac or pulmonary disease. Chest 1991;100:598–603.
3. Stein PD, Saltzman HA, Weg JG. Clinical characteristics of patients with acute pulmonary embolism. Am J Cardiol 1991;68:1723–1724.
4. Patil S, Henry JW, Rubenfire M, et al. Neural network in the clinical diagnosis of acute pulmonary embolism. Chest 1993;104:1685–1689.
5. Baxt WG. Use of an artificial neural network for the diagnosis of myocardial infarction. Ann Intern Med 1991;115:843–848.
6. Bounds DG, Lloyd PJ. A comparison of neural network and other pattern recognition approaches to the diagnosis of low back disorders. Neural Networks 1990;3:583–591.
7. Scott JA, Palmer EL. Neural network analysis of ventilation-perfusion lung scans. Radiology 1993;186:661–664.
8. Tourassi GD, Floyd CE, Sostman HD, et al. Artificial neural network for diagnosis of acute pulmonary embolism: effect of case and observer selection. Radiology 1995;194:889–893.
9. Fujita H, Katafuchi T, Uehara T, et al. Application of artificial neural network to computer-aided diagnosis of coronary artery disease in myocardial SPECT bull's-eye images. J Nucl Med 1992;33(2):272–76.
10. Hanley JA, McNeil BJ. The meaning and use of the area under a receiver operating characteristic (ROC) curve. Radiology 1982;143:29–36.

Ventilation-Perfusion Lung Scan

Techniques of Perfusion and Ventilation Imaging

Perfusion Imaging

Technology and ventilation imaging were reviewed by Stein and Gottschalk (1). In perfusion lung imaging, the amount of microembolization of radiolabeled particles is proportional to the pulmonary arterial blood flow to that region. Macroaggregated human albumin labeled with ^{99m}Tc is used. The aggregated albumin preparation typically contains 90% of particles within the 10 to 90 μm range. More than 600 million pulmonary arterioles are small enough to trap the administered particles (2). Because approximately 500,000 particles are routinely injected for an individual study, the effect is physiologically insignificant. The arterioles are only temporarily occluded because the material degrades into smaller particles, the biologic half-time being approximately six to eight hours (3). The fragments are then phagocytized by cells of the reticuloendothelial system.

The minimum toxic dose for albumin is 20 mg/kg (4). The usual imaging dose is about 0.14 μg/kg albumin. At least 60,000 particles should be injected for an adequate study, or the radioactivity is likely to be unevenly distributed in the vascular bed (5). Because the usual 2 to 4 mCi dose from most kits is distributed among approximately 500,000 particles, low-particle injections are rarely a problem.

Perfusion imaging is begun by an intravenous injection of macroaggregates, with the patient supine to permit an even distribution of flow from the base of the lung to the apex, although there is a ventral to posterior gradient (6). After injection, imaging is best performed with the patient erect, which allows maximum expansion of the lungs, especially at the lung bases. Anterior, poste-

101

rior, both laterals, and both posterior and anterior obliques have been advocated (7–9). Segmental delineation of the basal segments of both lower lobes is best seen in posterior oblique projections (9). Posterior oblique views separate the two lungs, thereby avoiding "shine through" artifacts sometimes present in the lateral images. Oblique images contributed to the definition and clarification of the abnormalities, and resulted in improved lesion localization in 73% of patients (10).

Single-photon emission computed tomography (SPECT) potentially may improve delineation of perfusion defects and permit more accurate analysis of their size, shape, and distribution, but this has not yet been proved (11).

Ventilation Imaging

Current methods for performing a ventilation study use a xenon gas, either ^{133}Xe or ^{127}Xe, radioactive krypton gas (^{81m}Kr), or a radioactive aerosol, usually the radioaerosol of ^{99m}Tc diethylenetriamine pentaacetic acid (DTPA) or ^{99m}Tc pyrophosphate (PYP). In addition, an ultra-fine dry dispersion of carbon "soot" that can be labeled with ^{99m}Tc has been used, particularly in Europe and Australia (12).

Some authorities believe the ventilation study with ^{133}Xe can be effectively performed after the perfusion portion of the ventilation-perfusion study (13). Carrying out the ventilation scan study after the perfusion scan would be convenient, because the ventilation scan needs to be performed only on those patients whose perfusion scans are indeterminate (14). The experience of others, however, indicates that scattered irradiation from the previously administered perfusion tracer significantly decreases the accuracy of the washout phase of the ventilation scan, particularly if ^{99m}Tc is used for ventilation imaging (6). ^{127}Xe has photon energies higher than that of ^{99m}Tc. As a consequence, ^{127}Xe ventilation studies can be performed after the perfusion scan. The uncertain availability of this tracer and its considerable cost have limited its general application (6).

Xenon Ventilation Studies

The preperfusion ^{133}Xe ventilation lung scan has three phases: the single-breath image, the equilibrium phase, and the washout phase. The single-breath image is obtained with the patient initially with his back to a wide field-of-view gamma camera (ideally erect, but often supine). A bolus of approximately 15 to 20 mCi of ^{133}Xe is injected into the mouthpiece of the spirometer system at a time when the patient begins a maximal inspiration. The patient holds his breath for the next 15 to 20 seconds and a single-breath image is obtained. Equilibrium phase imaging is obtained with the patient breathing in a closed spirometer for 4 to 5 minutes. During this interval, a posterior and both right and left posterior oblique images are obtained. Any areas of the lungs that xenon cannot reach will be demonstrated on these views. A tight-sealing face mask or mouthpiece must be used to ensure that complete equilibrium is reached (6). The washout phase is then begun by readjusting the intake valves of the spirometer system to permit the patient to inhale ambient air and exhale into a shielded charcoal trap that absorbs the expired radioactive gas. In general, the washout phase should last at least 5 minutes. Images are taken at 30- to 60-second intervals during the the washout. Posterior oblique views approximately halfway through the washout process enhance the ability to detect and locate xenon retention in the anterior-posterior plane.

The equilibrium image has an activity distribution that corresponds to the aerated lung. Images made during washout should show a rapid clearance of activity from the lungs, usually within 90 seconds. Often, there is slight retention in the upper zones compared with the lower zones. In contrast to the single-breath image, which displays an abnormality as a deficit in radioactivity, abnormal washout images show ^{133}Xe "hot spots" that characterize the uneven distribution of ventilation. In this situation, abnormally retained ^{133}Xe activity is superimposed on a background of decreasing activity from normally ventilated lung regions. A sufficiently long rebreathing equilibrium time (at least 4 minutes) is imperative to maximize the usefulness of the washout phase by permitting the radiotracer to enter abnormal lung zones by collateral air drift (6). The washout phase of the ^{133}Xe study is the most likely phase to show ventilation abnormalities (15). The major disadvantage of the xenon technique is that images of the lung are required in a preselected view, typically in the posterior projection, with some ancillary anteroposterior information added by oblique views. Additional information at times can be added by obtaining a "second-look" single-breath xenon study in a different view.

The typical analogue display of a Xe ventilation study for pulmonary embolism relies on a compromise intensity setting. The intensity is usually determined by experience, such that the early phases of the washout examination may be slightly intense relative to the later phases. The intensity of the later phases, at the time when the "unevenness" of abnormal xenon washout is best detected, will be set to optimize the abnormal appearance. In practice, however, it is sometimes difficult to adjust the washout intensity correctly, and other variables such as chest wall thickness, lung thickness (i.e., volume), and the depth and frequency of respiration may all affect the washout phase of the ventilation study. To avoid these problems, serial computerized washout images (e.g., 30- to 45-second intervals) may be modified by normalizing each image in the series. In this way, regions with delayed clearance become more prominent, particularly in the later phases of the washout.

Xenon clearance times have no absolute normal range because of the normal variability in the rate and depth of respiration between subjects. The normal lungs are homogeneous in horizontal appearance, although there may be changes from apex to base. Inhomogeneity of xenon lung clearance at any time during the washout phase indicates an abnormality.

Krypton Ventilation Studies

^{81m}Kr is a relatively insoluble inert gas with a 13-second half-life. It decays to ^{81}Kr by isomeric transition, emitting 190 keV gamma rays (65%) and internal conversion electrons. The gas is obtained by eluting a generator containing its parent ^{81}Rb, which has a 4.7-hour half-life. The short half-life of the ^{81}Rb generator is a disadvantage, since the generator contains only enough activity for clinical studies on the day it is delivered. This markedly increases cost, because a new generator is required for each day's work.

Inhalation of ^{81m}Kr results in images that demonstrate the distribution of regional tidal ventilation. Because of the ultrashort half-life of 13 seconds, by the time collateral air drift occurs, the ^{81m}Kr has decayed away. There is, therefore, no opportunity to obtain washout images. That inability is balanced by the fact that ventilation images can be obtained in multiple projections. This permits direct comparison with perfusion scans for the evaluation of ventilation-perfusion mismatches.

^{81m}Kr images provide a sensitive means for studying regional ventilation (16,17). If the minute ventilation becomes greater than normal, ^{81m}Kr regional count rates become more dependent on lung volume than on ventilation. This rarely, if ever, occurs in adults. Thus, ^{81m}Kr images tend to underestimate ventilation in regions with high airflow because of potential partial dependence on the regional lung volume. Furthermore, because ^{81m}Kr has a higher photon energy than ^{99m}Tc, a low energy collimator cannot be used without getting some septal penetration. This decreases the resolution of the ventilation scan. If a medium energy collimator is used to avoid septal penetration, the collimator resolution is inherently less than a low energy collimator, and resolution of both the perfusion and ventilation scans decreases.

Radioaerosol Inhalation Studies

Radioaerosols also provide a means for investigating regional ventilation and have recently become commercially available with the introduction of small, easily contained, and efficient aerosol nebulizers. Radioaerosols are small particles, rather than gases. The radioaerosols deposit in the lung by impaction in central airways, sedimentation in more distal airways, and random contact with alveolar walls during diffusion in the alveoli (18). The newer commercially available nebulizers produce submicron-size aerosols that penetrate relatively evenly to the lung periphery, whereas larger (3 to 5 μm) radioaerosols, which were used in the past, demonstrated substantial degrees of central airway deposition, resulting in poor images of peripheral ventilation patterns.

Currently, the radioaerosol most often employed is ^{99m}Tc-diethylenetriamine pentaacetate (DTPA). DTPA is a low molecular weight solute that is able to cross the respiratory epithelium and be removed from the lungs rapidly through the bloodstream. Because of its relatively short residence time in the lungs (whole lung half-time of approximately 55 minutes) the radiation dose from DTPA aerosol scintigraphy is lower than that of either ^{81m}Kr or ^{133}Xe. Good results have been shown with obtaining perfusion lung scans before ventilation scans when the ventilation scans were obtained with DTPA (19). Performing the perfusion scan before the ventilation scan permitted the ventilation study to be tailored for optimal positioning to determine if mismatched defects were present. Direct overlay of the ventilation image on the perfusion image allowed detection of some previously unrecognized perfusion defects. Ventilation scans were unnecessary in patients in whom the perfusion scans were normal and in patients who had matched chest radiographic and perfusion scan defects. ^{99m}Tc-pyrophosphate has also been used and has the advantage of a larger residence time, which is especially important in smokers (20).

To yield uniform apex-to-base deposition, the inhalation of radioaerosol can be performed with the patient supine. However, if post-perfusion aerosol images are obtained, and the perfusion defects are basilar, the erect position is often used. A nebulizer that generates submicron-size particles should be filled with approximately 30 mCi of ^{99m}Tc DTPA in 2 to 3 mL of saline, and the nebulizer should be aerated at a flow rate of 8 to 10 L/minute (21). After approximately 3 minutes of breathing, about 750 µCi of ^{99m}Tc aerosol will have been deposited in the lungs, yielding 100 K count images in approximately 2 minutes with a standard wide-field gamma camera with an all-purpose low-energy collimator. If post-perfusion aerosol scanning is done, the aerosol dose in the nebulizer is increased to as much as 45 mCi of ^{99m}Tc-pyrophosphate or DTPA and the inhalation of aerosol continues until the count rate obtained for the perfusion scan is doubled (20).

The various agents used for ventilation scans have no readily apparent difference from a diagnostic standpoint (21). Cost, patient logistics, and referral patterns determine which ventilation agent is best suited for a specific institution (6).

Regarding the distribution of ventilation, in upright normal subjects, the lung bases ventilate better than the apices. In the lateral decubitus position, the lower lung ventilates better per unit volume than the upper lung. When the subject is supine, there is little apex-to-base gradient, but there is still an anterior-posterior gradient, with the most dependent regions receiving more ventilation than the uppermost regions.

REFERENCES

1. Stein PD, Gottschalk A. Critical review of ventilation-perfusion lung scans in acute pulmonary embolism. Prog Cardiovasc Dis 1994;37:13–24.
2. Miller WS. The structure of the lungs. J Morphol 1893;8:165. Quoted by: Dalen JE, Haynes FW, Hoppin FG Jr, et al. Cardiovascular responses to experimental pulmonary embolism. Am J Cardiol 1967;20:3–9.
3. Neumann RD, Sostman HD, Gottschalk A. Current status of ventilation-perfusion imaging. Semin Nucl Med 1980;10:198–217.
4. Taplin GV, MacDonald NS. Radiochemistry of macroaggregated albumin and newer lung scanning agents. Semin Nucl Med 1971; 1:132–152.
5. Heck LL, Duley JW. Statistical considerations in lung imaging with ^{99m}Tc albumin particles. Radiology 1974;113:675–679.
6. Gottschalk A. Alderson PO, Sostman HD. Nuclear medicine techniques and applications. In: JF Murray and JA Nadel, eds. Textbook of respiratory medicine. 2nd ed. Philadelphia: WB Saunders, 1994:682–710.
7. Wellman HN, Mack JF, Saenger EL, et al. Clinical experience with oblique views in pulmonary perfusion scintiphotography in normal and pathological anatomy. J Nucl Med 1968;9:374. Abstract.
8. Mack JF, Wellman HN, Saenger EL. Oblique pulmonary scintiphotography in the analysis of perfusion abnormalities due to embolism. J Nucl Med 1969;10:420. Abstract.
9. Caride VJ, Puri S, Slavin JD, et al. The usefulness of posterior oblique views in perfusion lung imaging. Radiology 1976;121:669–671.
10. Nielson PE, Kirchner PT, Gerber FH. Oblique views in lung perfusion scanning: clinical utility and limitations. J Nucl Med 1977;18:967–971.
11. Osborne DR, Jaszczak RJ, Greer K, et al. Detection of pulmonary emboli in dogs: comparison of single photon emission computed tomography, gamma camera imaging, and angiography. Radiology 1983;146:493–497.

12. Fawdry RM, Gruenewald SM. Initial experience with technegas: a new ventilation agent. Australas Radiol 1988;32:232–238.
13. Kipper MS. Alazraki N. The feasibility of performing ^{133}Xe ventilation imaging following the perfusion study. Radiology 1982;144:581–586.
14. Stein PD, Terrin ML, Gottschalk A, et al. Value of ventilation-perfusion scans compared to perfusion scans alone in acute pulmonary embolism. Am J Cardiol 1992;69:1239–1241.
15. Alderson PO, Biello DR, Khan AR, et al. Comparison of ^{133}Xe single-breath and washout imaging in the scintigraphic diagnosis of pulmonary embolism. Radiology 1980;137:481–486.
16. Alderson PO, Line BR. Scintigraphic evaluation of regional pulmonary ventilation. Semin Nucl Med 1980;10:218–242.
17. Miller TR, Biello DR, Lee JI, et al. Ventilation imaging with ^{81m}Kr: a comparison with ^{133}Xe. Eur J Nucl Med 1981;6:11–16.
18. Stuart BO. Deposition of inhaled aerosols. Arch Intern Med 1973;131:60–73.
19. Freitas JE, Sarosi MG, Nagle CC, et al. Modified PIOPED criteria used in clinical practice. J Nucl Med 1995;36:1573–1578.
20. Krasnow AZ, Isitman AT, Collier BD, et al. Diagnostic applications of radioaerosols in nuclear medicine. In: Freeman LM, ed. Nuclear medicine annual 1993. New York: Raven Press Ltd, 1993:123–193.
21. Alderson PO, Biello DR, Gottschalk A, et al. ^{99m}Tc-DTPA aerosol and radioactive gases compared as adjuncts to perfusion scintigraphy in patients with suspected pulmonary embolism. Radiology 1984;153:515–521.

C H A P T E R
13

Ventilation-Perfusion Lung Scan Criteria Prior To PIOPED

Scintigraphic studies of normal lungs demonstrate homogeneous patterns of matched ventilation and perfusion (1). Nearly all pulmonary diseases, including neoplasms, infections, and chronic obstructive pulmonary disease, can produce decreased pulmonary blood flow to affected lung zones (2). Pulmonary consolidation, bronchial obstructive disease, and restrictive disease, as well as vascular occlusion disease, may cause abnormalities on both the perfusion lung scan and the ventilation lung scan. Vascular occlusion may result from neoplastic vascular compression and pulmonary vasculitis as well as pulmonary embolism. Other processes occurring in the pulmonary arterial lumen can cause a ventilation-perfusion mismatch, including embolism of material other than thrombus (fat embolism and foreign material injected by intravenous drug abusers), in situ thrombosis (sickle cell disease), and pulmonary artery tumors (3–7). Ventilatory defects may accompany the perfusion defect owing to bronchial constriction caused by substances released from emboli or by reductions in alveolar levels of carbon dioxide, a potent airway dilator. This response, however, is usually transient and uncommon in scintigraphic studies (8–10).

Pulmonary infection, hemorrhage, infarction, atelectasis, or other conditions associated with alveolar collapse and/or leakage of fluids into the alveolar space cause perfusion and ventilation abnormalities. The degree of impaired ventilation and perfusion can vary, but a matched ventilation and perfusion defect typically is present (11).

Emphysema caused by alpha$_1$-antitrypsin deficiency, and, presumably, emphysema resulting from other mechanisms, causes destructive loss of alveoli and the capillary bed, thereby affecting perfusion as well as ventilation (12). The pulmonary arterioles also constrict with hypoxia (12). Destruction of alveoli and the capillary bed and arteriolar constriction tend to cause matched ventilation and perfusion abnormalities (1).

Restrictive disease, particularly if caused by chronic fibrosis, usually results in a greater impairment of perfusion than ventilation (1).

107

A generalized abnormality on the chest radiograph, such as diffuse pulmonary edema or diffuse reticulonodular disease, may not cause the perfusion lung scan to be abnormal. Among 55 patients with diffuse radiographic opacities, 73% had normal or near normal perfusion images (13). A ventilation-perfusion scan in such patients, therefore, may assist in excluding pulmonary embolism, often guiding management decisions in these patients.

Diagnostic Criteria for Pulmonary Embolism

The scintigraphic hallmarks of pulmonary embolism are large, wedge-shaped, pleural-based perfusion defects in areas that ventilate normally and

Table 13–1.   CRITERIA FOR HIGH PROBABILITY V/Q LUNG SCAN PRIOR TO PIOPED

Biello, 1987[a]	Biello, et al.[b] 1979	Sullivan, et al.[c] Based on McNeil, 1980[d]	Hull, et al. 1983[e]
≥2 Large V/Q mismatches with Nl x-ray	≥1 Large V/Q mismatches with Nl x-ray	Multiple V/Q mismatches largest being ≥ segmental	≥1 Segmental V/Q mismatch
or	or		
≥2 Mod V/Q mismatches with Nl x-ray	≥2 mod V/Q mismatches with Nl x-ray		
or	or		
≥1 Q > x-ray[f]	≥1 Q > x-ray[f]		
Mod: 25–90% seg	Mod: 25–75% Seg		
Large: >90% seg	Large: >75% Seg		
V/Q mismatch = Nl V in region of Q defect	V/Q mismatch = Nl V in region of Q defect	V/Q mismatch = Nl or mildly reduced V with Nl x-ray in region of Q defect	
V/Q match = abnormal V in region of Q defect	V/Q match = abnormal V in region of Q defect		

Nl, normal
V/Q, ventilation-perfusion
x-ray, radiographic abnormality in region of perfusion abnormality
Mod, moderate
Seg, segment
[a] Biello DR. Radiological (scintigraphic) evaluation of patients with suspected pulmonary thromboembolism. JAMA 1987;257:3257–3259.
[b] Biello DR, Mattar AG, McKnight RC, et al. Ventilation-perfusion studies in suspected pulmonary embolism. Am J Radiol 1979;133:1033–1037.
[c] Sullivan DC, Coleman RE, Mills SR, et al. Lung scan interpretation: effect of different observers and different criteria. Radiology 1983;149:803–807.
[d] McNeil BJ. Ventilation-perfusion studies and the diagnosis of pulmonary embolism: concise communication. J Nucl Med 1980;21:319–323.
[e] Hull RD, Hirsh J, Carter CJ, et al. Pulmonary angiography, ventilation lung scanning, and venography for clinically suspected pulmonary embolism with abnormal perfusion lung scan. Ann Intern Med 1983;98:891–899.
[f] Our interpretation of criteria
Modified and reprinted with permission from Stein PD, Gottschalk A. Critical review of ventilation-perfusion lung scans in acute pulmonary embolism. Prog Cardiovasc Dis 1994;37:13–24.

Table 13–2.   CRITERIA FOR INTERMEDIATE PROBABILITY V/Q LUNG SCAN PRIOR TO PIOPED

Biello, 1987[a]	Biello, et al., 1978[b]	Sullivan, et al.[c] Based on McNeil, 1980[d]	Hull, et al. 1983[e]
≥1 Q = x-ray or 1 large V/Q mismatch or 1 mod V/Q mismatch or Severe COPD with Q defects	≥1 Q = x-ray or 1 mod V/Q mismatch with Nl x-ray or Severe COPD with Q defects	1 seg V/Q mismatch or ≥1 Q = x-ray[f] or Mixed V/Q mismatched and matched defects or 1 V/Q mismatch ≥ lobar size or Multiple subsegmental V/Q mismatches	≥1 subsegmental V/Q mismatch or ≥1 segmental V/Q match

N1, normal
V/Q, ventilation-perfusion
x-ray, radiographic abnormality in region of perfusion abnormality
Mod, moderate
Seg, segment
[a] Biello DR. Radiological (scintigraphic) evaluation of patients with suspected pulmonary thromboembolism. JAMA 1987;257:3257–3259.
[b] Biello DR, Mattar AG, McKnight RC, et al. Ventilation-perfusion studies in suspected pulmonary embolism. Am J Radiol 1979;133:1033–1037.
[c] Sullivan DC, Coleman RE, Mills SR, et al. Lung scan interpretation: effect of different observers and different criteria. Radiology 1983;149:803–807.
[d] McNeil BJ. Ventilation-perfusion studies and the diagnosis of pulmonary embolism: concise communication. J Nucl Med 1980;21:319–323.
[e] Hull RD, Hirsh J, Carter CJ, et al. Pulmonary angiography, ventilation lung scanning, and venography for clinically suspected pulmonary embolism with abnormal perfusion lung scan. Ann Intern Med 1983;98:891–899.
[f] Our interpretation of criteria
Modified and reprinted with permission from Stein PD, Gottschalk A. Critical review of ventilation-perfusion lung scans in acute pulmonary embolism. Prog Cardiovasc Dis 1994;37:13–24.

are radiographically clear (14). Wagner and associates (15) and DeNardo and associates (16) suggested combined ventilation-perfusion lung imaging as a way to improve the specificity of diagnosing pulmonary emboli by scintigraphy. McNeil and coworkers (17) highlighted the findings of numerous investigators. They pointed out that in regions where the chest radiograph is normal, abnormalities in the perfusion scan that are matched by zones of abnormal ventilation are less likely to represent pulmonary emboli than mismatched abnormalities (i.e., reduced perfusion with normal ventilation). Many studies have led to a gradual evolution of diagnostic criteria for scintigraphy. Tables 13–1 through 13–3 list diagnostic criteria for the interpretation of ventilation-perfusion lung scans that were employed by various investigators or seem to be suggested by their observations (18–21). This was reviewed by Stein and Gottschalk (22). The possible predictive values for pulmonary embolism with high, intermediate, low, and normal interpretations of ventilation-perfusion scans according to various proposed criteria were comparable (Table 13–4).

Table 13–3.   CRITERIA FOR LOW PROBABILITY V/Q LUNG SCAN PRIOR TO PIOPED

Biello, 1987[a]	Biello, et al., 1979[b]	Sullivan, et al.[c] Based on McNeil, 1980[d]	Hull et al., 1983[e]
Small V/Q mismatches or V/Q matches with NI x-ray or Q << x-ray	Small V/Q mismatches or V/Q matches with Nl x-ray or Q << x-ray	1 Subseg V/Q mismatch or ≥1 V/Q match	≥1 subsegmental V/Q match
Small: <25% seg	Small: <25% seg		

Nl, normal
V/Q, ventilation-perfusion
x-ray, radiographic abnormality in region of perfusion abnormality
Mod, moderate
Seg, segment
[a] Biello DR. Radiological (scintigraphic) evaluation of patients with suspected pulmonary thromboembolism. JAMA 1987;257:3257–3259.
[b] Biello DR, Mattar AG, McKnight RC, et al. Ventilation-perfusion studies in suspected pulmonary embolism. Am J Radiol 1979;133:1033–1037.
[c] Sullivan DC, Coleman RE, Mills SR, et al. Lung scan interpretation: effect of different observers and different criteria. Radiology 1983;149:803–807.
[d] McNeil BJ. Ventilation-perfusion studies and the diagnosis of pulmonary embolism: concise communication. J Nucl Med 1980;21:319–323.
[e] Hull RD, Hirsh J, Carter CJ, et al. Pulmonary angiography, ventilation lung scanning, and venography for clinically suspected pulmonary embolism with abnormal perfusion lung scan. Ann Intern Med 1983;98:891–899.
Modified and reprinted with permission from Stein PD, Gottschalk A. Critical review of ventilation-perfusion lung scans in acute pulmonary embolism. Prog Cardiovasc Dis 1994;37:13–24.

Table 13–4.   PROBABILITY OF PULMONARY EMBOLISM OBTAINED WITH V/Q CRITERIA PRIOR TO PIOPED

V/Q Prob.	Biello, 1987[a]	Biello, 1979[b]	Hull, et al. 1983[c]
High	90%	87–92%	86%
Intermed	30%	20–33%	21–40%
Low	10%	0–8%	13%
Normal	0%	0%	0%

V/Q, ventilation-perfusion
Intermed, intermediate
[a] Biello DR. Radiological (scintigraphic) evaluation of patients with suspected pulmonary thromboembolism. JAMA 1987;257:3257–3259.
[b] Biello DR, Mattar AG, McKnight RC, et al. Ventilation-perfusion studies in suspected pulmonary embolism. Am J Radiol 1979;133:1033–1037.
[c] Hull RD, Hirsh J, Carter CJ, et al. Pulmonary angiography, ventilation lung scanning, and venography for clinically suspected pulmonary embolism with abnormal perfusion lung scan. Ann Intern Med 1983;98:891–899.
Modified and reprinted with permission from Stein PD, Gottschalk A. Critical review of ventilation-perfusion lung scans in acute pulmonary embolism. Prog Cardiovasc Dis 1994;37:13–24.

A "normal" chest radiograph refers to the radiographic appearance in the region of the ventilation or perfusion defect and not necessarily the entire radiograph. Similarly, a chest radiographic defect indicates a radiographic opacity in the region related to the ventilation or perfusion defect. A lung zone is one-third of a lung divided craniocaudally (i.e., upper, middle, and lower zones). Definitions of a mismatched defect, matched defect, large segmental defect, and moderate size segmental defect varied among investigators (Table 13–1).

McNeil showed likelihood ratios for several ventilation-perfusion scan patterns (18). Based upon her data, others developed criteria for the interpretation of ventilation-perfusion scans (23,24). These criteria differ somewhat from one another. None of these developed criteria showed areas under receiver operating characteristic curves that differed significantly from criteria suggested by Biello and Biello and associates (19,20,23,24).

A common cause of ventilation-perfusion mismatched defects not owing to acute pulmonary embolism is persistent mismatched defects from prior pulmonary embolism. Pulmonary thromboemboli resolve because of natural thrombolytic processes (25,26). A residual ($\pm 10\%$) defect 1 year after acute pulmonary embolism was reported on perfusion lung scans in 8 of 50 (16%) treated with anticoagulants in the Urokinase Pulmonary Embolism Trial (25). Perfusion lung scans in patients with no prior cardiopulmonary disease who were treated with anticoagulants showed incomplete resolution in 3 of 32 (9%) (25). Those with prior cardiopulmonary disease showed incomplete resolution in 5 of 18 (28%). Others showed incomplete clearing of the perfusion scan in 3 of 10 (30%) with no prior cardiopulmonary disease (27), and incomplete resolution in 11 of 33 (33%) patients, many of whom had prior cardiopulmonary disease (28).

The Urokinase Pulmonary Embolism Trial, although a landmark investigation, and the strongest literature published to date on resolution of the perfusion lung scan, may be inconclusive regarding the extent of natural clearing of the perfusion scan for two reasons. First, the techniques of perfusion scintigraphy in 1973 were archaic relative to today's standards (22), and second, the trial included patients who had massive or submassive pulmonary embolism, because the UPET was a therapeutic trial (25). As intended, the patients were not a cross-section of patients with pulmonary embolism. The mean rate of resolution of perfusion defects after 24 hours was 7.4% (25). This suggests that diagnostic studies within 24 hours would be likely to show the defect of pulmonary embolism.

REFERENCES

1. Gottschalk A, Alderson PO, Sostman HD. Nuclear medicine techniques and applications. In: Murray JF, Nadel JA, eds. Textbook of Respiratory Medicine. 2nd ed. Philadelphia: WB Saunders, 1994:862–710.
2. Secker-Walker RH, Siegel BA. The use of nuclear medicine in the diagnosis of lung disease. Radiol Clin North Am 1973;11:215–241.
3. McNeil BJ. A diagnostic strategy using ventilation-perfusion studies in patients suspect for pulmonary embolism. J Nucl Med 1976;17:613–616.
4. Smith RRL, Hutchins GM. Pulmonary focal embolization complicating the Budd-Chiari syndrome. N Engl J Med 1978;298:1069–1070.
5. Sostman HD, Brown M, Toole A, et al. Perfusion scan in pulmonary vascular/lymphangitic carcinomatosis: the segmental contour pattern. AJR 1981;137:1072–1074.

6. Myerson PJ, Myerson DA, Katz R, et al. Gallium imaging in pulmonary artery sarcoma mimicking pulmonary embolism. J Nucl Med 1976;17:893–895.
7. Velchik MG, Tobin M, McCarthy K. Nonthromboembolic causes of high-probability lung scans. Am J Physiol Imaging 1989;4:32–38.
8. Thomas D, Stein M, Tanabe G, et al. Mechanism of bronchoconstriction produced by thromboemboli in dogs. Am J Physiol 1964;206:1207–1212.
9. Kessler RM, McNeil BJ. Impaired ventilation in a patient with angiographically demonstrated pulmonary emboli. Radiology 1975;114:111–112.
10. Epstein J, Taylor A, Alazraki N, et al. Acute pulmonary embolus associated with transient ventilatory defect. J Nucl Med 1976;16:1017–1020.
11. Finley TN, Tooley WH, Swenson EW, et al. Pulmonary surface tension in experimental atelectasis. Am Rev Respir Dis 1964;89:372–378.
12. Stein PD, Leu JD, Welch MH, et al. Pathophysiology of the pulmonary circulation in emphysema associated with alpha$_1$ antitrypsin deficiency. Circulation 1971;43:227–239.
13. Newman GE, Sullivan DC, Gottschalk A, et al. Scintigraphic perfusion patterns in patients with diffuse lung disease. Radiology 1982;143:227–231.
14. Neumann RD, Sostman HD, Gottschalk A. Current status of ventilation-perfusion imaging. Semin Nucl Med 1980;10:198–217.
15. Wagner HN JR, Lopez-Majano V, Langan JK, et al. Radioactive xenon in the differential diagnosis of pulmonary embolism. Radiology 1968;91:1168–1174.
16. DeNardo GL, Goodwin DA, Ravasini R, et al. The ventilatory lung scan in the diagnosis of pulmonary embolism. N Engl J Med 1970;282:1334–1336.
17. McNeil BJ, Holman L, Adelstein J. The scintigraphic definition of pulmonary embolism. JAMA 1974;227:753–756.
18. McNeil BJ. Ventilation-perfusion studies and the diagnosis of pulmonary embolism: concise communication. J Nucl Med 1980;21:319–323.
19. Biello DR, Mattar AG, McKnight RC, et al. Ventilation-perfusion studies in suspected pulmonary embolism. Am J Radiol 1979;133:1033–1037.
20. Biello DR. Radiological (scintigraphic) evaluation of patients with suspected pulmonary thromboembolism. JAMA 1987;257:3257–3259.
21. Hull RD, Hirsh J, Carter CJ, et al. Pulmonary angiography, ventilation lung scanning, and venography for clinically suspected pulmonary embolism with abnormal perfusion lung scan. Ann Intern Med 1983;98:891–899.
22. Stein PD, Gottschalk A. Critical review of ventilation-perfusion lung scans in acute pulmonary embolism. Prog Cardiovasc Dis 1994;37:13–24.
23. Webber MM, Gomes AS, Roe D, et al. Comparison of Biello, McNeil, and PIOPED criteria for the diagnosis of pulmonary emboli on lung scans. Am J Roentgenol 1990;154:975–981.
24. Sullivan DC, Coleman RE, Mills SR, et al. Lung scan interpretation: effect of different observers and different criteria. Radiology 1983;149:803–807.
25. Urokinase Pulmonary Embolism Trial. Perfusion lung scanning. Circulation 1973;47(Supp):II-46–II-50.
26. Dalen JE, Banas JS, Brooks HL, et al. Resolution rate of acute pulmonary embolism in man. N Engl J Med 1969;280:1194–1199.
27. Wimalaratna HSK, Farrell J, Lee HY. Measurement of diffusing capacity in pulmonary embolism. Resp Med 1989;83:481–485.
28. Paraskos JA, Adelstein SJ, Smith RE, et al. Late prognosis of acute pulmonary embolism. N Engl J Med 1973;289:55–58.

14

Observations from PIOPED: Value of Ventilation-Perfusion Lung Scans Alone and in Combination with Clinical Assessment

The Prospective Investigation of Pulmonary Embolism Diagnosis (PIOPED) was a national collaborative study designed to determine the sensitivities and specificities of ventilation-perfusion lung scans in patients with suspected acute pulmonary embolism (1). All patients in whom attending physicians suspected acute pulmonary embolism were asked to consent to undergo obligatory angiography if their ventilation-perfusion lung scan was abnormal. Among those who consented for participation in PIOPED, a random sample was selected for investigation.

Pulmonary embolism was diagnosed by visualization of an intraluminal filling defect on the pulmonary angiogram, or by identification of a thromboembolism at autopsy. Pulmonary embolism was excluded by a good quality bilateral pulmonary angiogram that failed to show an intraluminal filling defect. In patients in whom the pulmonary angiogram was inadequate, pulmonary embolism was excluded by the absence of an adverse event over the course of 1 year while not receiving anticoagulants. Patients with a normal ventilation-perfusion scan were not required to undergo pulmonary angiography. Pulmonary embolism also was excluded in such patients by the absence of an adverse event that suggested recurrent pulmonary embolism during one year of follow-up while not receiving anticoagulant therapy.

In addition to the randomized patients described in the primary PIOPED report (1), an arm of PIOPED included patients who were referred for pulmonary angiography by attending physicians. These non-randomized patients were not included in the analysis of sensitivity and specificity reported in PIOPED (1), and these patients are not included in the data described in this chapter unless specifically stated. Useful information, however, was obtained from data in

113

these patients. A number of secondary investigations based on PIOPED data included both arms of PIOPED.

Because of the pivotal nature of PIOPED, the scintigraphic methods will be described in detail. The protocol strongly preferred ventilation and perfusion studies with the patient in the upright position, but other positions were acceptable. Ventilation studies were performed with 5.6×10^8 to 11.1×10^8 Bq of ^{133}xe using a 20% symmetric window set over the 80-keV energy peak. They started with a 100,000-count, posterior-view, first-breath image and then posterior equilibrium (wash-in) images for two consecutive 120-second periods. Washout consisted of three serial 45-second posterior views, 45-second left and right posterior oblique views, and a final 45-second posterior view. Then, perfusion scans were obtained with 1.5×10^8 Bq of technetium ^{99m}Tc macroaggregated albumin that contained 100,000 to 700,000 particles using a 20% symmetric windows set over the 140-keV energy peak. Particles were injected into an antecubital vein over 5 to 10 respiratory cycles, with the patient supine or at most semierect. The perfusion images consisted of anterior, posterior, both posterior oblique, and both anterior oblique views, with 750,000 counts per image for each. For the lateral view with the best perfusion, 500,000 counts per image were collected; the other lateral view was obtained for the same length of time. Scintillation cameras with a wide field of view (38.1 cm in diameter) were used with parallel-hole, low-energy, all-purpose collimators.

Two nuclear medicine readers, not from the center that performed the scan, independently interpreted the lung scans with chest roentgenograms according to pre-established study criteria. If the two readers disagreed, the interpretations were adjudicated by readers who were selected randomly from the remaining clinical centers. If adjudicating readers did not agree with either of the first two readers, scans went to panels of nuclear medicine readers. The final adjudicated ventilation-perfusion scan readings consisted of four categories: high probability, intermediate probability (indeterminate), low probability, and near normal/normal.

The criteria for the interpretation of ventilation-perfusion scans developed for the Prospective Investigation of Pulmonary Embolism Diagnosis (PIOPED) have become widely used (1). These are shown in Table 14–1.

The PIOPED criteria were developed on the basis of two or more mismatched segmental equivalent defects being indicative of a high probability of PE. A mismatched segmental equivalent defect is one large mismatched segmental defect or two moderate-size segmental defects. A large segmental defect is >75% of a segment. A moderate size segmental defect is ≥25% of a segment but ≤75% of a segment (Figs. 14–1,14–2). These criteria assume that a mismatched moderate-size segmental equivalent defect is of less diagnostic value than a mismatched large segmental defect (2). One of the difficulties with this system of grading is the interpretation of the size of the mismatched defect. The distinguishability of large versus moderate-size segmental defects requires skill and judgment. Experienced readers of radionuclide lung scans often underestimate the size of segmental defects (3).

The PIOPED criteria for interpretation of ventilation-perfusion lung scans defined a "very low probability" ventilation-perfusion scan, but the results of PIOPED reported "nearly normal/normal" interpretations. The latter interpretation includes nearly normal ventilation-perfusion lung scans and entirely normal

Table 14–1. PIOPED CENTRAL SCAN INTERPRETATION CATEGORIES AND CRITERIA

High probability

≥2 large (>75% of a segment) segmental perfusion defects without corresponding ventilation or roentgenographic abnormalities or substantially larger than either matching ventilation or chest roentgenogram abnormalities

≥2 moderate segmental (≥25% and ≤75% of a segment) perfusion defects without matching ventilation or chest roentgenogram abnormalities and 1 large mismatched segmental defect

≥4 moderate segmental perfusion defects without ventilation or chest roentgenogram abnormalities

Intermediate probability (indeterminate)

Not falling into normal, very low, low, or high probability categories

Borderline high or borderline low

Difficult to categorize as low or high

Low probability

Nonsegmental perfusion defects (e.g., very small pleural effusion causing blunting of the costophrenic angle, cardiomegaly, enlarged aorta, hila, and mediastinum, and elevated diaphragm)

Single moderate mismatched segmental perfusion defect with normal chest roentgenogram
Large or moderate segmental perfusion defects involving no more than 4 segments in 1 lung and no more than 3 segments in 1 lung region with matching ventilation defects either equal to or larger in size and chest roentgenogram either normal or with abnormalities substantially smaller than perfusion defects

>3 Small segmental perfusion defects (<25% of a segment) with a normal chest roentgenogram

Very low probability

≤3 Small segmental perfusion defects with a normal chest roentgenogram

Normal

No perfusion defects present
Perfusion outlines exactly the shape of the lungs as seen on the chest roentgenogram (hilar and aortic impressions may be seen, chest roentgenogram and/or ventilation study may be abnormal)

Reprinted with permission from A Collaborative Study by the PIOPED Investigators: Value of the ventilation-perfusion scan in acute pulmonary embolism: results of the Prospective Investigation of Pulmonary Embolism Diagnosis (PIOPED). JAMA 1990;263:2753–2759.

ventilation-perfusion lung scans. A nearly normal ventilation-perfusion lung scan category included readings of very low probability by one central scan reader and low probability by the other, very low probability by both, very low probability by one and normal by the other. An entirely normal ventilation-perfusion lung scan was one that was agreed upon by both central scan readers as being normal (Fig. 14–3).

Agreement among scan readers was excellent in PIOPED for high probability (95%), very low probability (92%), and normal (94%) scan categories (1). For intermediate probability (indeterminate) and low probability scan categories, the readers agreed less frequently (75% and 70%, respectively).

The sensitivity of a high probability ventilation-perfusion lung scan interpretation among 251 patients in PIOPED with angiographically diagnosed pulmonary embolism was 41% (1). Sensitivity was defined as the percentage of

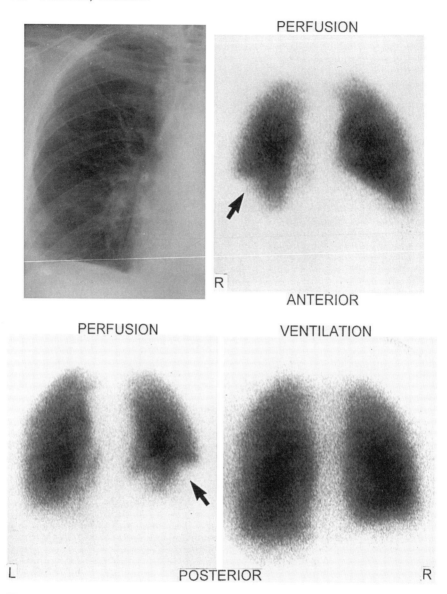

Figure 14–1. Top left. Chest radiograph, right lower zone, showing a mild parenchymal abnormality. **Top right.** Perfusion scan, anterior view, showing a perfusion defect (arrow) that is much larger than the radiographic abnormality. **Bottom left.** Perfusion scan, posterior view, showing the same large perfusion defect seen in the anterior view (arrow). **Bottom right.** Ventilation scan, posterior view, equilibrium phase, showing nearly normal ventilation. The washout phase was normal. The ventilation-perfusion lung scan was interpreted as high probability for pulmonary embolism. A pulmonary angiogram showed a large embolism in the right lower zone. The perfusion scan was obtained with ^{99m}Tc macroaggregated albumin. The ventilation scan was obtained with ^{133}xe.

patients with pulmonary embolism who had a high probability ventilation-perfusion lung scan. The specificity of a high probability ventilation-perfusion lung scan among 480 patients with negative pulmonary angiograms was 97% (1). Specificity was defined as the percentage of patients with pulmonary angiograms free of signs of pulmonary embolism who had non-high probability interpretations of the ventilation-perfusion lung scans.

The frequency of pulmonary embolism among patients in whom the diagnosis was made or excluded entirely by pulmonary angiography differed somewhat from the frequency in patients in whom outcome analysis as well as pulmonary angiography were employed (Table 14–2). A larger number of patients were included in the database of those with low probability or nearly normal interpretations of the ventilation-perfusion scans, and probably a more representative portion of the population was included in the group in whom outcome analysis was used. The following results refer to patients in whom outcome analysis in combination with pulmonary angiography was employed, although both sets of data are shown in Figure 14–4.

Among the general population of patients suspected of pulmonary embolism, a high probability ventilation-perfusion scan using original PIOPED criteria was indicative of pulmonary embolism in 87% (Table 14–2) (1). Among patients in whom the ventilation-perfusion scan probability interpretation was intermediate, pulmonary embolism was present in 30%. Therefore, the intermediate or indeterminate interpretation was uninformative.

Among patients whom a low probability interpretation of the ventilation-perfusion lung scan was made, pulmonary embolism was present in 14%. Some physicians believe that this percentage of patients with pulmonary embolism who have a low probability ventilation-perfusion scan is too high to adequately exclude pulmonary embolism (4). Therefore, patients with low probability ventilation-perfusion scans require further diagnostic studies (4–6).

A nearly normal or normal ventilation-perfusion lung scan by original PIOPED criteria showed pulmonary embolism in only 4% of patients (Table

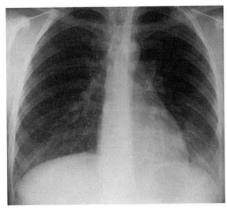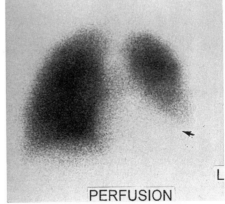

Figure 14–2A. **Left.** Chest radiograph, showing mild linear atelectasis at the left base. **Right.** Perfusion scan, anterior view, showing a massive perfusion defect (arrow) that is much larger than the radiographic abnormality.

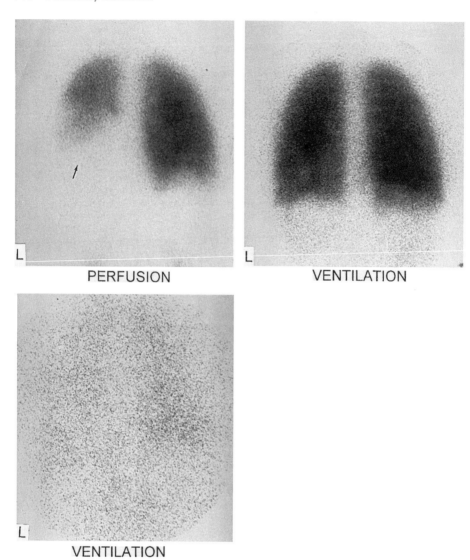

PERFUSION

VENTILATION

VENTILATION

Figure 14–2B. **Top Left.** Perfusion scan, posterior view, showing the same large perfusion defect (arrow) seen in the anterior view of Figure 14–2A, right. **Top Right.** Ventilation scan, posterior view, equilibrium phase, showing nearly normal ventilation. **Bottom.** Ventilation scan, washout phase, showing normal washout. The ventilation-perfusion lung scan was interpreted as high probability for pulmonary embolism. A pulmonary angiogram showed pulmonary embolism. Technique of ventilation-perfusion scans was as in Figure 14–1.

14–2). Conversely, such an interpretation excluded pulmonary embolism in 96% of patients.

Among patients with nearly normal ventilation-perfusion lung scans included in both arms of PIOPED (patients who volunteered for random assign-

ANTERIOR   POSTERIOR

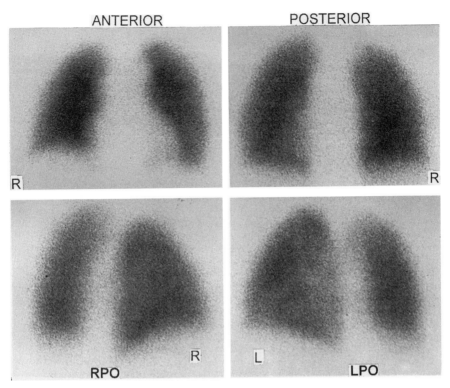

Figure 14–3.   Normal perfusion lung scan in a patient with borderline cardiomegaly and a prominent aorta. **Top left.** Anterior view. **Top right.** Posterior view. **Bottom left.** Right posterior oblique (RPO) view. **Bottom right.** Left posterior oblique (LPO) view. A pulmonary angiogram was negative for pulmonary embolism. The perfusion scan was obtained with ^{99m}Tc macroaggregated albumin.

ment to obligatory angiography and patients referred for angiography), the frequency of pulmonary embolism was 8 of 165 (5%) (7). Pulmonary embolism was diagnosed more frequently among patients with nearly normal ventilation-perfusion lung scans who underwent pulmonary angiography, 8 of 75 (11%) than in those in whom pulmonary embolism was diagnosed on the basis of an adverse outcome while receiving no anticoagulant therapy, 0 of 90 (0%) (7). At first glance, this may suggest that recurrent pulmonary embolism was not apparent in patients with pulmonary embolism of such mild severity that the ventilation-perfusion scan was nearly normal. There is no evidence that this was the case, however (7). In patients with nearly normal ventilation-perfusion scans who were assessed by outcome events versus patients assessed by angiography, the ventilation-perfusion scan showed fewer mismatched segmental perfusion defects, very low probability or normal ventilation-perfusion interpretations by 1 of the 2 ventilation-perfusion readers, and a generally lower clinical assessment (7). The observed lower frequency of pulmonary embolism in patients evaluated by outcome events compared with those who underwent angiography, therefore, can be attributed to a lower likelihood of pulmonary embolism.

Table 14–2.   VENTILATION-PERFUSION LUNG SCAN RESULTS: ALL
RANDOMIZED PATIENTS USING ORIGINAL PIOPED
CRITERIA

V/Q Scan Probability Category	Pulmonary Angio and Outcome Analysis[a*]		Pulmonary Angio Only	
	PE/Pts	(%)	PE/Pts	(%)
High prob	103/118	(87)	102/116	(88)
Intermediate prob	104/345	(30)	105/322	(33)
Low prob	40/296	(14)	39/238	(16)
Near normal/normal prob	5/128	(4)	5/55	(9)
Total	252/887	(28)	251/731	(34)

[a*] Pulmonary embolism was diagnosed by pulmonary angiography in 248 patients and by autopsy in 4 patients.
*Pulmonary embolism was excluded by pulmonary angiography in 465 patients. Pulmonary embolism was excluded by outcome assessment (the absence of adverse events during 1 year follow-up while not receiving antibiotics) in 170 patients.
Data reprinted with permission from A Collaborative Study by the PIOPED Investigators: Value of the ventilation-perfusion scan in acute pulmonary embolism: results of the Prospective Investigation of Pulmonary Embolism Diagnosis (PIOPED). JAMA 1990;263:2753–2759.

PIOPED ALL PATIENTS

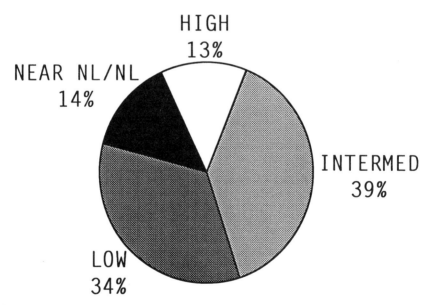

Figure 14–4.   Distribution of interpretations of ventilation-perfusion lung scans in all patients randomized for investigation in PIOPED. Intermed, Intermediate; Near NL/NL, Near normal/normal.

A normal ventilation-perfusion scan entirely excluded pulmonary embolism in the experience of PIOPED and others (1,8–10). There were 21 patients in PIOPED who had ventilation-perfusion scans read as normal by both central readers. Three underwent angiography and none showed thromboemboli. None of the remaining 18 patients received anticoagulants and none had clinically evident pulmonary embolism on follow-up. Sporadic case reports suggest that pulmonary embolism may occur in the presence of a normal perfusion lung scan. If these reports are correct, such cases are extremely rare. The major theoretical reasons for pulmonary embolism associated with a normal perfusion scan are central, nonobstructing, nonlateralized pulmonary embolism or minimal defects on the perfusion scan that are not appreciated (11). Patients with a single, small, or partially occluding embolus may not show a perfusion defect because of limitations of perfusion scanning.

A history of prior pulmonary embolism diminished the positive predictive value of a ventilation-perfusion lung scan for acute pulmonary embolism. Among 19 patients with histories of prior pulmonary embolism and a high probability ventilation-perfusion scan, the positive predictive value of the high probability ventilation-perfusion scan was only 74% compared with 91% for those without a history of pulmonary embolism. This difference of positive predictive values reflected a loss of specificity in the high probability ventilation-perfusion scan diagnosis for patients with histories of pulmonary embolism. The specificity of the ventilation-perfusion scan was only 88% among patients with a history of pulmonary embolism, whereas it was 98% among patients with no prior pulmonary embolism (1).

In PIOPED, only 13% of patients had high probability ventilation-perfusion scans. Intermediate ventilation-perfusion scan readings occurred in 39% of patients. Low probability ventilation-perfusion scans occurred in 34% and nearly normal ventilation/perfusion scans in 14% (Fig. 14–1).

Clinical Assessment in Combination with Lung Scans

One of the important contributions of PIOPED was demonstrating the value of clinical assessment in combination with ventilation-perfusion lung scan. Clinical assessment used in combination with the findings of ventilation-perfusion lung scans strengthened the diagnostic value of the ventilation-perfusion scan (1). In PIOPED, if both the independent clinical assessment and findings by ventilation-perfusion lung scans were high probability for pulmonary embolism, the diagnosis was correct in 96% of patients (Table 14–3) (1). If both the independent clinical assessment and findings by ventilation-perfusion lung scanning were low probability, pulmonary embolism was present in only 4% of patients. Unfortunately, these concordant diagnostic combinations were uncommon, occurring in only 28% of patients with clinically suspected pulmonary embolism. Either clinical uncertainty or uncertainty regarding the ventilation-perfusion lung scan findings (i.e., intermediate ventilation-perfusion scan pattern) was present in 72% of patients. The probability of pulmonary embolism with various ventilation-perfusion scan probabilities combined with various concordant and discordant clinical suspicions is shown in Table 14–3.

A history of immobilization within 3 months of the suspected acute pulmonary embolism among patients in PIOPED markedly affected the positive pre-

Table 14–3. CLINICAL ASSESSMENT AND VENTILATION-PERFUSION
SCAN PROBABILITY IN PIOPED

| V/Q Scan | Clinical Assessment | | | | | |
| | Highly Likely | | Uncertain | | Unlikely Probability | |
	PE/Pts	%	PE/Pts	%	PE/Pts	%
High prob	28/29	96	70/80	88	5/9	56
Intermediate prob	27/41	66	66/236	28	11/68	16
Low prob	6/15	40	30/191	16	4/90	4
Near Normal/Normal prob	0/5	0	4/62	6	1/61	2
Total	61/90	68	170/569	30	21/228	9

Highly likely = 80–100% likelihood of PE based on clinical assessment.
Uncertain = 20–79% likelihood of PE based on clinical assessment.
Unlikely = 0–19% likelihood of PE based on clinical assessment.
PE = pulmonary embolism.
V/Q = ventilation-perfusion scan.
Pulmonary embolism was diagnosed by pulmonary angiography in 248 patients and by autopsy in 4 patients.
Pulmonary embolism was excluded by pulmonary angiography in 465 patients. Pulmonary embolism was excluded by outcome assessment (the absence of adverse events during 1 year follow-up while not receiving antibiotics) in 170 patients.
Modified and reprinted with permission from A Collaborative Study by the PIOPED Investigators: Value of the ventilation-perfusion scan in acute pulmonary embolism: results of the Prospective Investigation of Pulmonary Embolism Diagnosis (PIOPED). JAMA 1990;263:2753–2759.

dictive value of intermediate and low probability ventilation-perfusion lung scans (Grant BJB, Lincheng W., Nasrabadi NM, et al. Personal communication). Among patients with intermediate probability ventilation-perfusion lung scans, the probability of pulmonary embolism was 41% in those who were immobilized and 24% in those who were not. Among patients with low probability ventilation-perfusion lung scans, the probability of pulmonary embolism was 24% in those who were immobilized and 10% in those who were not.

REFERENCES

1. A Collaborative Study by the PIOPED Investigators. Value of the ventilation-perfusion scan in acute pulmonary embolism: results of the Prospective Investigation of Pulmonary Embolism Diagnosis (PIOPED). JAMA 1990;263:2753–2759.
2. Neumann RD, Sostman HD, Gottschalk A. Current status of ventilation-perfusion imaging. Semin Nucl Med 1980;10:198–217.
3. Morrell NW, Nijran KS, Jones BE, et al. The underestimation of segmental defect size in radionuclide lung scanning. J Nucl Med 1993;34:370–374.
4. Hull RD, Raskob GE. Low-probability lung scan findings: A need for change. Ann Internal Med 1991;114:142–143.
5. Stein PD, Hull RD, Saltzman, HA, et al. Strategy for diagnosis of patients with suspected acute pulmonary embolism. Chest 1993;103:1553–1559.
6. Stein PD, Hull RD, Pineo G. Strategy that includes serial and noninvasive leg tests for diagnosis of thromboembolic disease in patients with suspected acute pulmonary embolism: estimated percentage of patients, based on data from PIOPED, in whom a noninvasive diagnosis or exclusion of thromboembolic disease might be safely made. Arch Intern Med 1995;155:2101–2104.

7. Henry JW, Stein PD, Gottschalk A, et al. Pulmonary embolism among patients with a nearly normal ventilation-perfusion lung scan. Chest (in press).
8. Stein PD. Low-dose heparin for prevention of pulmonary embolism and significance of normal lung scan. ACCP Bulletin 1982;21:12–14.
9. Hull RD, Raskob GE, Coates G, et al. Clinical validity of a normal perfusion lung scan in patients with suspected pulmonary embolism. Chest 1990;97:23–26.
10. Kipper MS, Moser KM, Kortman KE, et al. Long-term follow-up of patients with suspected pulmonary embolism and a normal lung scan. Chest 1982;82:411–415.
11. Stein PD, Gottschalk A. Critical review of ventilation-perfusion lung scans in acute pulmonary embolism. Prog Cardiovasc Dis 1994;37:13–24.

CHAPTER

15

Lung Scans in Patients with a Normal Chest Radiograph, Patients with No Prior Cardiopulmonary Disease, and Patients with Prior Cardiopulmonary Disease

The original criteria for the evaluation of ventilation-perfusion scans from the Prospective Investigation of Pulmonary Embolism Diagnosis (PIOPED) were tested in patients with a normal chest radiograph, patients with no prior cardiopulmonary disease, and patients with any prior cardiopulmonary disease (1,2). As the complexity of associated cardiopulmonary disease increased, the likelihood that the ventilation-perfusion lung scan interpretation would be intermediate probability (indeterminate) also increased. Using the original PIOPED criteria, an intermediate probability interpretation of the ventilation-perfusion lung scan was 13% in patients with a normal chest radiograph, 33% in patients with no prior cardiopulmonary disease, and 43% in patients with any prior cardiopulmonary disease (Fig. 15–1). With even more complex disease (chronic obstructive pulmonary disease, COPD), 60% of patients had intermediate probability interpretations of the ventilation-perfusion lung scans. (Patients with COPD are discussed in detail in Chapter 28.) Among each of these categories of patients, the positive predictive value of high, low, and nearly normal ventilation-perfusion lung scans was similar (1,2). As indicated in Chapter 28, the positive predictive value of high, low, and nearly normal ventilation-perfusion lung scans in patients with COPD was also comparable with the other categories of patients (3).

The number of patients with a normal chest radiograph and a high probability ventilation-perfusion scan was small and therefore of little meaning (Table 15–1) (1,2). A high probability ventilation-perfusion lung scan in patients with no prior cardiopulmonary disease had a positive predictive value for pulmonary

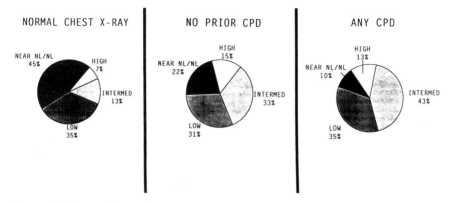

Figure 15–1.   Distribution of interpretations of ventilation-perfusion scans among patients with a normal chest radiograph (Left) no prior cardiopulmonary disease (CPD) (Center), and patients with any prior cardiopulmonary disease (Right). As the complexity of disease increased, the percent of patients with ventilation-perfusion scan interpretations of intermediate (intermed) probability increased from 13% to 43%. Some of the distributions do not add to exactly 100% because percentages were rounded off.

Table 15–1.   V/Q SCAN FINDINGS IN PATIENTS WITH VARIOUS DEGREES OF COMPLEXITY OF ASSOCIATED CARDIOPULMONARY DISEASE

V/Q Scan Probability	Normal Chest Radiograph[1] PE/n	(%)	No Prior CPD[2] PE/n	(%)	Any Prior CPD[2] PE/n	(%)
High	6/9	(67)	5/54	(93)	55/66	(83)
Intermediate	4/17	(24)	47/119	(39)	58/227	(26)
Low	8/47	(17)	17/113	(15)	25/182	(14)
Near Normal/NL	2/60	(3)	3/79	(4)	2/51	(4)

V/Q = ventilation perfusion; PE = pulmonary embolism; NL = normal.
[1] Stein et al, Am J Cardiol 1991 (1).
[2] Stein et al, Chest 1991 (2).

embolism of 93%. In patients with prior cardiopulmonary disease, the positive predictive value was 83%, which did not differ to a statistically significant extent.

In patients with a low-probability interpretation of the ventilation-perfusion lung scan, pulmonary embolism was present in 17% of patients with a normal chest radiograph, 15% of patients with no prior cardiopulmonary disease, and 14% of patients with any prior cardiopulmonary disease (Table 15–1).

In patients with a near/normal or normal interpretation of ventilation-perfusion scan, pulmonary embolism was present in 3% with a normal chest radiograph, 4% with no prior cardiopulmonary disease, and 4% with any prior cardiopulmonary disease.

The sensitivities and specificities of high probability ventilation-perfusion scans were similar in patients with a normal chest radiograph, patients with no

Table 15–2. SENSITIVITY AND SPECIFICITY OF V/Q SCANS IN PATIENTS
WITH A NORMAL CHEST RADIOGRAPH, PATIENTS WITH
NO PRIOR CARDIOPULMONARY DISEASE, AND PATIENTS
WITH ANY PRIOR CARDIOPULMONARY DISEASE

	Sensitivity High Prob V/Q Test+ PE+ (%)	Specificity High Prob V/Q Test – /PE– (%)
Normal chest radiograph	6/20 (30)	110/113 (97)
No prior cardiopulmonary disease	50/117 (43)	244/248 (98)
Any prior cardiopulmonary disease	55/140 (39)	375/386 (97)

PE = pulmonary embolism
Prob = probability
All differences NS
Data reprinted from Stein PD, Alavi A, Gottschalk A, et al. Usefulness of non-invasive diagnostic tools for diagnosis
of acute pulmonary embolism in patients with a normal chest radiograph. Am J Cardiol 1991;67:1117–1120; and
Stein PD, Coleman RE, Gottschalk A, et al. Diagnostic utility of ventilation-perfusion lung scans in acute pulmonary
embolism is not diminished by pre-existing cardiac or pulmonary disease. Chest 1991;100:604–606.

prior cardiopulmonary disease, and patients with any prior cardiopulmonary
disease (1,2). The sensitivities in these categories of patients ranged from 30%
to 43% (Table 15–2). The specificities were 97% to 98% (Table 15–2).

Dyspnea and a low partial pressure of oxygen in arterial blood in a patient
with a normal chest radiograph suggested the diagnosis of pulmonary embolism
and was seen more often among patients with pulmonary embolism than in
patients in whom pulmonary embolism was excluded. A PaO_2 ≤70 mm Hg in a
patient with a normal chest radiograph occurred in 9 of 17 (53%) with pulmonary
embolism and in 22 of 93 (24%) with no pulmonary embolism (1). Neither this
combination nor other combinations, however, were diagnostic. This combination, nevertheless, draws attention to the likelihood of pulmonary embolism
and suggests the need for further diagnostic studies.

REFERENCES

1. Stein PD, Alavi A, Gottschalk A, et al. Usefulness of non-invasive diagnostic tools for
   diagnosis of acute pulmonary embolism in patients with a normal chest radiograph.
   Am J Cardiol 1991;67:1117–1120.
2. Stein PD, Coleman RE, Gottschalk A, et al. Diagnostic utility of ventilation-perfusion
   lung scans in acute pulmonary embolism is not diminished by pre-existing cardiac
   or pulmonary disease. Chest 1991;100:604–606.
3. Lesser BA, Leeper KV, Stein PD, et al. The diagnosis of pulmonary embolism in
   patients with chronic obstructive pulmonary disease. Chest 1992;102:17–22.

CHAPTER 16

Perfusion Lung Scans Alone in Acute Pulmonary Embolism

Ventilation lung scans are obtained in combination with perfusion lung scans with the thought that ventilation would be abnormal in areas of pneumonia or local hypoventilation, but would be normal in pulmonary embolism (1). We looked at the value of perfusion scans alone, using original criteria for ventilation-perfusion scan interpretation from the Prospective Investigation of Pulmonary Embolism Diagnosis (PIOPED) (2). Perfusion defects, in the absence of a ventilation scan, were interpreted on the basis of regional findings on the plain chest radiograph. The positive predictive values of high probability, intermediate probability, low probability, and near normal/normal interpretations of perfusion scans alone were comparable with the positive predictive values of ventilation-perfusion scans (Table 16–1) (3).

Ninety-eight patients in PIOPED with suspected acute pulmonary embolism were randomly selected to have perfusion scans read independently of, as well as in combination with, the ventilation scans. These lung scans were read without knowledge of the clinical manifestations or results of the pulmonary angiograms. Pulmonary embolism was diagnosed by pulmonary angiography in 29 of these patients. Pulmonary embolism was excluded by angiography in 33 patients and by outcome committee classification in 5 patients. The diagnosis was uncertain (angiogram or outcome classification not performed) in 31 patients. Therefore, the diagnosis of pulmonary embolism was established or excluded in 67 patients. The diagnostic validity of ventilation-perfusion scans compared with that of perfusion scans alone was evaluated in these 67 patients. Comparisons of the frequency of various scan interpretations (high probability, intermediate probability, low probability, and near normal/normal scans) were obtained in all 98 patients (3).

The characteristics of the 98 patients selected for analysis of their perfusion scans alone were compared with those remaining patients who were not selected for comparative analyses. Age, gender, hospital service in which the patient was located, associated diagnoses, pulmonary artery mean pressure, and partial pressure of oxygen in arterial blood (PaO_2) showed no statistically significant difference between the two groups.

127

Table 16–1.   POSITIVE PREDICTIVE VALUES OF PERFUSION SCANS
ALONE COMPARED WITH VENTILATION-PERFUSION SCANS

Scan Interpretation	Perfusion Scan PE/n (%)	V/Q Scan PE/n (%)
High	14/15 (93)	15/16 (94)
Intermediate	14/38 (37)	9/25 (36)
Low	0/12 (0)	5/25 (20)
Near normal/normal	1/2 (50)	0/1 (0)

All differences between perfusions scan alone and ventilation-perfusion (V/Q) scans were not significant.
PE = pulmonary embolism
n = number of patients
V/Q = ventilation-perfusion
Modified and reprinted with permission from Stein PD, Terrin ML, Gottschalk A, et al. Value of ventilation-perfusion scans compared to perfusion scans alone in acute pulmonary embolism. Am J Cardiol 1992;69:1239–1241.

Table 16–2.   DISTRIBUTION OF LUNG SCAN INTERPRETATIONS IN 98
PATIENTS WITH PERFUSION SCANS ALONE AND
VENTILATION-PERFUSION SCANS

Scan Interpretation	Perfusion Scan (%)	V/Q Scan (%)
High	17	18
Intermediate	49	35
Low	23[a*]	38
Near normal/normal	10	9

[a*] p < 0.05 Perfusion scan versus V/Q scan
PE, pulmonary embolism
n, number of patients
V/Q, ventilation-perfusion
Modified and reprinted with permission from Stein PD, Terrin ML, Gottschalk A, et al. Value of ventilation-perfusion scans compared to perfusion scans alone in acute pulmonary embolism. Am J Cardiol 1992;69:1239–1241.

The positive predictive value of high probability interpretations of perfusion scans alone was 93%, which did not differ significantly from that of high probability interpretations of ventilation-perfusion scans, 94% (Table 16–1) (3).

The positive predictive value for pulmonary embolism among patients with low probability interpretations of perfusion lung scans alone, 0%, did not differ significantly from that of low probability interpretations of ventilation-perfusion scans, 20% (3).

Few patients had nearly normal/normal ventilation-perfusion or perfusion scans. Comparisons in this category, therefore, were not meaningful.

Fewer patients who had perfusion scans alone had low probability interpretations than did those with ventilation-perfusion scans (23% versus 38%), and a trend suggested that more patients with perfusion scans alone had intermediate probability interpretations than did those with ventilation-perfusion scans (Table 16–2) (3).

The sensitivity of high probability perfusion scans alone, 48%, was comparable with that of high probability ventilation-perfusion scans, 52%. The specificity of high probability perfusion scans alone, 97%, was identical to that of high probability ventilation-perfusion scans (3).

We showed that a high probability perfusion scan had no less positive predictive value for acute pulmonary embolism than did a high probability ventilation-perfusion scan. Similarly, a low probability or near normal/normal perfusion scan excluded pulmonary embolism with no less validity than did a low probability or near normal/normal ventilation-perfusion scan. Somewhat more patients who had only perfusion scans had intermediate (indeterminate) probability interpretations than did those with ventilation-perfusion scans, but this difference was not statistically significant. Fewer patients with low probability perfusion scans alone had low probability interpretations. The data indicate that if ventilation scans cannot be performed, useful information can be obtained if the interpretation of the perfusion is high or low probability, or near normal/normal. If the perfusion scan is interpreted as intermediate probability for pulmonary embolism, a subsequent ventilation-perfusion scan may change the interpretation to a more definitive probability. A promptly obtained perfusion scan may spare patients an unnecessary hospitalization or unnecessary anticoagulant therapy while awaiting further diagnostic tests (4).

Investigators in the PISA-PED study used only perfusion lung scans (5). A perfusion scan compatible with pulmonary embolism was defined as a scan with a single or multiple wedge-shaped perfusion defects of any size. Diversion of blood away from an underperfused area usually resulted in associated overperfused single or multiple wedge-shaped areas. A perfusion scan was considered negative for pulmonary embolism if single or multiple perfusion defects did not exhibit a wedge shape. Positive perfusion scans had a positive predictive value of 95%. A negative perfusion scan had a negative predictive value of 81%. Combining clinical assessment with the perfusion scan showed good results when clinical assessment and the perfusion scan reading were concordant. Only a minority of patients (21%) had discordant clinical and perfusion scan assessments, and these patients required pulmonary angiography. These results, at first glance, appear better than the results of PIOPED. In the PISA-PED study, however, 24% of patients had normal perfusion scans; in PIOPED, only 2% had normal scintiscans. The two study populations, therefore, were dissimilar.

REFERENCES

1. Wagner HN JR, Lopez-Majano V, Langan JK, et al. Radioactive xenon in the differential diagnosis of pulmonary embolism. Radiology 1968;91:1168–1174.
2. A Collaborative Study by the PIOPED Investigators. Value of the ventilation-perfusion scan in acute pulmonary embolism: results of the prospective investigation of pulmonary embolism diagnosis (PIOPED). JAMA 1990;263:2753–2759.
3. Stein PD, Terrin ML, Gottschalk A, et al. Value of ventilation-perfusion scans compared to perfusion scans alone in acute pulmonary embolism. Am J Cardiol 1992;69:1239–1241.
4. van Beek EJR, Kuyer PMM, Schenk BE, et al. A normal perfusion lung scan in patients with clinically suspected pulmonary embolism. Chest 1995;108:170–173.
5. PISA-PED Investigators. Invasive and noninvasive diagnosis of pulmonary embolism. Chest 1995;107:33S–38S.

CHAPTER 17

Revised Criteria for Evaluation of Ventilation-Perfusion Lung Scans Recommended by Nuclear Physicians in PIOPED

After the Prospective Investigation of Pulmonary Embolism Diagnosis (PIOPED) was concluded, nuclear physicians in PIOPED re-evaluated the original criteria for interpreting ventilation-perfusion lung scans (1). They correlated probability estimates of pulmonary embolism based on the ventilation-perfusion lung scans with the actual frequency of pulmonary embolism as determined by pulmonary angiography.

The nuclear physicians in PIOPED determined that most of the original PIOPED criteria appropriately categorized ventilation-perfusion scans (1). However, they recommended that three criteria be reconsidered (see Table 17–3):

1. Two segmental mismatches may not be the optimum threshold for high probability, and in some cases, two mismatches should be considered for intermediate probability. Because of the small number of cases with this finding, however, no definite, statistically founded recommendation could be made.
2. A single, moderate mismatched perfusion defect is appropriately categorized as intermediate, rather than as low, probability.
3. Extensive matched ventilation-perfusion abnormalities are appropriate for low probability, provided that the chest radiograph is clear. Single-matched defects may be better categorized as intermediate probability. Owing to the small number of cases with this finding, no definite, statistically founded recommendation could be made.

The nuclear physicians suggested that the revised criteria resulting from these adjustments now be used for interpreting ventilation-perfusion scans (1).

130

Table 17–1. FREQUENCY OF PULMONARY EMBOLISM IN PATIENTS WITH VARIOUS PATTERNS OF MISMATCHED PERFUSION DEFECTS

Type of Mismatch	Number of Patients	PE (%)
1 segmental equivalent	33	52
One large defect	24	46
Two moderate defects	9	67
1.5 segmental equivalents	18	72
One large + one moderate defect	11	73
Three moderate defects	7	71
2 segmental equivalents	7	71
Two large defects	5	80
One large + two moderate defects	1	0
Four moderate defects	1	100
2.5 segmental equivalents	10	100
Two large + one moderate defect	8	100
One large + three moderate defects	1	100
Five moderate defects	1	100

defect = mismatched perfusion defect
Modified and reprinted with permission from Gottschalk A, Sostman HD, Coleman RE, et al. Ventilation-perfusion scintigraphy in the PIOPED study. Part II. Evaluation of the scintigraphic criteria and interpretations. J Nucl Med 1993;34:1119–1126.

Analyses focused upon individual PIOPED criteria. In many instances, combined patterns were excluded. Combined patterns involving mismatched defects were considered in the analysis of criteria for "high probability," since mismatched defects and high probability diagnoses took priority over other patterns in the PIOPED criteria. For example, a patient with three segmental mismatches (which meets criteria for high probability) and matched ventilation-perfusion defects (which meet the criteria for low probability) should have been assigned to the high probability category. Therefore, all patients with mismatched perfusion defects, including those with combined patterns, were considered in the analysis of high probability (1). Because low-probability criteria did not take precedence in scan categorization, it was necessary to isolate analyses of those criteria to patients who did not have scan findings that would place them in a higher category (1).

Correlations of scintigraphic patterns that fulfilled individual PIOPED criteria were made with pulmonary angiograms read as definitely positive or definitely negative for pulmonary embolism (1). There were 731 patients in PIOPED in the randomized obligatory pulmonary angiography group who had definitive angiographic results (2). Correlations of ventilation-perfusion scans with pulmonary angiograms were made in 393 of those patients (54%) who satisfied pertinent individual PIOPED criteria on their ventilation-perfusion lung scans (1).

Analyses of the PIOPED criteria for evaluating ventilation-perfusion scans arbitrarily defined the following ranges:

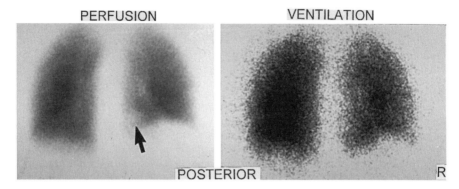

PERFUSION   VENTILATION

POSTERIOR   R

Figure 17–1. **Left.** Perfusion scan, posterior view, showing solitary perfusion defect (arrow), in the posterior basal segment of the right lower lobe. **Right.** Ventilation scan, posterior view, initial breath showing no ventilation defect. Equilibrium and washout phases also showed no ventilation defect. According to original PIOPED criteria, this single mismatched moderate-size perfusion defect should have been interpreted as low probability for pulmonary embolism, but according to the revised PIOPED criteria, this ventilation-perfusion scan should be interpreted as intermediate probability. Pulmonary embolism was shown on the pulmonary angiogram.

Table 17–2. PATIENTS WITH ONLY MATCHED DEFECTS ON THE VENTILATION-PERFUSION SCAN

	Numbers of Pts.	PE (%)
Single matched defect (any size)	23	26
Multiple matched defects (any size)	66	14
All matched defects	89	17

Data from Gottschalk A, Sostman HD, Coleman RE, et al. Ventilation-perfusion scintigraphy in the PIOPED study. Part II. Evaluation of the scintigraphic criteria and interpretations. J Nucl Med 1993;34:1119–1126.

1. High probability = 80 to 100% likelihood of PE.
2. Intermediate probability = 20 to 79% likelihood of PE.
3. Low probability = 0 to 19% likelihood of PE.

Two large mismatched perfusion defects did not provide a reliable interpretation of high probability, whereas 2.5 mismatched segmental equivalent perfusion defects provided a more accurate categorization (Table 17–1) (1). A mismatched segmental equivalent perfusion defect is 1 large (>75% of a segment) mismatched perfusion defect or 2 moderate-size (25% to 75% of a segment) perfusion defects. The nuclear physicians in PIOPED could not definitely recommend changing the threshold for high probability, however, because the number of patients with this pattern was small.

Ten of 28 patients (36%) with a single, moderate mismatched perfusion defect had pulmonary embolism (1). It was clear that this was not a valid criterion for low probability. Scans with this finding should be considered intermediate probability for pulmonary embolism (Fig. 17–1).

Table 17–3. ORIGINAL PIOPED CRITERIA FOR VENTILATION/PERFUSION LUNG SCANS COMPARED WITH PROPOSED REVISED CRITERIA

HIGH PROBABILITY		INTERMEDIATE PROBABILITY		LOW PROBABILITY	
PIOPED (2)	PIOPED Revised (1)	PIOPED (2)	PIOPED Revised (1)	PIOPED (2)	PIOPED Revised (1)
≥2 Large V/Q mismatches or 1 large V/Q and ≥2 moderate V/Q mismatches or ≥4 Moderate V/Q mismatches	2 large V/Q mismatches (2 large V/Q are borderline high probability or 1 large V/Q and ≥2 moderate V/Q mismatches or ≥4 moderate V/Q mismatches	1 large V/Q mismatch ± 1 moderate V/Q mismatch or 2 or 3 moderate V/Q mismatches	1 large ± 1 moderate V/Q mismatch or 1 to 3 moderate V/Q mismatches or 1 matched V/Q with Nl x-ray (2 large V/Q mismatches are borderline intermediate to high probability)	1 Moderate V/Q mismatch with Nl x-ray or Q << x-ray or V/Q matches with Nl x-ray or x-ray << Q involving ≤4 segments in 1 lung and ≤3 segment in 1 lung region or Perfusion defects due to pleural effusion, cardiomegaly, enlarged aorta, hilum, mediastinum, and elevated diaphragm or >3 small Q with Nl x-ray or Very low probability ≤3 small Q with Nl x-ray	≥1 Q << x-ray defect or ≥2 V/Q matches with Nl x-ray and some areas of normal perfusion in lung or Perfusion defects due to pleural effusion, cardiomegaly, enlarged aorta, hilum, mediastinum, and elevated diaphragm or ≥1 small Q with Nl x-ray

Nl, normal; V/Q = ventilation/perfusion; x-ray = radiographic abnormality in region of perfusion abnormality; Mod = moderate; Seg = segment. Moderate = 25–75% Segment. Large = >75% Segment

V/Q mismatch = Nl V and Ni x-ray or Q > V or x-ray in region of Q defect.

Data from PIOPED (2) and Gottschalk and associates (1).

Patients with a single matched perfusion defect appeared to have a higher likelihood of pulmonary embolism than patients with 2 or more matched perfusion defects (1). A single matched defect was associated with pulmonary embolism in 26% of patients (Table 17–2). Two or more matched perfusion defects were associated with pulmonary embolism in 14% of patients. A single matched perfusion defect, therefore, should be considered for intermediate probability.

REFERENCES

1. Gottschalk A, Sostman HD, Coleman RE, et al. Ventilation-perfusion scintigraphy in the PIOPED study. Part II. Evaluation of the scintigraphic criteria and interpretations. J Nucl Med 1993;34:1119–1126.
2. A Collaborative Study by the PIOPED Investigators. Value of the ventilation-perfusion scan in acute pulmonary embolism: results of the prospective investigation of pulmonary embolism diagnosis (PIOPED). JAMA 1990;263:2753–2759.

C H A P T E R 18

Criteria for Very Low Probability Interpretation of Ventilation-Perfusion Lung Scans

The criteria used for the interpretation of low probability ventilation-perfusion lung scans in PIOPED patients with suspected acute pulmonary embolism (1) have been modified since the conclusion of the Prospective Investigation of Pulmonary Embolism Diagnosis (PIOPED) (2) (Chapter 17). In PIOPED, using the original criteria, 14% of patients with ventilation-perfusion scans interpreted as low probability had pulmonary embolism (1). The PIOPED criteria for low probability included (1):

1. Nonsegmental perfusion defects ≤ radiographic abnormality.
2. Perfusion defects ≤ ventilation defects with normal chest radiograph.
3. Perfusion defects < radiographic defect.
4. More than 3 small perfusion defects with a normal chest radiograph.
5. A single moderate-size mismatched perfusion defect with a normal chest radiograph.

The Nuclear Medicine Working Group of PIOPED recommended that the following modifications be made for low probability interpretations (2):

1. A single, moderate mismatched perfusion defect should be categorized as intermediate rather than as low probability.
2. Multiple and relatively extensive matched ventilation-perfusion abnormalities are appropriate for low probability, provided that the chest radiograph is clear.
3. Single matched defects may be better categorized as intermediate probability, although this cannot be definitely validated statistically.

These revised PIOPED criteria were found to be more accurate than the original PIOPED criteria (3). The modified PIOPED criteria, however, were tested

135

prospectively in a population of patients that differed significantly from the population of patients investigated in PIOPED (4).

A single, moderate-size segmental perfusion mismatch was categorized as intermediate probability for pulmonary embolism instead of low probability. Patients with a low probability interpretation using the modified criteria had a 6% frequency of pulmonary embolism (4); in PIOPED, such patients had a 14% frequency of pulmonary embolism. In the population of patients investigated, 36% had normal pulmonary scintiscans, compared with 2% in PIOPED. The prevalence of pulmonary embolism was also lower, 10% versus 28% in PIOPED.

The modifications of the PIOPED criteria for low probability were made on the assumption that patients with low probability interpretations of ventilation-perfusion scans should have a positive predictive value of pulmonary embolism <20% (2). A "very low probability" interpretation with a positive predictive value less than 10% would be more useful than a "low probability" interpretation (5). In view of this, we evaluated the individual characteristics and combinations of characteristics of the low probability ventilation-perfusion lung scan to identify criteria for a "very low probability" interpretation (<10% positive predictive value) (6). To do this, we maximized the useful PIOPED database by evaluating individual lungs rather than individual patients. We also evaluated the arm of PIOPED that included patients referred for pulmonary angiography as well as patients randomized for pulmonary angiography. The analysis identified some ventilation-perfusion scan criteria that seem appropriate for a "very low probability" interpretation (<10% positive predictive value) in patients with suspected acute pulmonary embolism (6). The data were limited, however, and statistically significant differences were not shown between positive predictive values of ventilation-perfusion scan criteria we categorized as "very low probability" and criteria we categorized as "low probability." Nevertheless, this is the largest database on this subject, and larger databases, studied in the detail of the data acquired for PIOPED, are unlikely to be acquired in the near future. We believe that the trends suggested by the following data can be applied in a useful fashion.

Criteria Suited for Very Low Probability (<10% Positive Predictive Value for Pulmonary Embolism)

Some nonsegmental perfusion abnormalities were associated with a very low positive predictive value for pulmonary embolism. These were enlargement of the heart, hila, or mediastinum, or elevated hemidiaphragm (Fig. 18–1).

A pleural effusion with obliteration of the costophrenic angle showed a higher positive predictive value for pulmonary embolism than other nonsegmental perfusion abnormalities, and was not included among the nonsegmental perfusion abnormalities associated with a very low probability of pulmonary embolism (Fig. 18–2). As shown in Table 18–1, lungs with a nonsegmental perfusion abnormality that included enlargement of the heart, hila, mediastinum, or elevated hemidiaphragm had a positive predictive value for pulmonary embolism of 8% (6). Lungs with a pleural effusion that caused obliteration of the costophrenic angle had a positive predictive value for pulmonary embolism of 29%.(Table 18–1, Fig. 18–3) (6). This criterion had been used previously for the interpretation of ventilation-perfusion scans as low probability (1,7,8).

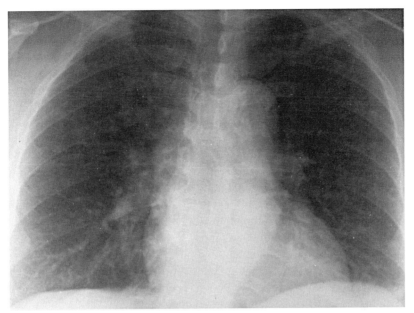

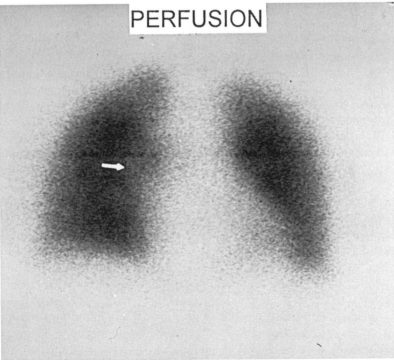

PERFUSION

Figure 18–1. **Top.** Plain chest radiograph showing mild cardiomegaly and prominence of hila. **Bottom.** Perfusion lung scan, anterior view, showing nonsegmental perfusion abnormalities. The scan shows prominence of the hila, more clearly shown on the right (arrow) and cardiomegaly. These types of nonsegmental perfusion abnormalities were associated with a very low positive predictive value for pulmonary embolism.

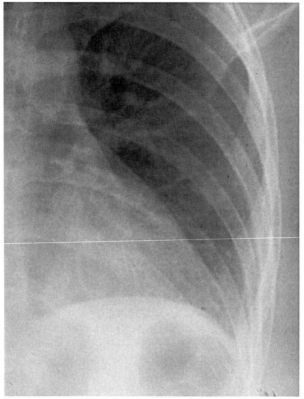

PERFUSION   VENTILATION

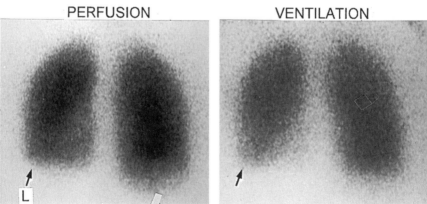

POSTERIOR

Figure 18–2. **Top.** Plain chest radiograph showing small pleural effusion. **Bottom Left.** Perfusion lung scan, posterior view, showing a nonsegmental perfusion defect (arrow) in the region of the pleural effusion. **Bottom.** Ventilation lung scan, equilibrium phase, posterior view, showing a ventilation defect (arrow)in the region of the pleural effusion. Pulmonary embolism was found in 29% of patients with such nonsegmental perfusion abnormalities.

Table 18–1. POSITIVE PREDICTIVE VALUE OF INDIVIDUAL CRITERIA USED FOR LOW PROBABILITY ASSESSMENT OF VENTILATION-PERFUSION LUNG SCANS

	PE/Total (%)	95% CI
Lungs with Only One Type of Perfusion Defect		
Costophrenic angle effusion	4/14 (29)[a]	8–58
Nonsegmental abnormality	8/103 (8)	3–15
Perfusion defect < x-ray		
1 zone	2/24 (8)	1–27
2 or 3 zones	1/16 (6)	0–30
All zones	3/48 (8)	2–20
Matched V/Q (x-ray normal)		
1 zone	4/34 (12)	3–27
2 or 3 zones	1/30 (3)	0–17
All zones	5/64 (8)	3–17
Lungs with Two Types of Perfusion Defects		
Costophrenic angle effusion	1/10 (10)	0–45
+		
Nonsegmental abnormality		
Costophrenic angle effusion	1/8 (13)	0–53
+		
Matched V/Q (x-ray normal)		
Nonsegmental abnormality	3/34 (9)	2–24
+		
Perfusion defect < x-ray		
Nonsegmental abnormality	4/29 (14)	4–12
+		
Matched V/Q (x-ray normal)		

[a] Costophrenic angle effusion vs nonsegmental abnormality P < 0.02
Costophrenic angle effusion vs parenchymal x-ray P < 0.05
Costophrenic angle effusion vs matched V/Q P < 0.05
Combinations of two perfusion defects were excluded from the table if the combination was observed in only 4 or fewer lungs.
Costophrenic angle effusion = pleural effusion with obliteration of the costophrenic angle with the perfusion defect ≤ x-ray abnormality.
Nonsegmental abnormality = nonsegmental perfusion abnormality including enlargement of the hilum, mediastinum, or heart or elevated diaphragm with the perfusion defect ≤ x-ray abnormality.
Perfusion defect < x-ray, = parenchymal abnormality on the chest radiograph with the perfusion defect < radiographic abnormality.
Matched V/Q (x-ray normal) = Matched ventilation-perfusion defect with normal chest radiograph and perfusion defect ≤ ventilation defect.
Reprinted with permission from Stein PD, Relyea B, Gottschalk A. Evaluation of the positive predictive value of specific criteria used for the assessment of low probability ventilation-perfusion lung scans. J Nucl Med 1996;37:577–581.

Matched ventilation-perfusion abnormalities, in the presence of a regionally normal chest radiograph, when occurring as the only type of perfusion defect in 2 or 3 zones of a single lung, showed a positive predictive value for pulmonary embolism of 3% (Table 18–1) (6). A matched ventilation-perfusion defect occurring as the only type of perfusion defect in 1 zone of a single lung showed

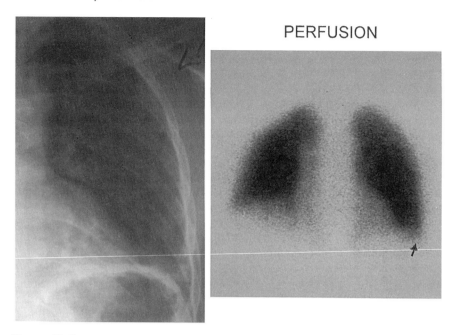

PERFUSION

Figure 18–3. **Left.** Plain chest radiograph showing linear atelectasis in the left lower zone. **Right.** Perfusion lung scan, anterior view, showing small perfusion defect (arrow) in the region of the atelectasis. Perfusion defects smaller than associated parenchymal abnormalities on the chest radiograph, when occurring as the only type of perfusion defect, showed a positive predictive value for pulmonary embolism of 8%. The pulmonary angiogram in this patient showed no pulmonary embolism.

a trend toward a higher positive predictive value for pulmonary embolism than matched perfusion defects in 2 or 3 zones in a single lung (Fig. 18–4). The positive predictive value for pulmonary embolism with matched perfusion defects in 1 zone was 4 of 34 (12%); in 2 zones, 1 of 20 (5%); and in 3 zones, 0 of 10 (0%) (Table 18–1) (6). A matched ventilation-perfusion defect in the presence of a normal chest radiograph was one of the criteria used by PIOPED and others to assess low probability (1,7–11). In PIOPED, a zone of the lung was defined as the upper, middle, or lower third of the lung, divided in the cranial-caudal direction without regard to lung volume (12).

A nonsegmental perfusion defect in combination with a perfusion defect smaller than the abnormality on the chest radiograph showed a positive predictive value for pulmonary embolism of 9% (Table 18–1) (6).

Criteria Suited for Low Probability (10% to 19% Positive Predictive Value for Pulmonary Embolism), but not Suited for Very Low Probability

A pleural effusion with blunting of the costophrenic angle in combination with a nonsegmental perfusion defect (enlargement of the heart, hila, or medias-

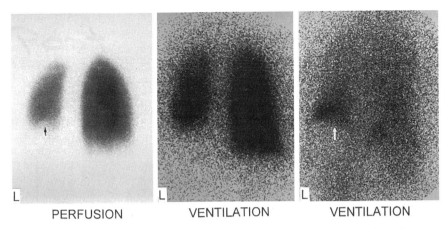

PERFUSION   VENTILATION   VENTILATION

Figure 18–4. **Left.** Perfusion lung scan, posterior view, showing a perfusion defect (arrow) in the left lower zone. **Center.** Ventilation scan, posterior view, initial breath, showing impaired ventilation in the left lower zone. **Right.** Ventilation scan, posterior view, 240 sec washout, showing impaired washout in the left lower zone (arrow). A matched ventilation-perfusion defect occurring as the only type of perfusion defect in 1 zone of a single lung showed a trend toward a higher positive predictive value for pulmonary embolism than matched perfusion defects in 2 zones or 3 zones in a single lung. This patient showed no pulmonary embolism on the pulmonary angiogram.

tinum, or elevated hemidiaphragm) showed a positive predictive value for pulmonary embolism of 10% (Table 18–1) (6). Note that a small pleural effusion alone is associated with a higher positive predictive value for pulmonary embolism (29%).

A pleural effusion with blunting of the costophrenic angle in combination with a matched ventilation-perfusion abnormality and a regionally normal chest radiograph showed a positive predictive value for pulmonary embolism of 13% (Table 18–1) (6).

A nonsegmental perfusion defect (enlargement of the heart, hila, or mediastinum, or elevated hemidiaphragm) in combination with a matched ventilation-perfusion defect showed a positive predictive value for pulmonary embolism of 14% (Table 18–1) (6).

Some combinations of 2 types of perfusion defects had too few patients to analyze. Data were insufficient to analyze 3 or 4 types of perfusion defects in combination (6).

Stratification of patients according to the presence or absence of prior cardiopulmonary disease suggested that some criteria suited for the general population as "very low probability" (positive predictive value <10%) might only be "low probability" (positive predictive value 10% to 19%) in patients with no prior cardiopulmonary disease (Table 18–2) (6).

In summary, analysis of PIOPED data identified some V/Q scan criteria (Table 18–3) that seem appropriate for a "very low probability" interpretation (<10% positive predictive value) in patients with suspected acute PE. The data were limited, and statistically significant differences were not shown between positive predictive values of V/Q criteria we categorize as "very low probability" and criteria we categorize as "low probability." We believe, nevertheless, that

Table 18–2. POSITIVE PREDICTIVE VALUE OF INDIVIDUAL CRITERIA USED FOR LOW PROBABILITY ASSESSMENT OF V/Q SCANS IN LUNGS OF PATIENTS WITH AND PATIENTS WITHOUT PRIOR CARDIOPULMONARY DISEASE

	No Prior CPD PE/Total (%)	Prior CPD PE/Total (%)
Lungs with Only One Type of Perfusion Defect		
Costophrenic angle effusion	2/6 (33)	2/8 (25)
Nonsegmental abnormality	1/44 (2)	7/56 (13)
Perfusion defect < x-ray	2/17 (12)	1/23 (4)
Matched V/Q (x-ray normal)	4/22 (18)[a]	1/40 (3)
Lungs with Two Types of Perfusion Defects		
Nonsegmental abnormality + Perfusion defect < x-ray	1/8 (13)	2/25 (8)
Nonsegmental abnormality + Matched V/Q (x-ray normal)	1/8 (13)	2/19 (11)

Combination of two perfusion defects were excluded from the table if the combination was observed in only 4 or fewer lungs.
Some patients had no information regarding CPD or no CPD. Therefore, the totals in this table do not equal the values in Table 18–1.
CPD = cardiopulmonary disease
Costophrenic angle effusion, pleural effusion with obliteration of the costophrenic angle with the perfusion defect ≤ x-ray abnormality
Nonsegmental abnormality = nonsegmental perfusion abnormality including enlargement of the hilum, mediastinum, or heart, or elevated diaphragm with the perfusion defect ≤ x-ray abnormality
Perfusion defect < x-ray = parenchymal abnormality on the chest radiograph with the perfusion defect < radiographic abnormality
Matched V/Q (x-ray normal) = matched ventilation-perfusion defect with normal chest radiograph and perfusion defect ≤ ventilation defect
[a] $P < 0.05$ no CPD versus CPD
Reprinted with permission from Stein PD, Relyea B, Gottschalk A. Evaluation of the positive predictive value of specific criteria used for the assessment of low probability ventilation-perfusion lung scans. J Nucl Med 1996;37:577–581.

the trends suggested by the data can be applied in a useful fashion. Nonsegmental perfusion abnormalities, perfusion defects smaller than opacities on the chest radiograph, these 2 types of perfusion abnormalities in combination, and matched ventilation-perfusion abnormalities in 2 or 3 zones of a single lung showed a positive predictive value <10%. These criteria, therefore, can be used for a very low probability interpretation. A matched ventilation-perfusion defect in only 1 zone of the lung showed a positive predictive value for pulmonary embolism higher than 10% and should be not be considered a criterion for very low probability, but can be considered a criterion for low probability. Perfusion defects associated with small pleural effusions (obliteration of the costophrenic angle) showed a positive predictive value of 29% and should be considered a criterion for intermediate probability.

Table 18–3. CATEGORIZATION OF CRITERIA USED FOR
INTERPRETATION OF VENTILATION-PERFUSION SCANS IN
PIOPED AS LOW PROBABILITY BASED ON INDIVIDUAL
POSITIVE PREDICTIVE VALUES

**Criteria Appropriate for Very Low Probability Interpretation of V/Q Scan
(Positive Predictive Value <10%)**
Nonsegmental abnormality
Perfusion defect < x-ray
Matched V/Q (x-ray normal) in 2 or 3 zones of a single lung
Nonsegmental abnormality + perfusion defect < x-ray

**Criteria Appropriate for Low Probability Interpretation of V/Q Scan
(Positive Predictive Value 10–19%)**
Matched V/Q (x-ray normal) in 1 zone of a single lung
Costophrenic angle effusion + nonsegmental abnormality
Costophrenic angle effusion + matched V/Q (x-ray normal)
Nonsegmental abnormality + matched V/Q (x-ray normal)

**Criteria Appropriate for Intermediate Probability Interpretation of V/Q Scan
(Positive Predictive Value 20–79%)**
Costophrenic angle effusion

V/Q = ventilation-perfusion
Costophrenic angle effusion = pleural effusion with obliteration of the costophrenic angle with the perfusion defect ≤ x-ray abnormality
Nonsegmental abnormality = nonsegmental perfusion abnormality including enlargement of the hilum, mediastinum, or heart, or elevated diaphragm with the perfusion defect ≤ x-ray abnormality
Perfusion defect < x-ray = parenchymal abnormality on the chest radiograph with the perfusion defect < radiographic abnormality
Matched V/Q (x-ray normal) = matched ventilation-perfusion defect with normal chest radiograph and perfusion defect ≤ ventilation defect
Reprinted with permission from Stein PD, Relya B, Gottschalk A. Evaluation of the positive predictive value of specific criteria used for the assessment of low probability ventilation-perfusion lung scans. J Nucl Med. 1996;37:577–581.

REFERENCES

1. A Collaborative Study by the PIOPED Investigators. Value of the ventilation-perfusion scan in acute pulmonary embolism: results of the Prospective Investigation of Pulmonary Embolism Diagnosis (PIOPED). JAMA 1990;263:2753–2759.
2. Gottschalk A, Sostman HD, Coleman RE, et al. Ventilation-perfusion scintigraphy in the PIOPED study. Part II. Evaluation of the scintigraphic criteria and interpretations. J Nucl Med 1993;34:1119–1126.
3. Sostman HD, Coleman RE, DeLong DM, et al. Evaluation of revised criteria for ventilation-perfusion scintigraphy in patients with suspected pulmonary embolism. Radiology 1994;193:103–107.
4. Freitas JE, Sarosi MG, Nagle CC, et al. Modified PIOPED criteria used in clinical practice. J Nucl Med 1995;36:1573–1578.
5. Hull RD, Raskob GE. Low-probability lung scan findings: a need for change. Ann Internal Med 1991;114:142–143.
6. Stein PD, Relyea B, Gottschalk A. Evaluation of the positive predictive value of specific criteria used for the assessment of low probability ventilation-perfusion lung scans. J Nucl Med 1996;37:577–581.
7. Biello DR, Mattar AG, McKnight RC, et al. Ventilation-perfusion studies in suspected pulmonary embolism. Am J Radiol 1979;133:1033–1037.

8. Biello DR. Radiological (scintigraphic) evaluation of patients with suspected pulmonary thromboembolism. JAMA 1987;257:3257–3259.
9. McNeil BJ. Ventilation-perfusion studies and the diagnosis of pulmonary embolism: concise communication. J Nucl Med 1980;21:319–323.
10. Sullivan DC, Coleman RE, Mills SR, et al. Lung scan interpretation: effect of different observers and different criteria. Radiology 1983;149:803–807.
11. Webber MM, Gomes AS, Roe D, et al. Comparison of Biello, McNeil, and PIOPED criteria for the diagnosis of pulmonary emboli on lung scans. Am J Roentgenol 1990;154:975–981.
12. Gottschalk A, Juni J, Sostman HD, et al. Ventilation-perfusion scintigraphy in the PIOPED study. Part I: data collection and tabulation. J Nucl Med 1993;34:1109–1118.

Pulmonary Embolism in Patients with Small Perfusion Defects

If the only scintigraphic abnormality on ventilation-perfusion lung scans in the Prospective Investigative Pulmonary Embolism Diagnosis (PIOPED) was 1 to 3 small segmental perfusion defects in the presence of a normal regional chest radiograph, the lung scan was interpreted as very low probability for pulmonary embolism (PE) (1). A small subsegmental perfusion defect was defined as less than 25% of a segment in the presence of a regionally normal chest radiograph (1). Evaluation of this criterion was independent of findings on the ventilation scan, and a regionally normal chest radiograph was required. Analysis of some of the data from PIOPED showed that patients with any small subsegmental perfusion defects with a regionally normal chest radiograph showed pulmonary embolism in 2 of 29 (7%) (2). Based on these data, any number of small subsegmental perfusion defects with a regionally normal chest radiograph, in the revised ventilation-perfusion criteria resulting from PIOPED, were assigned to a low probability interpretation (an interpretation with a positive predictive value of <20% for pulmonary embolism) (2).

Alderson and Martin, using pooled data, calculated a positive predictive value of 0 of 33 (0%) for small ventilation-perfusion mismatches defined as <25% of a segment (3). (The PIOPED criteria differed because PIOPED indicated that ventilation scan findings were irrelevant when only small perfusion defects were present.) The number of small defects was unstated. Silberstein and associates, based on data from PIOPED, showed pulmonary embolism in 2 of 80 (2.5%) patients with 1 to 3 small subsegmental perfusion defects (4). They did not evaluate the positive predictive value for pulmonary embolism of more than 3 subsegmental defects. Findings on the ventilation scan were irrelevant in this study.

One to Three Small Perfusion Defects

We further assessed the diagnostic value of small subsegmental perfusion defects on lung scans of patients with suspected acute pulmonary embolism

145

(5). The positive predictive value for pulmonary embolism of lung scans with 1 to 3 small subsegmental perfusion defects with a regionally normal chest radiograph was 1% to 3%, depending on the group analyzed. This satisfied the criterion for a very low probability interpretation (<10% positive predictive value) (6). This low positive predictive value for pulmonary embolism is comparable to the positive predictive value reported by Silberstein (4). Among patients in whom pulmonary embolism was diagnosed or excluded by pulmonary angiography, 1 of 29 (3%) with 1 to 3 small subsegmental perfusion defects showed pulmonary embolism (Table 19–1, Fig. 19–1, Fig. 19–2) (5). Among patients in

Table 19–1. PULMONARY EMBOLISM WITH LUNG SCANS SHOWING ONLY SMALL SUBSEGMENTAL PERFUSION DEFECTS

Number of Small Subsegmental Perfusion Defects	Diagnosis by Pulmonary Angiography PE/Total (%)	Diagnosis by Pulmonary Angiography or Follow-Up PE/Total (%)
1–3	1/29 (3)	1/68 (1)[a]
>3	3/18 (17)	3/27 (11)
Any	4/47 (9)	4/95 (4)

[a] $P < .05$ 1–3 Defects versus >3 Defects
Reprinted with permission from Stein PD, Henry JW, Gottschalk A. Small segmental perfusion defects in the assessment of lung scans of patients with suspected pulmonary embolism. J Nucl Med 1996;37:1313–1315.

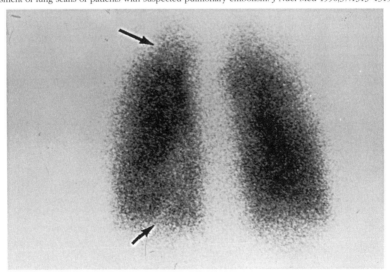

Figure 19–1. Posterior view of a perfusion lung scan. Both the round lesion in the left apex (arrow) and the retrocardiac lesion in the base of the left lung (arrow) were small segmental perfusion defects (<25% of a segment). The patient showed no pulmonary embolism on pulmonary angiography. (Reprinted with permission from from Stein PD, Henry JW, Gottschalk A. Small segmental perfusion defects in the assessment of lung scans of patients with suspected pulmonary embolism. J Nucl Med 1996;37:1313–1315.)

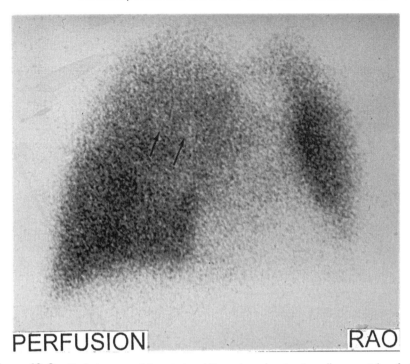

Figure 19–2. Perfusion scan, right anterior oblique view, showing 2 small segmental perfusion defects (arrows), both <25% of a segment. Outcome analysis showed no evidence of pulmonary embolism.

whom pulmonary embolism was diagnosed or excluded by pulmonary angiography or follow-up, 1 of 68 (1%) showed pulmonary embolism. Angiographic findings in patients who had pulmonary embolism are shown in Table 19–2. Most vessels with pulmonary embolism showed partial filling.

More Than Three Small Perfusion Defects

The positive predictive value for pulmonary embolism of lung scans with more than 3 small subsegmental perfusion defects with a regionally normal chest radiograph was 11% to 17%, depending on the group analyzed (5). Among patients in whom pulmonary embolism was diagnosed or excluded by pulmonary angiography, 3 of 18 (17%) with 3 or more small subsegmental perfusion defects showed pulmonary embolism (Table 19–1). Among patients in whom pulmonary embolism was diagnosed or excluded by pulmonary angiography or follow-up, 3 of 27 (11%) showed pulmonary embolism. A perfusion lung scan with more than 3 small subsegmental defects, therefore, satisfied the criteria for a low probability interpretation (<20% positive predictive value for pulmonary embolism) (2, 6).

Any Small Perfusion Defects

Among patients in whom pulmonary embolism was diagnosed or excluded by pulmonary angiography, 4 of 47 (9%) with any small subsegmental perfusion

Table 19–2. PULMONARY ANGIOGRAPHIC FINDINGS IN PATIENTS WHO SHOWED PULMONARY EMBOLISM AND SMALL SUBSEGMENTAL PERFUSION DEFECTS

Pt #	Number of Defects	Artery in Which PE Was Visualized	Partial Filling	100% Occlusion
1	1–3	RLL, 1[a]* seg	X	
		RLL, peripheral	X	
2	>3	LLL, peripheral	X	
3	>3	RLL	X	
		RLL, 2 seg	X	
		RLL, 1 seg		X
4	>3	LML, peripheral	X	
		LLL, peripheral	X	

PT #, patient number
LLL, left lower lobar artery
RLL, right lower lobar artery
LML, left middle lobar artery
Seg, segmental artery
PE, pulmonary embolism
[a]* the number indicates the number of segmental arteries showing PE
Reprinted with permission from the Stein PD, Henry JW, Gottschalk A. Small segmental perfusion defects in the assessment of lung scans of patients with suspected pulmonary embolism. J Nucl Med 1996;37:1313–1315.

defects showed pulmonary embolism (Table 19–1) (5). Among patients in whom pulmonary embolism was diagnosed or excluded by pulmonary angiography or follow-up, 4 of 95 (4%) with any small perfusion defects showed pulmonary embolism.

A trend suggested a higher positive predictive value for pulmonary embolism with more than 3 small subsegmental perfusion defects in patients with no prior cardiopulmonary disease than in patients with prior cardiopulmonary disease (5). Few patients with prior cardiopulmonary disease, however, had perfusion scans that showed only small subsegmental defects because the criteria for inclusion required no regional parenchymal abnormalities on the chest radiograph (5).

In summary, perfusion lung scans with 1 to 3 small subsegmental defects satisfy the criterion for a very low probability (<10% positive predictive value) for pulmonary embolism, and perfusion lung scans with >3 small subsegmental defects satisfy the criterion for a low probability (<20% positive predictive value) for pulmonary embolism.

REFERENCES

1. The PIOPED Investigators. Value of the ventilation-perfusion scan in acute pulmonary embolism: results of the Prospective Investigation of Pulmonary Embolism Diagnosis (PIOPED). JAMA 1990;263:2753–2759.

2. Gottschalk A, Sostman HD, Coleman RE, et al. Ventilation-perfusion scintigraphy in the PIOPED study. Part II. Evaluation of the scintigraphic criteria and interpretations. J Nucl Med 1993;34:1119–1126.
3. Alderson PO, Martin EC. Pulmonary embolism: diagnosis with multiple imaging modalities. Radiology 1987;164:297–312.
4. Silberstein E, Worsley DF, Alavi A, et al. The clinical significance of the very low probability (PIOPED) lung scan pattern. J Nucl Med 1995;36:113P. Abstract.
5. Stein PD, Henry JW, Gottschalk A. Small segmental perfusion defects in the assessment of patients with suspected pulmonary embolism. J Nucl Med 1996;37:1313–1315.
6. Stein PD, Relyea B, Gottschalk A. Evaluation of the positive predictive value of specific criteria used for the assessment of low probability ventilation-perfusion lung scans. J Nucl Med 1996;37:577–581.

Matched Defects of Ventilation, Perfusion and the Chest Radiograph: The Triple Matched Defect

A matched ventilation-perfusion defect with associated matching chest radiographic opacity (the triple match) has been reported to be an intermediate (indeterminate) finding, with a positive predictive value for acute pulmonary embolism of 26% (Fig. 20–1) (1). This was similar to the positive predictive value for pulmonary embolism of a perfusion defect that matched the chest radiograph, 27% (2). The triple match can be caused by pulmonary embolism creating a pulmonary "infarction" (usually pulmonary hemorrhage), but other etiologies are more common (1). Worsley and associates showed that pulmonary embolism was present more frequently with triple matches in the lower zones of the lung compared with the upper or middle zones (1). They indicated that matching ventilation-perfusion defects and chest radiographic opacities isolated to the upper and middle zones represent a low probability of pulmonary embolism (less than 20% positive predictive value), whereas triple matched defects in the lower zone represent an intermediate probability for pulmonary embolism (20% to 79% positive predictive value) (1).

We further explored the diagnostic value of triple matched defects by using a subset of patients from the collaborative study Prospective Investigation of Pulmonary Embolism Diagnosis (PIOPED) (3). We included data only from patients who were randomized for obligatory pulmonary angiography, because nonrandomized patients had a higher positive predictive value of triple matched defects in the upper plus middle zones than randomized patients. A zone of the lung was defined as the upper, middle, or lower third of the lung, divided in the cranial-caudal direction. Lungs with mismatched perfusion defects were excluded because even the smallest number of mismatched perfusion defects indicate at least an intermediate probability for pulmonary embolism (4, 5). Lungs with triple matched defects that had a pleural effusion were also eliminated. Small pleural effusions that caused blunting of the costophrenic angle

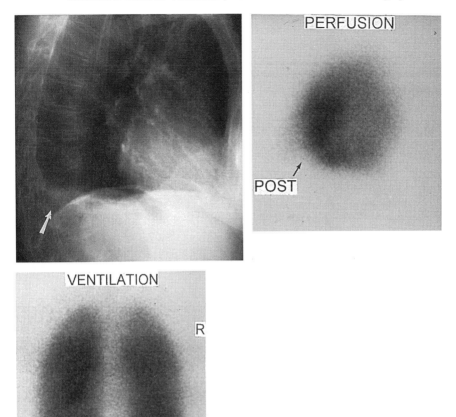

Figure 20–1. **Top.** Chest radiograph, lateral view, showing an infiltrate in the posterior portion of the base of the right lung (arrow). **Top Right.** Perfusion scan, lateral view of right lung, showing perfusion defect in posterior inferior portion (arrow). **Bottom.** Ventilation scan, posterior view, equilibrium phase, showing absent ventilation in base of right lung. The finding of a matched ventilation-perfusion defect with associated matching chest radiographic opacity (the triple match) in a lower lung zone has an intermediate probability with a positive predictive value for acute pulmonary embolism of 23%. This patient had pulmonary embolism.

were associated with pulmonary embolism in more than 20% of patients (6). Observations with these refined data, in general, confirmed the observations of Worsley and associates, although some important differences existed (1).

Pulmonary embolism with triple matched defects was infrequent in the upper or middle lung zones, 1 of 27 (4%) (Table 20–1) (3). The positive predictive value in the lower lung zone, 13 of 57 (23%), was higher than in the upper plus middle zones (Table 20–1). The positive predictive value of triple matched defects in the left lung was comparable to the right lung, 13% versus 20%.

Table 20–1. POSITIVE PREDICTIVE VALUE OF TRIPLE MATCHED
DEFECTS ACCORDING TO LUNG ZONE

	Gottschalk[a] PE/No.	Worsley[b] PE/No.
Upper zone	0/13 (0)	4/36 (11)
Middle zone	1/14 (7)	6/52 (12)
Lower zone	13/57 (23)[c]	61/187 (33)[d]
Total	14/84 (17)	71/275 (26)

PE = pulmonary embolism. No = number
[a] Data from Gottschalk A, Stein PD, Henry JW, et al. Matched ventilation-perfusion defects and chest radiographic abnormalities: re-evaluation of the triple matched defect in the assessment of acute pulmonary embolism. 1996;37:(10)In Press.[b] Data from Worsley DF, Kim CK, Alavi A, et al. Detailed analysis of patients with matched ventilation-perfusion defects and chest radiographic opacities. J Nucl Med 1993;34:1851–1853.
[c] P < .05 upper + middle zone vs lower zone
[d] P < .005 upper zone vs lower zone; middle zone vs lower zone
Reprinted with permission from Gottschalk A, Stein PD, Henry JW, et al. Matched ventilation-perfusion defects and chest radiographic abnormalities: re-evaluation of the triple matched defect in the assessment of acute pulmonary embolism. J Nucl Med 1996;37(10).

Pulmonary embolism was more frequent in patients with triple matches that involved 25% to 50% of a zone than in patients with either larger or smaller triple matched defects (Table 20–2)(3). Triple matched defects that involved 25% to 50% of a zone showed a positive predictive value for pulmonary embolism of 12 of 38 (32%). Triple matched defects smaller than 25% of a zone showed a lower positive predictive, 2 of 23 (9%). Triple matched defects larger than 50% of a zone also showed a lower positive predictive value, 0 of 23 (0%). Triple matched defects that involved <25% of a zone tend to represent a linear opacity, whereas triple matched defects >50% tended to be large areas of consolidation. The category of 25% to 50% of a zone represents a segmental appearance.

Stratification according to prior cardiopulmonary disease showed a comparable positive predictive value for pulmonary embolism of triple matched defects in the lower zones of patients with prior cardiopulmonary disease and patients without prior cardiopulmonary disease, 8 of 37 (22%) versus 5 of 20 (25%) (3). The positive predictive value for pulmonary embolism was also comparable in the upper plus middle zones in patients with prior cardiopulmonary disease and patients with no prior cardiopulmonary disease, 0 of 19 (0%) versus 1 of 8 (13%).

A triple matched defect in the upper lung zone satisfied the criterion for a very low probability interpretation defined as <10% positive predictive value (3). A triple matched defect in the lower lung zone did not satisfy the criteria either for very low or low probability interpretations. Such defects indicated an intermediate (indeterminate) probability for pulmonary embolism, defined as a 20 to 79% positive predictive value (3).

The pulmonary diagnoses in 25 patients with triple matched defects who did not have pulmonary embolism were pneumonia (n=11), pulmonary carcinoma (n=5), pulmonary fibrosis (n=2), atelectasis (n=2), chronic obstructive pulmonary disease (n=2), tuberculosis (n=1), pulmonary eosinophilia (n=1),

Table 20–2. POSITIVE PREDICTIVE VALUE OF TRIPLE MATCHED
DEFECTS ACCORDING TO SIZE

Size of Triple Match (Percent of Zone)	Gottschalk[a] PE/No.	Worsley[b] PE/No.
<25	2/23 (9)	23/86 (27)
25–50	12/38 (32)[c]	34/125 (27)
51–75	0/11 (0)	8/36 (22)
>75	0/12 (0)	6/28 (21)

[a] Data from Gottschalk A, Stein PD, Henry JW, et al. Matched ventilation-perfusion defects and chest radiographic abnormalities: re-evaluation of the triple matched defect in the assessment of acute pulmonary embolism. J Nucl Med 1996;37(10) (in press).
[b] Data from Worsley DF, Kim CK, Alavi A, et al. Detailed analysis of patients with matched ventilation-perfusion defects and chest radiographic opacities. J Nucl Med 1993;34:1851–1853.
[c] P < .05, 25–50% vs < 25%; 25–50% vs 51–75%; 25–50% vs >75%
PE = pulmonary embolism
Reprinted with permission from Gottschalk A, Stein PD, Henry JW, et al. Matched ventilation-perfusion defects and chest radiographic abnormalities: re-evaluation of the triple matched defect in the assessment of acute pulmonary embolism. J Nucl Med 1996;37(10).

and heart failure (n=1) (3). In 29 patients who did not have pulmonary embolism, the cause of the triple matched defect was not indicated.

In summary, refinement of the PIOPED data for evaluation of triple matched defects was made by eliminating nonrandomized patients, lungs with mismatched perfusion defects and lungs with a pleural effusion. These refined data indicated that triple matched defects with pulmonary embolism (radiographic pulmonary infarcts) are uncommon in the upper lung zone or middle lung zone, the positive predictive value of combined upper and middle zones being 4%. In the lower lung zone, however, the positive predictive value of a triple matched defect was 23%. When a triple matched defect with pulmonary embolism occurred, it was most likely to be 1 to 2 segments in size (25 to 50% of a zone).

REFERENCES

1. Worsley DF, Kim CK, Alavi A, et al. Detailed analysis of patients with matched ventilation-perfusion defects and chest radiographic opacities. J Nucl Med 1993;34:1851–1853.
2. Biello DR, Mattar AG, McKnight RC, et al. Ventilation-perfusion studies in suspected pulmonary embolism. Amer J Radiol 1979;133:1033–1037.
3. Gottschalk A, Stein PD, Henry JW, et al. Matched ventilation-perfusion defects and chest radiographic abnormalities: re-evaluation of the triple matched defect in the assessment of acute pulmonary embolism. J Nucl Med 1996;37(10) (in press).
4. Stein PD, Gottschalk A, Henry JW, et al. Stratification of patients according to prior cardiopulmonary disease and probability assessment based upon the number of mismatched segmental equivalent perfusion defects: approaches to strengthen the

diagnostic value of ventilation-perfusion lung scans in acute pulmonary embolism. Chest 1993;104:1461–1467.

5. Stein PD, Henry JW, Gottschalk A. Mismatched vascular defects: an easy alternative to mismatched segmental equivalent defects for the interpretation of ventilation-perfusion lung scans in pulmonary embolism. Chest 1993;104:1468–1472.

6. Stein PD, Relyea B, Gottschalk A. Evaluation of the positive predictive value of specific criteria used for the assessment of low probability ventilation-perfusion lung scans. J Nucl Med 1996;37:577–581.

CHAPTER **21**

Pulmonary Embolism in a Single Lung with a Normal Scan and an Abnormal Contralateral Side

The ventilation-perfusion (V/Q) lung scan is often used to guide the angiographer to the area most suspicious for pulmonary embolism. Some patients cannot safely undergo bilateral pulmonary angiograms. In such patients, it might be desirable to have a non-angiographic benchmark that would indicate whether it is reasonable to perform an angiogram only in the most suspicious lung rather than bilaterally.

We evaluated whether a single lung that is normal on ventilation-perfusion scan has a sufficiently low positive predictive value of pulmonary embolism to allow the angiographer to terminate a pulmonary angiogram after the contralateral abnormal lung is studied (1). Contrary to experience with bilaterally normal ventilation-perfusion scans, a lung scan that was normal in a single lung did not entirely exclude pulmonary embolism.

Normal single lungs had no mismatched perfusion defects, defined as moderate or large segmental perfusion defects ≥ 25% of a segment without corresponding ventilation or radiographic abnormalities, or perfusion defects substantially larger than either matching ventilation or chest radiographic abnormalities (1). Normal single lungs also had no matched ventilation and perfusion abnormalities where the regional chest radiograph was clear and a ventilation abnormality was present, with the perfusion defect equivalent in size or smaller, and there was no perfusion defect smaller than the radiographic abnormality. In addition, patients with normal single lungs had no pleural effusion and no small subsegmental defects (<25% of a segment). Normal single lungs showed no nonsegmental abnormalities defined as enlarged mediastinum, heart, or hilum, or elevated hemidiaphragm.

Patients were excluded if both lungs were normal (normal ventilation-perfusion scan) (1). A bilaterally normal ventilation-perfusion lung scan entirely excluded pulmonary embolism in the experience of PIOPED and others (2–4).

155

Table 21–1. SCAN FINDINGS ON SIDE OF ABNORMAL VENTILATION/
PERFUSION SCAN IN PATIENTS WHO HAD PULMONARY
EMBOLISM

Patient Number	PE, Side ABN V/Q	PE, Side NL V/Q	Mismatch V/Q	Nonsegmental	Pleural Effusion	Matched V/Q
1	No	Yes	0	0	CPA	RUZ, RMZ
2	Yes	Yes	0	0	CPA	RLZ
3	Yes	No	0	0	≤1/3	0

ABN = abnormal; NL = normal; CPA = costophrenic angle obscured; ≤1/3 = pleural effusion obscured diaphragm
and extended ≤1/3 up thorax.
Reproduced from Gottschalk A, Stein PD, Henry JW, et al with permission.

Table 21–2. SCAN FINDINGS ON SIDE OF ABNORMAL VENTILATION/
PERFUSION SCAN IN PATIENTS WHO DID NOT HAVE
PULMONARY EMBOLISM

Mismatch V/Q n/N (%)	Nonsegmental n/N (%)	Pleural Effusion n/N (%)	Matched V/Q n/N (%)
1/16 (6)*	0/16 (0)	CPA 8/16 (50)	1 Zone 3/16 (19)
		OBS DIAP 3/16 (19)	2 Zones 2/16 (13)
		≤1/3 3/16 (19)	3 Zones 1/16 (6)
		1/2 1/16 (6)	

* Single moderate size mismatched perfusion defect
CPA = costophrenic angle obscured; OBS DIAP = obscured diaphragm; ≤1/3 = pleural effusion obscured diaphragm
and extended ≤1/3 up thorax; 1/2 = pleural effusion extended 1/2 up thorax.
n = number with finding; N = number evaluated.
Reproduced from Gottschalk A, Stein PD, Henry JW, et al with permission

Pulmonary embolism on the side of a normal V/Q scan occurred in 2 of 19 (11%), which was within the range of probabilities defined as a low probability ventilation-perfusion scan (1,5). If pulmonary embolism was excluded by angiography on the side of the abnormal ventilation-perfusion scan, the pulmonary embolism on the side of the normal ventilation-perfusion scan occurred in 1 of 19 (5%). This was in the range of probabilities defined as very low probability for pulmonary embolism (5). It was the same probability of pulmonary embolism as a nearly normal ventilation-perfusion scan in PIOPED (6), but higher than the probabiltiy of pulmonary embolism in patients with an entirely normal ventilation-perfusion scan (1). Findings on the side of the abnormal ventilation-perfusion scan among patients with pulmonary embolism are shown in Table 21–1. Findings on the side of the abnormal V/Q scan among patients who did not have pulmonary embolism are shown in Table 21–2.

Reasons why pulmonary embolism could be present with a normal perfusion scan are central, nonobstructing, nonlateralized pulmonary embolism or

Table 21–3. PULMONARY ANGIOGRAPHIC FINDINGS IN SINGLE LUNGS
THAT SHOWED PULMONARY EMBOLISM ON THE SIDE OF
A NORMAL VENTILATION/PERFUSION LUNG SCAN

Patient Number	Artery in Which PE Was Visualized	Partial Occlusion	100% Occlusion
1	LLL, 1 Segmental Branch	O	X
	LLL, 1 Segmental Branch	X	O
	LLL, Peripheral	X	O
2	LLL, Peripheral	X	O

LLL = left lower lobar artery.
Reproduced from Gottschalk A, Stein PD, Henry JW, et al with permission.

minimal defects on the perfusion scan that are not appreciated. A single, small, or partially occluding embolus may not show a perfusion defect because of limitations of perfusion scanning (7,8). The pulmonary embolism in one patient caused only partial occlusion of peripheral branches of the lower lobe pulmonary artery. The pulmonary embolism in another patient involved two segmental branches and peripheral branches of the lower lobe pulmonary artery. One of the segmental branches was completely occluded. The other vessels with pulmonary embolism showed only partial occlusion (Table 21–3).

In summary, a normal ventilation-perfusion scan of a single lung, the contralateral lung being non-high probability for pulmonary embolism, did not entirely exclude pulmonary embolism in that lung. The probability of pulmonary embolism on the side of a normal ventilation-perfusion scan, if the angiogram did not show pulmonary embolism on the side of the abnormal ventilation-perfusion scan, was 5%. This observation in patients undergoing pulmonary angiography may assist in determining whether the pulmonary angiogram should be bilateral.

REFERENCES

1. Gottschalk A, Stein PD, Henry JW, et al. Can pulmonary angiography be limited to the most suspicious side if the contralateral side appears normal on the ventilation-perfusion lung scan? Data from PIOPED. Chest 1996;110:392–394.
2. The PIOPED Investigators. Value of the ventilation/perfusion scan in acute pulmonary embolism: results of the Prospective Investigation of Pulmonary Embolism Diagnosis (PIOPED). JAMA 1990;263:2753–2759.
3. Hull RD, Raskob GE, Coates G, et al. Clinical validity of a normal perfusion lung scan in patients with suspected pulmonary embolism. Chest 1990;97:23–26.
4. Stein PD. Low-dose heparin for prevention of pulmonary embolism and significance of normal lung scan. ACCP Bulletin 1982;21:12–14.
5. Stein PD, Relyea B, Gottschalk A. Evaluation of the positive predictive value of specific criteria used for the assessment of low probability ventilation/perfusion lung scans. J Nucl Med 1996;37:577–581.
6. Henry JW, Stein PD, Gottschalk A, et al. Pulmonary embolism among patients with a nearly normal ventilation/perfusion lung scan. Chest 1996;110:395–398.

7. Alderson PO, Rujanavech N, Secker-Walker RH, et al. The role of ^{133}Xe ventilation studies in the scintigraphic detection of pulmonary embolism. Radiology 1976;120:633–640.
8. Alderson PO, Doppman JL, Diamond SS, et al. Ventilation-perfusion lung imaging and selective pulmonary angiography in dogs with experimental pulmonary embolism. J Nucl Med 1978;19:164–171.

CHAPTER 22

Probability Assessment Based on the Number of Mismatched Segmental Equivalent Perfusion Defects and Stratification According to Prior Cardiopulmonary Disease

The sensitivity and specificity of ventilation-perfusion lung scans in acute pulmonary embolism were assessed in the Prospective Investigation of Pulmonary Embolism Diagnosis (PIOPED) and in subsequent studies of data from PIOPED based upon preassigned diagnostic criteria for high, intermediate and low probabilities (1–4). Such categorical diagnoses encompass a spectrum of diagnostic probabilities of pulmonary embolism that is not communicated to the referring physician. We strengthened the diagnostic value of ventilation-perfusion lung scans by creating a table of positive predictive values and specificities based on the observed number of mismatched segmental equivalent perfusion defects (Table 22–1, Fig. 22–1) (5). This table was more informative than categorical assessments, and permitted the nuclear scan reader to assign specific risks of pulmonary embolism to individual patients. In addition, we showed that stratification of patients according to the presence or absence of prior cardiopulmonary disease enhanced the ventilation-perfusion scan assessment of the probability of pulmonary embolism among patients in both of these clinical categories (5).

One segmental equivalent was defined as one large segment or two moderate-size segments (6). For example, 1.5 mismatched segmental equivalents can be obtained with either 1 large and 1 moderate mismatched segmental perfusion defect or 3 moderate mismatched segmental perfusion defects. With increasing numbers of mismatched segmental equivalent perfusion defects, there was a continuum of gradually increasing specificities and positive predictive values, and decreasing sensitivities (Table 22–1, Fig. 22–1) (5). No discrete criterion

Table 22-1.   POSITIVE PREDICTIVE VALUE OF CUMULATIVE NUMBER
OF MISMATCHED SEGMENTAL EQUIVALENT PERFUSION
DEFECTS AMONG PATIENTS WITH NO PRIOR
CARDIOPULMONARY DISEASE AND PATIENTS WITH PRIOR
CARDIOPULMONARY DISEASE

Segmental Equivalents	Patients with No Prior Cardiopulmonary Disease (n = 421) #PE/#Pts (%)	Patients with Prior Cardiopulmonary Disease (n = 629) #PE/#Pts (%)	All Patients (n = 1050) #PE/#Pts (%)
≥0.0	173/421 (41)	205/629 (33)[a]	378/1050 (36)
≥0.5	123/154 (80)	130/192 (68)[b]	253/346 (73)
≥1.0	102/118 (86)	113/155 (73)[a]	215/273 (79)
≥1.5	91/102 (89)	99/128 (77)[b]	190/230 (83)
≥2.0	79/87 (91)	91/114 (80)[c]	170/201 (85)
≥2.5	72/80 (90)	87/105 (83)	159/185 (86)
≥3.0	65/73 (89)	81/97 (84)	146/170 (86)
≥3.5	60/67 (90)	77/88 (88)	137/155 (88)
≥4.0	57/63 (90)	74/84 (88)	131/147 (89)
≥4.5	50/53 (94)	70/78 (90)	120/131 (92)
≥5.0	49/52 (94)	65/72 (90)	114/124 (92)
≥5.5	47/50 (94)	61/66 (92)	108/116 (93)
≥6.0	42/44 (95)	59/64 (92)	101/108 (94)
≥6.5	40/42 (95)	56/61 (92)	96/103 (93)
≥7.0	38/40 (95)	51/56 (91)	89/96 (93)
≥7.5	34/36 (94)	43/47 (91)	77/83 (93)

[a] P < .01
[b] P < .02
[c] P < .05, no prior cardiopulmonary disease versus prior cardiopulmonary disease
These probabilities were calculated with chi square and are higher than reported in Stein PD, Gottschalk A, Henry JW, et al. Stratification of patients according to prior cardiopulmonary disease and probability assessment based upon the number of mismatched segmental equivalent perfusion defects: approaches to strengthen the diagnostic value of ventilation-perfusion lung scans in acute pulmonary embolism. Chest 1993;104:1461–1467, because Yates' correction, which was unnecessarily conservative, was used in the previous analysis.
Modified and reprinted with permission from Stein PD, Gottschalk A, Henry JW, et al. Stratification of patients according to prior cardiopulmonary disease and probability assessment based upon the number of mismatched segmental equivalent perfusion defects: approaches to strengthen the diagnostic value of ventilation-perfusion lung scans in acute pulmonary embolism. Chest 1993;104:1461–1467.

for "high probability" can be clearly identified from the data. Rather than define an arbitrary number of mismatched segmental equivalent defects as "high probability" for all patients, use of Table 22-1 enables readers of ventilation-perfusion scans to assign a positive predictive value and specificity to individual patients.

Stratification of patients according to the presence or absence of prior cardiopulmonary disease enhanced the ventilation-perfusion scan assessment of pulmonary embolism among both clinical categories of patients (5). Among patients with no prior cardiopulmonary disease, ≥0.5 mismatched segmental equivalent perfusion defects were associated with a positive predictive value for pulmonary embolism of 80% (Fig. 22-2, Table 22-1). With ≥1.5 mismatched segmental equivalents, the positive predictive value for pulmonary embolism was 89% in patients with no prior cardiopulmonary disease.

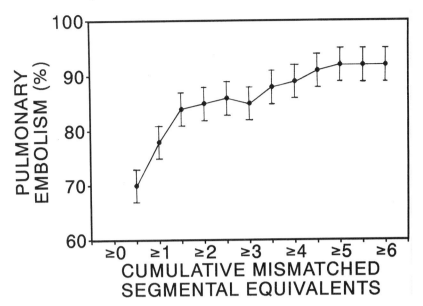

Figure 22–1. Positive predictive value for pulmonary embolism according to the number of mismatched segmental equivalent perfusion defects on the ventilation-perfusion lung scan. Bars represent standard error.

Among patients with prior cardiopulmonary disease, more mismatched segmental equivalent perfusion defects were required to give a particular positive predictive value and specificity than among patients with no prior cardiopulmonary disease. Among patients with prior cardiopulmonary disease, ≥ 2 mismatched segmental equivalent perfusion defects were required for an 80% positive predictive value of pulmonary embolism, and ≥ 4.5 mismatched segmental equivalents were required for a 90% positive predictive value of pulmonary embolism (5).

Further stratification of patients with prior cardiopulmonary disease into those with prior cardiac disease (exclusive of prior pulmonary disease) and those with prior pulmonary disease (exclusive of prior cardiac disease) did not strengthen the positive predictive value of either group. No significant differences were shown between patients with prior cardiac disease and patients with prior lung disease (Fig. 22–3).

As shown in Table 22–1, some patients with pulmonary embolism had no mismatched large or moderate-size segmental defects. The patients who had pulmonary embolism and no mismatched segmental lesions had either small perfusion defects, mediastinal abnormalities, pleural effusions, a variety of parenchymal radiographic abnormalities, ventilation-perfusion matched defects, or any combination of these. None had an entirely normal ventilation-perfusion scan.

A higher area under the receiver operating characteristic (ROC) curve occurred for patients with no prior cardiopulmonary disease versus patients with prior cardiopulmonary disease (0.8905 versus 0.8215) (p=0.026) (Fig.

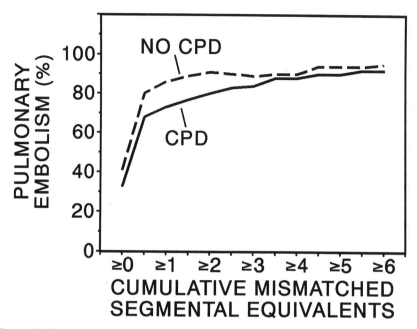

Figure 22–2. Positive predictive value of pulmonary embolism relative to the cumulative number of mismatched segmental equivalent perfusion defects. Broken line indicates patients with no prior cardiopulmonary disease (NO CPD). Unbroken line indicates patients with any prior cardiopulmonary disease (CPD). Significant differences occurred with ≥0.5 (P<.02), ≥1.0 segmental equivalents (P<.01), ≥1.5 (P<.02) and ≥2.0 (P<.05) segmental equivalents. These probabilites were calculated by chi square and are higher than reported by Stein PD, Gottschalk A, Henry JW, et al. Stratification of patients according to prior cardiopulmonary disease and probability assessment based upon the number of mismatched segmental equivalent perfusion defects: approaches to strengthen the diagnostic value of ventilation-perfusion lung scans in acute pulmonary embolism. Chest 1993;104:1461–1467, because Yates' correction, which was unnecessarily conservative, was used in the previous calculations. (Reprinted with permission from Stein PD, Gottschalk A, Henry JW, et al. Stratification of patients according to prior cardiopulmonary disease and probability assessment based upon the number of mismatched segmental equivalent perfusion defects: approaches to strengthen the diagnostic value of ventilation-perfusion lung scans in acute pulmonary embolism. Chest 1993;104:1461–1467.)

22–4). This indicates that ventilation-perfusion scans had a greater ability to distinguish between normal and abnormal in patients with no prior cardiopulmonary disease (7).

Sensitivity and specificity according to the number of mismatched segmental equivalent perfusion defects among patients stratified according to the presence or absence of prior cardiopulmonary disease is shown in Table 22–2. With stratification, among patients with no prior cardiopulmonary disease, the presence of 1.0 or more mismatched segmental equivalent perfusion defects was more sensitive for pulmonary embolism than the PIOPED criteria for high probability (≥2 segmental equivalent defects) applied to unstratified patients (59% versus 41%)(P<.001) (1, 5). This increased sensitivity was associated with a comparable positive predictive value (86% versus 87%) and specificity (94% versus 97%) (1, 5).

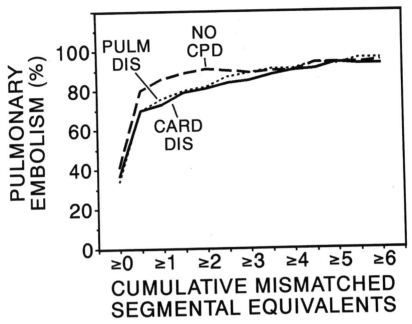

Figure 22–3. Positive predictive value of pulmonary embolism relative to the cumulative number of mismatched segmental equivalent perrfusion defects among patients with no prior cardiopulmonary disease (NO CPD), any prior cardiac disease (CARD DIS) and any prior pulmonary disease (PULM DIS). There were no significant differences between patients with prior cardiac disease and patients with prior pulmonary disease. (Reprinted with permission from Stein PD, Gottschalk A, Henry JW, et al. Stratification of patients according to prior cardiopulmonary disease and probability assessment based upon the number of mismatched segmental equivalent perfusion defects: approaches to strengthen the diagnostic value of ventilation-perfusion lung scans in acute pulmonary embolism. Chest 1993;104:1461–1467.)

In summary, tables are shown that can be used by readers of ventilation-perfusion lung scans to assign to their patients an individualized percentage probability of pulmonary embolism and specificity based on the observed number of mismatched segmental equivalent defects. This strengthens the diagnostic value of ventilation-perfusion lung scans and gives more useful information than "high," "intermediate," and "low" probability categories. Stratification of patients by prior disease status enhances the ability of ventilation-perfusion scan readers to assign an accurate positive predictive value to both clinical categories of patients. Among patients with no prior cardiopulmonary disease, stratification reduces the number of inconclusive ventilation-perfusion readings by showing a high positive predictive value of pulmonary embolism with fewer mismatched segmental equivalent defects than were required in PIOPED.

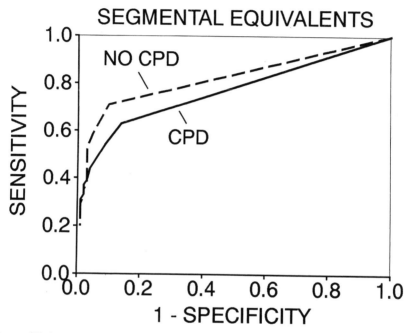

Figure 22–4. Receiver operating characteristic (ROC) curves showing relation of sensitivity to false positives (1-specificity) among patients with no prior cardiopulmonary disease (NO CPD) and patients with prior CPD. The area under the ROC curve of patients with no prior CPD was greater than the area under the curve of patients with prior CPD (.8905/.8215)(P<.05).

Table 22–2. NUMBER OF MISMATCHED SEGMENTAL EQUIVALENT PERFUSION DEFECTS, SENSITIVITY AND SPECIFICITY AMONG PATIENTS WITH NO PRIOR CARDIOPULMONARY DISEASE AND PATIENTS WITH PRIOR CARDIOPULMONARY DISEASE

Segmental Equivalents	Patients with No Prior Cardiopulmonary Disease (n = 421)		Patients with Prior Cardiopulmonary Disease (n = 629)		All Patients (n = 1050)	
	SENS (%)	SPEC (%)	SENS (%)	SPEC (%)	SENS (%)	SPEC (%)
≥0.0	100	0	100	0	100	0
≥0.5	71	88	63	85	67	86
≥1.0	59	94	55	90	57	91
≥1.5	53	96	48	93	50	94
≥2.0	46	97	44	95	45	95
≥2.5	42	97	42	96	42	96
≥3.0	38	97	40	96	39	96
≥3.5	35	97	38	97	36	97
≥4.0	33	98	36	98	35	98
≥4.5	29	99	34	98	32	98
≥5.0	28	99	32	98	30	99
≥5.5	27	99	30	99	29	99
≥6.0	24	99	29	99	27	99
≥6.5	23	99	27	99	25	99
≥7.0	22	99	25	99	24	99
≥7.5	20	99	21	99	20	99

SENS, sensitivity
SPEC, specificity
Reprinted with permission from Stein PD, Gottschalk A, Henry JW, et al. Stratification of patients according to prior cardiopulmonary disease and probability assessment based upon the number of mismatched segmental equivalent perfusion defects: approaches to strengthen the diagnostic value of ventilation-perfusion lung scans in acute pulmonary embolism. Chest 1993;104:1461–1467.

REFERENCES

1. A collaborative study by the PIOPED Investigators. Value of the ventilation/perfusion scan in acute pulmonary embolism: results of the Prospective Investigation of Pulmonary Embolism Diagnosis (PIOPED). JAMA 1990;263:2753–2759.
2. Stein PD, Alavi A, Gottschalk A, et al. Usefulness of noninvasive diagnostic tools for diagnosis of acute pulmonary embolism in patients with a normal chest radiograph. Am J Cardiol 1991;67:1117–1120.
3. Stein PD, Coleman RE, Gottschalk A, et al. Diagnostic utility of ventilation/perfusion lung scans in acute pulmonary embolism is not diminished by pre-existing cardiac or pulmonary disease. Chest 1991;100:604–606.
4. Lesser BA, Leeper KV, Stein PD, et al. The diagnosis of acute pulmonary embolism in patients with chronic obstructive pulmonary disease. Chest 1992;102:17–22.
5. Stein PD, Gottschalk A, Henry JW, et al. Stratification of patients according to prior cardiopulmonary disease and probability assessment based upon the number of

mismatched segmental equivalent perfusion defects: approaches to strengthen the diagnostic value of ventilation/perfusion lung scans in acute pulmonary embolism. Chest 1993;104:1461–1467.

6. Neumann RD, Sostman HD, Gottschalk A. Current status of ventilation/perfusion imaging. Semin Nucl Med 1980;10:198–217.

7. Hanley JA, McNeil BJ. The meaning and use of the area under a receiver operating characteristic (ROC) curve. Radiology 1982;143:29–36.

CHAPTER 23

Probability Assessment Based on the Number of Mismatched Vascular Perfusion Defects and Stratification According to Prior Cardiopulmonary Disease

The diagnosis of pulmonary embolism from ventilation-perfusion lung scans, according to criteria in the Prospective Investigation of Pulmonary Embolism Diagnosis (PIOPED), is made on the basis of the number of mismatched segmental equivalent perfusion defects (1). One segmental equivalent has been defined as 1 large segment or 2 moderate-size segments (2). The diagnosis of pulmonary embolism on the basis of the number of mismatched segmental equivalents assumes that a mismatched moderate-size segmental perfusion defect is of less diagnostic value than a mismatched large-size segmental perfusion defect (2). This assumption has not been fully tested. Considerable skill and judgment are required to distinguish a moderate-size mismatched segmental perfusion defect (25% to 75% of a segment) from a large-size mismatched segmental perfusion defect (>75% of a segment). Experienced readers of radionuclide lung scans often underestimate the size of segmental defects (3). We showed that ventilation-perfusion lung scans can be assessed without the need to distinguish large mismatched segmental defects from moderate-size mismatched segmental defects (4). This makes the interpretation of ventilation-perfusion lung scans easier and more objective.

The positive predictive value of pulmonary embolism relative to the number of mismatched large segmental perfusion defects was similar to the positive predictive value of pulmonary embolism relative to the number of mismatched moderate-size segmental perfusion defects. The positive predictive value of pulmonary embolism based upon the cumulative number of mismatched large segmental defects, irrespective of the number of mismatched moderate-size segmental defects, is shown in Figure 23–1 and Table 23–1.

167

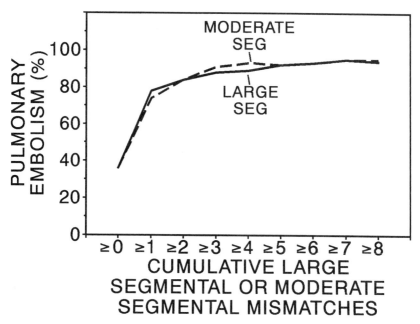

Figure 23–1. Positive predictive value of pulmonary embolism according to the cumulative number of large segmental (SEG) perfusion defects (irrespective of the number of moderate-size segmental defects) (unbroken line) and according to the number of moderate-size segmental perfusion defects (irrespective of the number of large segmental defects) (broken line). (Reprinted with permission from Stein PD, Henry JW, Gottschalk A. Mismatched vascular defects: an easy alternative to mismatched segmental equivalent defects for the interpretation of ventilation-perfusion lung scans in pulmonary embolism. Chest 1993;104:1468–1472.)

The positive predictive value of pulmonary embolism based upon the cumulative number of mismatched moderate-size segmental perfusion defects, irrespective of the number of mismatched large segmental perfusion defects, is also shown in Figure 23–1 and Table 23–1. Based on the similarity of the positive predictive value of large mismatched perfusion defects and moderate-size mismatched perfusion defects, we defined a mismatched vascular perfusion defect as a mismatched large or moderate segmental perfusion defect. The number of mismatched vascular perfusion defects, therefore, was the number of large and/or moderate-size mismatched perfusion defects (4).

The size of the mismatched defect, providing it was ≥25 percent of a segment, was of no consequence. The positive predictive value of the cumulative number of mismatched vascular defects (mismatched large and/or moderate-size segments) is shown in Table 23–2 and Figure 23–2. The sensitivity and specificity of various numbers of mismatched vascular defects are shown in Table 23–3.

The cumulative number of mismatched segmental equivalent perfusion defects and the cumulative number of vascular defects were of comparable diagnostic value, as indicated by similar values of the maximum likelihood estimates of the areas under the receiver operating characteristics (ROC) curves (Table 23–4, Fig. 23–3).

Table 23-1.   POSITIVE PREDICTIVE VALUE OF PULMONARY EMBOLISM
IN RELATION TO THE CUMULATIVE NUMBER OF
MISMATCHED LARGE SEGMENTAL PERFUSION DEFECTS
AND MODERATE-SIZE SEGMENTAL PERFUSION DEFECTS

Cumulative Number of Defects	Mismatched Large Segmental Defects (n = 1064)		Mismatched Moderate-Size Segmental Defects (n = 1064)	
	#PE/#Pts	%PE	#PE/#Pts	%PE
≥0	383/1064	36	383/1064	36
≥1	197/251	78	205/277	74
≥2	161/191	84	119/141	84
≥3	135/153	88	89/98	91
≥4	119/133	89	64/69	93
≥5	108/117	92	48/52	92
≥6	92/99	93	40/43	93
≥7	78/82	95	36/38	95
≥8	62/66	94	35/37	95

PE, pulmonary embolism
Pts, patients
Modified and reprinted with permission from Stein PD, Henry JW, Gottschalk A. Mismatched vascular defects: an easy alternative to mismatched segmental equivalent defects for the interpretation of ventilation-perfusion lung scans in pulmonary embolism. Chest 1993;104:1468–1472.

Stratification of patients according to the presence or absence of prior cardiopulmonary disease enhanced the positive predictive value of the number of mismatched vascular defects in each category (Table 23–2, Fig. 23–4). Among patients with no prior cardiopulmonary disease, ≥1 vascular defect indicated a positive predictive value for pulmonary embolism of 80%, and ≥2 mismatched vascular defects indicated a positive predictive value of 89% (Fig. 23–5). Among patients with prior cardiopulmonary disease, ≥1 mismatched vasular perfusion defect indicated a positive predictive value of 68%, and ≥2 mismatched vascular perfusion defects indicated a positive predictive value of 77%. Tables 23–2 and 23–3 can be used to assess a positive predictive value and specificity for individual patients stratified according to prior cardiopulmonary disease and according to the number of mismatched vascular perfusion defects.

Patients with prior cardiac disease and those with prior pulmonary disease showed a comparable positive predictive value (Fig. 23–6). There was, therefore, no advantage in stratification according to the specific prior cardiac or pulmonary disease.

We previously showed that the positive predictive value and specificity of pulmonary embolism can be determined from tables that show the cumulative number of mismatched segmental equivalent perfusion defects (5) (Chapter 22). Stratification according to prior cardiopulmonary disease was shown to be advantageous. The number of mismatched vascular defects is as powerful for the assessment of ventilation-perfusion scans as the number of mismatched segmental equivalents. The number of mismatched vascular defects is easier to interpret, and permits a more objective evaluation (4).

Table 23–2.   POSITIVE PREDICTIVE VALUE OF PULMONARY EMBOLISM IN RELATION TO THE CUMULATIVE NUMBER OF MISMATCHED VASCULAR PERFUSION DEFECTS (LARGE AND/OR MODERATE-SIZE SEGMENTAL PERFUSION DEFECTS)

Cumulative Prior Number of Defects	All Patients (n = 1064)	%	No Prior CPD (n = 421)	%	Any CPD (n = 629)	%
>0 33	383/1064	36	173/421	41	205/629	33[a]
≥1 68	255/350	73	123/154	80	130/190	68[b]
≥2 77	200/244	82	94/106	89	105/136	77[c]
≥3 80	170/201	85	79/87	91	90/112	80[c]
≥4 84	149/172	87	67/75	89	81/96	84
≥5 89	130/144	90	55/60	92	75/84	89
≥6 93	116/124	94	49/52	94	67/72	93
≥7 92	103/110	94	43/45	96	60/65	92
≥8 91	93/100	93	41/43	95	52/57	91

CPD, cardiopulmonary disease
[a] P < .01
[b] P < .02
[c] P < .05, prior cardiopulmonary disease versus no prior cardiopulmonary disease
These probabilities are higher than reported by Stein PD, Henry JW, Gottschalk A. Mismatched vascular defects: an easy alternative to mismatched segmental equivalent defects for the interpretation of ventilation-perfusion lung scans in pulmonary embolism. Chest 1993;104:1468–1472, because the chi square probabilities previously calculated used the unnecessarily conservative Yates' correction.
Modified and reprinted with permission from Stein PD, Henry JW, Gottschalk A. Mismatched vascular defects: an easy alternative to mismatched segmental equivalent defects for the interpretation of ventilation-perfusion lung scans in pulmonary embolism. Chest 1993;104:1468–1472.

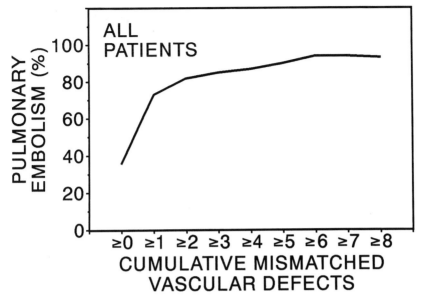

Figure 23–2.   Positive predictive value of pulmonary embolism based on the cumulative number of mismatched vascular defects (the number of mismatched large and/or moderate-size segmental defects). (Reprinted with permission from Stein PD, Henry JW, Gottschalk A. Mismatched vascular defects: an easy alternative to mismatched segmental equivalent defects for the interpretation of ventilation-perfusion lung scans in pulmonary embolism. Chest 1993;104:1468–1472.)

Table 23–3.   SENSITIVITY AND SPECIFICITY IN RELATION TO THE NUMBER OF MISMATCHED VASCULAR PERFUSION DEFECTS (LARGE SEGMENTAL AND/OR MODERATE-SIZE SEGMENTAL PERFUSION DEFECTS)

Cumulative Number of Defects	All Patients		No Prior CPD		Prior CPD	
	SENS (%)	Spec (%)	SENS (%)	Spec (%)	SENS (%)	Spec (%)
≥0	100	0	100	0	100	0
≥1	67	86	71	88	63	86
≥2	52	94	54	95	51	93
≥3	44	95	46	97	44	95
≥4	39	97	39	97	40	96
≥5	34	98	32	98	37	98
≥6	30	99	28	99	33	99
≥7	27	99	25	99	29	99
≥8	24	99	24	99	25	99

SENS, sensitivity
SPEC, specificity
CPD, cardiopulmonary disease
All differences between no prior cardiopulmonary disease and prior cardiopulmonary disease were not significant
Reprinted with permission from Stein PD, Henry JW, Gottschalk A. Mismatched vascular defects: an easy alternative to mismatched segmental equivalent defects for the interpretation of ventilation-perfusion lung scans in pulmonary embolism. Chest 1993;104:1468–1472.

Table 23–4. MAXIMUM LIKELIHOOD ESTIMATES OF THE AREAS UNDER
RECEIVER OPERATING CHARACTERISTIC CURVES BASED
ON THE NUMBER OF MISMATCHED VASCULAR PERFUSION
DEFECTS AND THE NUMBER OF MISMATCHED SEGMENTAL
EQUIVALENT PERFUSION DEFECTS

	Mismatched Vascular Defects (Area)	Mismatched Segmental Equivalents (Area)
All patients (n = 1064)	0.8512	0.8530
Patients with no prior cardiopulmonary disease (n = 421)	0.8875[a]	0.8905[b]
Patients with any prior cardiopulmonary disease (n = 629)	0.8280	0.8215

[a] P = .051, no prior cardiopulmonary disease versus any prior cardiopulmonary diseases; mismatched vascular defects

[b] P = .026, no prior cardiopulmonary disease versus any prior cardiopulmonary disease; mismatched segmental equivalents

Differences between mismatched vascular defects and mismatched segmental equivalent defects were not significant

Reprinted with permission from Stein PD, Henry JW, Gottschalk A. Mismatched vascular defects: an easy alternative to mismatched segmental equivalent defects for the interpretation of ventilation-perfusion lung scans in pulmonary embolism. Chest 1993;104:1468–1472.

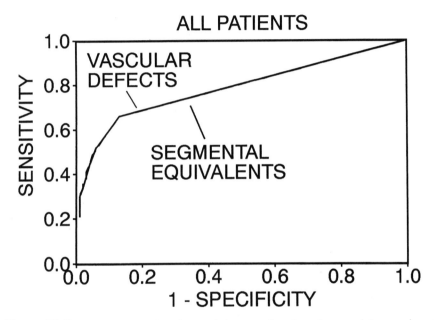

Figure 23–3. Receiver operating characteristic curves based on the cumulative number of mismatched segmental equivalent perfusion defects and on the cumulative number of mismatched vascular perfusion defects. The curves are superimposed.

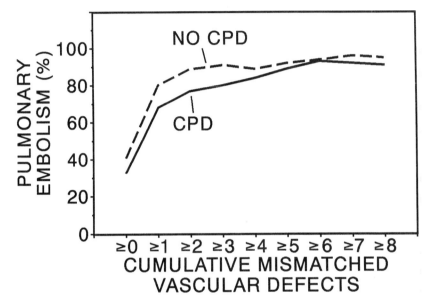

Figure 23–4. Positive predictive values of pulmonary embolism based on the cumulative number of mismatched vascular defects among patients with no prior cardiopulmonary disease (NO CPD) and among patients with any prior cardiopulmonary disease (CPD). Differences between patients with CPD and NO CPD occurred with ≥ 1 mismatched vascular defect (P<.02), ≥ 2 defects (P<.05), and ≥ 3 defects (P<.05). Probabilities are based on chi square without Yates' correction. (Reprinted with permission from Stein PD, Henry JW, Gottschalk A. Mismatched vascular defects: an easy alternative to mismatched segmental equivalent defects for the interpretation of ventilation-perfusion lung scans in pulmonary embolism. Chest 1993;104:1468–1472.)

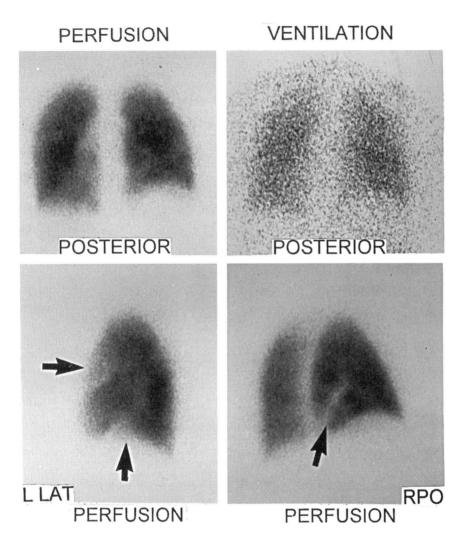

Figure 23–5.   **Top left.** Perfusion scan, posterior view, showing suggestion of perfusion defects, seen better in left lateral view. **Top right.** Ventilation scan, posterior view, washout phase, showing no abnormality. **Bottom left.** Perfusion scan in left lateral view showing moderate-size perfusion defects (arrows) in left anterior segment of left upper lobe and anterior basal segment of left lower lobe. **Bottom right.** Perfusion scan, right posterior oblique (RPO) view, showing a nonsegmental perfusion abnormality associated with atelectasis (arrow). Among patients with no prior cardiopulmonary disease, two or more mismatched vascular perfusion defects indicated a positive predictive value for pulmonary embolism of 89%. Pulmonary embolism was shown on the pulmonary angiogram in this patient.

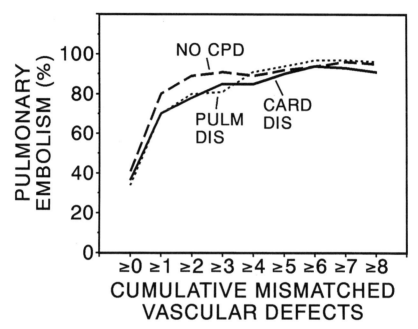

Figure 23–6. Positive predictive value of pulmonary embolism according to the cumulative number of mismatched vascular perfusion defects among patients with no prior cardiopulmonary disease (NO CPD), prior pulmonary disease (PULM DIS), and prior cardiac disease (CARD DIS). The positive predictive value of pulmonary embolism among patients with prior cardiac disease and those with prior pulmonary disease was similar. (Reprinted with permission from Stein PD, Henry JW, Gottschalk A. Mismatched vascular defects: an easy alternative to mismatched segmental equivalent defects for the interpretation of ventilation-perfusion lung scans in pulmonary embolism. Chest 1993;104:1468–1472.)

REFERENCES

1. A collaborative study by the PIOPED Investigators. Value of the ventilation/perfusion scan in acute pulmonary embolism: results of the Prospective Investigation of Pulmonary Embolism Diagnosis (PIOPED). JAMA 1990;263:2753–2759.
2. Neumann RD, Sostman HD, Gottschalk A. Current status of ventilation/perfusion imaging. Semin Nucl Med 1980;10:198–217.
3. Morrell NW, Nijran KS, Jones BE, et al. The underestimation of segmental defect size in radionuclide lung scanning. J Nucl Med 1993;34:370–374.
4. Stein PD, Henry JW, Gottschalk A. Mismatched vascular defects: an easy alternative to mismatched segmental equivalent defects for the interpretation of ventilation/perfusion lung scans in pulmonary embolism. Chest 1993;104:1468–1472.
5. Stein PD, Gottschalk A, Henry JW, et al. Stratification of patients according to prior cardiopulmonary disease and probability assessment based upon the number of mismatched segmental equivalent perfusion defects: approaches to strengthen the diagnostic value of ventilation/perfusion lung scans in acute pulmonary embolism. Chest 1993;104:1461–1467.

Addition of Clinical Assessment to Stratification According to Prior Cardiopulmonary Disease Further Optimizes Interpretation of Lung Scans

The diagnostic value of ventilation-perfusion lung scans was enhanced by showing the positive predictive value for pulmonary embolism relative to the cumulative number of mismatched segmental equivalent perfusion defects (1) (Chapter 22), where one segmental equivalent is one large segmental defect (>75% of a segment) or two moderate-size segmental defects (25% to 75% of a segment) (2). The positive predictive value for pulmonary embolism, relative to the cumulative number of mismatched vascular perfusion defects (large and/or moderate-size segmental defects), was also shown (3) (Chapter 23). Interpreting ventilation-perfusion scans on the basis of mismatched vascular defects eliminated the need to estimate whether a segmental defect was large or moderate in size, and made scan interpretation easier. Stratification according to the presence or absence of prior cardiopulmonary disease enhanced the accuracy of the ventilation-perfusion scan interpretation, irrespective of whether the scans were interpreted on the basis of mismatched segmental equivalent defects or mismatched vascular defects (1,3).

The diagnostic value of ventilation-perfusion lung scans was further enhanced by combining prior clinical assessment in patients stratified according to the presence of prior cardiopulmonary disease (4). By combining prior clinical assessment with stratification of patients according to the presence or absence of prior cardiopulmonary disease, a family of curves was derived that allowed an accurate assessment of the positive predictive value of pulmonary embolism based upon the number of mismatched segmental equivalent defects or upon the number of mismatched vascular defects (4). The families of curves were

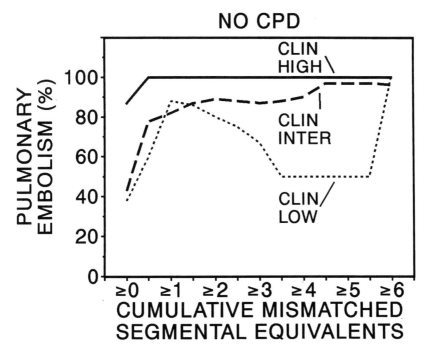

Figure 24–1.   Positive predictive value of pulmonary embolism relative to the cumulative number of mismatched segmental equivalent perfusion defects among patients with no prior cardiopulmonary disease (NO CPD). Patients were categorized according to a high likelihood clinical assessment (CLIN HIGH), intermediate likelihood clinical assessment (CLIN INTER), or low likelihood clinical assessment (CLIN LOW). Only few patients had a low likelihood clinical assessment and ≥1 mismatched segmental equivalent perfusion defect. The CLIN LOW curve, therefore, fluctuated. (Reprinted with permission from Stein PD, Henry JW, Gottschalk A. The addition of clinical assessment to stratification according to prior cardiopulmonary disease further optimizes the interpretation of ventilation-perfusion lung scans in pulmonary embolism. Chest 1993;104:1472–1476.)

comparable, irrespective of whether assessment was based upon segmental equivalent defects or vascular defects. The primary advantage of using vascular equivalent defects, as indicated previously (3) (Chapter 23), is the ability to assess ventilation-perfusion lung scans without differentiating large segmental defects from moderate-size segmental defects.

Patients with No Prior Cardiopulmonary Disease

Patients with no prior cardiopulmonary disease, irrespective of whether they were evaluated on the basis of mismatched segmental equivalent perfusion defects (Fig. 24–1) or mismatched vascular pefusion defects (Fig. 24–2), showed comparable families of curves. A high likelihood clinical assessment, in patients with no prior cardiopulmonary disease, in combination with ≥ 0.5 mismatched segmental equivalent perfusion defects or ≥ 1 mismatched vascular perfusion defect, resulted in a positive predictive value for pulmonary embolism of 100% (Table 24–1, Table 24–2) (4).

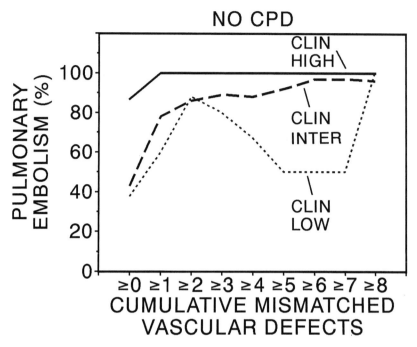

Figure 24–2.   Positive predictive value of pulmonary embolism relative to the cumulative number of mismatched vascular perfusion defects among patients with no prior cardiopulmonary disease (NO CPD). Abbreviations as in Figure 24–1. Only few patients had a low likelihood clinical assessment and ≥1 mismatched vascular defect. The CLIN LOW curve, therefore, fluctuated. (Reprinted with permission from Stein PD, Henry JW, Gottschalk A. The addition of clinical assessment to stratification according to prior cardiopulmonary disease further optimizes the interpretation of ventilation-perfusion lung scans in pulmonary embolism. Chest 1993;104:1472–1476.)

Among patients with no prior cardiopulmonary disease and an intermediate likelihood clinical assessment, a positive predictive value for pulmonary embolism ≥ 80% was shown with ≥ 1 mismatched segmental equivalent perfusion defect and ≥ 2 mismatched vascular perfusion defects. To achieve ≥ 90% positive predictive value for pulmonary embolism, ≥ 4 mismatched segmental equivalent perfusion defects or ≥ 5 mismatched vascular perfusion defects were required (Table 24–1, Table 24–2) (4).

Among patients with no prior cardiopulmonary disease who had a low likelihood clinical assessment, ≥ 1 mismatched segmental equivalent perfusion defect or ≥ 2 mismatched vascular perfusion defects resulted in a positive predictive value for pulmonary embolism of ≥ 80%. With a larger number of mismatched defects, data were inconsistent because of small numbers of patients (Table 24–1, Table 24–2) (4).

Patients with Prior Cardiopulmonary Disease

Among patients with a high probability clinical assessment and prior cardiopulmonary disease, ≥ 0.5 mismatched segmental equivalent perfusion defects

Table 24–1. POSITIVE PREDICTIVE VALUE OF PULMONARY EMBOLISM
IN RELATION TO THE CUMULATIVE NUMBER OF
MISMATCHED SEGMENTAL EQUIVALENT PERFUSION
DEFECTS AND CLINICAL ASSESSMENT AMONG PATIENTS
WITH NO PRIOR CARDIOPULMONARY DISEASE (N = 324)

Mismatched Segmental Equivalents	High Clinical Likelihood #PE/#Pts (%)	Intermed Clin LIkelihood #PE/#Pts (%)	Low Clinical Likelihood #PE/#Pts (%)
≥0	27/31 (87)[a]	107/251 (43)	16/42 (38)[c]
≥0.5	19/19 (100)[b]	79/101 (78)	9/15 (60)[d]
≥1	18/18 (100)	64/78 (82)	7/8 (88)
≥1.5	16/16 (100)	58/67 (87)	6/7 (86)
≥2	15/15 (100)	51/57 (89)	4/5 (80)
≥2.5	14/14 (100)	46/52 (88)	3/4 (75)
≥3	14/14 (100)	41/47 (87)	2/3 (67)
≥3.5	13/13 (100)	38/43 (88)	1/2 (50)
≥4	13/13 (100)	35/39 (90)	1/2 (50)
≥4.5	11/11 (100)	31/32 (97)	1/2 (50)
≥5	11/11 (100)	30/31 (97)	1/2 (50)
≥5.5	10/10 (100)	29/30 (97)	1/2 (50)
≥6	8/8 (100)	26/27 (96)	1/1 (100)
≥6.5	8/8 (100)	26/27 (96)	1/1 (100)
≥7	8.8 (100)	24/25 (96)	1/1 (100)
≥7.5	7/7 (100)	21/22 (95)	1/1 (100)

PE, pulmonary embolism
Pts, patients
Intermed, intermediate
Clin, clinical
[a] P < .001
[b] P < .05, high versus intermediate clinical likelihood
[c] P < .001
[d] P < .01, high versus low clinical likelihood
Probabilities are higher than reported by Stein PD, Henry JW, Gottschalk A. The addition of clinical assessment to stratification according to prior cardiopulmonary disease further optimizes the interpretation of ventilation-perfusion lung scans in pulmonary embolism. Chest 1993;104:1472–1476, because chi square probabilities previously were calculated using Yates' correction, which was unnecessarily conservative.
Modified and reprinted with permission from Stein PD, Henry JW, Gottschalk A. The addition of clinical assessment to stratification according to prior cardiopulmonary disease further optimizes the interpretation of ventilation-perfusion lung scans in pulmonary embolism. Chest 1993;104:1472–1476.

and ≥ 1 mismatched vascular perfusion defect resulted in a positive predictive value for pulmonary embolism ≥ 88% (Fig. 24–3, Fig. 24–4, Table 24–3, Table 24–4) (4).

Among patients with an intermediate probability clinical assessment, ≥ 1.5 mismatched segmental equivalent defects and ≥ 3 mismatched vascular defects indicated a positive predictive value ≥ 80%. To achieve ≥ 90% positive predictive value for pulmonary embolism, ≥ 3.5 mismatched segmental equivalent defects or ≥ 5 mismatched vascular defects were required (Fig. 24–3, Fig. 24–4, Table 24–3, Table 24–4) (4).

Among patients with a low probability clinical assessment, and prior cardiopulmonary disease, the positive predictive value for pulmonary embolism did

Table 24–2.   POSITIVE PREDICTIVE VALUE OF PULMONARY EMBOLISM
IN RELATION TO THE CUMULATIVE NUMBER OF
MISMATCHED VASCULAR PERFUSION DEFECTS AND
CLINICAL ASSESSMENT AMONG PATIENTS WITH NO PRIOR
CARDIOPULMONARY DISEASE (n = 324)

Mismatched Vascular Defects	High Clinical Likelihood #PE/#Pts (%)	Intermed Clin Likelihood #PE/#Pts (%)	Low Clinical Likelihood #PE/#Pts (%)
≥0	27/31 (87)[a]	107/251 (43)	16/42 (38)[c]
≥1	19/19 (100)[b]	79/101 (78)	9/15 (60)[d]
≥2	16/16 (100)	60/70 (86)	7/8 (88)
≥3	16/16 (100)	50/56 (89)	4/5 (80)
≥4	15/15 (100)	42/48 (88)	2/3 (67)
≥5	11/11 (100)	36/39 (92)	1/2 (50)
≥6	10/10 (100)	31/32 (97)	1/2 (50)
≥7	8/8 (100)	28/29 (97)	1/2 (50)
≥8	8/8 (100)	26/27 (96)	1/1 (100)

PE, pulmonary embolism
Pts, patients
Clin, clinical
[a] P < .001
[b] P < .05, high versus intermediate
[c] P < .001
[d] P < .01, high versus low
Probabilities are higher than reported by Stein PD, Henry JW, Gottschalk A. The addition of clinical assessment to stratification according to prior cardiopulmonary disease further optimizes the interpretation of ventilation-perfusion lung scans in pulmonary embolism. Chest 1993;104:1472–1476, because chi square probabilities previously were calculated using Yates' correction, which was unnecessarily conservative.
Modified and reprinted with permission from Stein PD, Henry JW, Gottschalk A. The addition of clinical assessment to stratification according to prior cardiopulmonary disease further optimizes the interpretation of ventilation-perfusion lung scans in pulmonary embolism. Chest 1993;104:1472–1476.

not exceed 33% (Fig. 24–2, Fig. 24–4, Table 24–2, Table 24–4). Few patients, however, had ≥ 1 mismatched segmental equivalent or ≥ 2 mismatched vascular defects (4).

Presentation of the data as continuous numbers of mismatched defects provided a positive predictive value for pulmonary embolism based upon the ventilation-perfusion scan characteristics of any particular patient. This flexibility was not possible with the criteria used for ventilation-perfusion scan interpretation data as presented in PIOPED, which employed fixed numbers of defects for various probabilities of pulmonary embolism (5).

Clinical assessment was important (4). Among patients with no prior cardiopulmonary disease, a high likelihood clinical assessment was indicative of pulmonary embolism in > 85% of patients, irrespective of the findings on the ventilation-perfusion lung scan. Also, a sufficiently large numbers of mismatched segmental equivalent perfusion defects or mismatched vascular perfusion defects negated a low or intermediate likelihood clinical impression.

Among patients with prior cardiopulmonary disease, larger numbers of mismatched perfusion defects were required to negate an intermediate likelihood clinical assessment than among patients with no prior cardiopulmonary

ANY CPD

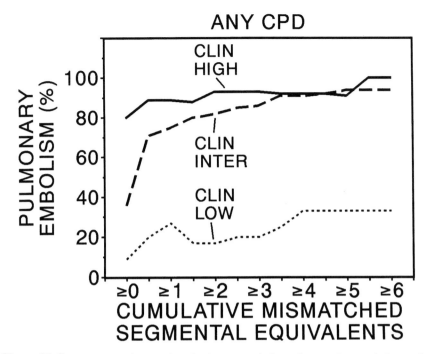

Figure 24–3. Positive predictive value of pulmonary embolism relative to the cumulative number of mismatched segmental equivalent perfusion defects among patients with prior cardiopulmonary disease (ANY CPD). Abbreviations as in Figure 24–1. Only few patients had a low likelihood clinical assessment and ≥1 mismatched segmental equivalent perfusion defect. The CLIN LOW curve, therefore, fluctuated. (Reprinted with permission from Stein PD, Henry JW, Gottschalk A. The addition of clinical assessment to stratification according to prior cardiopulmonary disease further optimizes the interpretation of ventilation-perfusion lung scans in pulmonary embolism. Chest 1993;104:1472–1476.)

disease (4). A low likelihood clinical assessment among patients with prior cardiopulmonary disease indicated a low positive predictive value for pulmonary embolism, irrespective of the number of mismatched defects, although there were few patients in this category.

Prior clinical assessment in PIOPED was made by physicians who were experienced in pulmonary embolism. Objective clinical information can be obtained by any physician or physician's assistant, however, and processed with neural network computer intelligence (6). This gives a clinical assessment as accurate as that of physicians experienced with pulmonary embolism (Chapter 11).

In summary, stratification of patients according to the presence or absence of prior cardiopulmonary disease, the addition of prior clinical assessment, and the use of continuous cumulative data in regard to the number of mismatched defects enhanced the assessment of the positive predictive value of pulmonary embolism in individual patients. Assessment on the basis of mismatched vascular defects, rather than mismatched segmental equivalent defects, made the interpretation easier, and added objectivity.

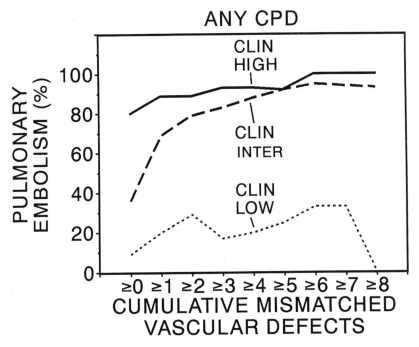

Figure 24–4.   Positive predictive value of pulmonary embolism relative to the cumulative number of mismatched vascular perfusion defects among patients with prior cardiopulmonary disease (ANY CPD). Abbreviations as in Figure 24–1. Only few patients had a low likelihood clinical assessment and ≥1 mismatched vascular defect. The CLIN LOW curve, therefore, fluctuated. (Reprinted with permission from Stein PD, Henry JW, Gottschalk A. The addition of clinical assessment to stratification according to prior cardiopulmonary disease further optimizes the interpretation of ventilation-perfusion lung scans in pulmonary embolism. Chest 1993;104:1472–1476.)

Table 24–3. POSITIVE PREDICTIVE VALUE OF PULMONARY EMBOLISM IN RELATION TO THE CUMULATIVE NUMBER OF MISMATCHED SEGMENTAL EQUIVALENT PERFUSION DEFECTS AND CLINICAL ASSESSMENT AMONG PATIENTS WITH PRIOR CARDIOPULMONARY DISEASE (n = 569)

Mismatched Segmental Equivalents	High Clinical Likelihood #PE/#Pts (%)	Intermed Clin Likelihood #PE/#Pts (%)	Low Clinical Likelihood #PE/#Pts (%)
≥ 0	24/30 (80)[a]	144/396 (36)[c]	13/143 (9)[b]
≥0.5	17/19 (89)	99/139 (71)[c]	3/15 (20)[b]
≥1.0	16/18 (89)	86/115 (75)[c]	3/11 (27)[b]
≥1.5	15/17 (88)	78/98 (80)	1/6 (17)
≥2.0	13/14 (93)	72/88 (82)	1/6 (17)
≥2.5	13/14 (93)	68/80 (85)	1/5 (20)
≥3.0	13/14 (93)	63/73 (86)	1/5 (20)
≥3.5	12/13 (92)	61/67 (91)	1/4 (25)
≥4.0	11/12 (92)	59/65 (91)	1/3 (33)
≥4.5	11/12 (92)	55/60 (92)	1/3 (33)
≥5.0	10/11 (91)	51/54 (94)	1/3 (33)
≥5.5	10/10 (100)	47/50 (94)	1/3 (33)
≥6.0	10/10 (100)	45/48 (94)	1/3 (33)
≥6.5	9/9 (100)	44/47 (94)	1/3 (33)
≥7.0	8/8 (100)	41/44 (93)	0/2 (0)
≥7.5	7/7 (100)	39/41 (95)	0/2 (0)

PE = pulmonary embolism; Pts = patients; Intermed = intermediate
Clin = clinical
[a] P < .001 high vs intermediate
[b] P < .001 high vs low
[c] P < .001 intermediate vs low
Probabilities are higher than reported by Stein and associates (4) because chi square probabilities previously were calculated using Yates' correction, which was unnecessarily conservative.
Modified and reproduced from Stein PD, Henry JW, Gottschalk A, with permission.

186 Pulmonary Embolism

Table 24-4. POSITIVE PREDICTIVE VALUE OF PULMONARY EMBOLISM IN RELATION TO THE CUMULATIVE NUMBER OF MISMATCHED VASCULAR PERFUSION DEFECTS AND CLINICAL ASSESSMENT AMONG PATIENTS WITH PRIOR CARDIOPULMONARY DISEASE (n = 569)

Mismatched Vascular Defects	High Clinical Likelihood #PE/#Pts (%)	Intermed Clin Likelihood #PE/Pts (%)	Low Clinical Likelihood #PE/Pts (%)
≥0	24/30 (80)[a]	144/396 (36)[d]	13/143 (9)[b]
≥1	17/19 (89)	99/139 (71)[d]	3/15 (20)[b]
≥2	16/18 (89)	81/103 (79)[e]	2/7 (29)[c]
≥3	13/14 (93)	71/86 (83)	1/6 (29)
≥4	13/14 (93)	63/72 (88)	1/5 (20)
≥5	12/13 (92)	59/64 (92)	1/4 (25)
≥6	11/11 (100)	52/55 (95)	1/3 (33)
≥7	10/10 (100)	46/49 (94)	1/3 (33)
≥8	7/7 (100)	42/45 (93)	0/2 (0)

PE = pulmonary embolism; Pts = patients; Intermed = intermediate; Clin = clinical
[a] P < .001 high vs intermediate
[b] P < .001 high vs low
[c] P < .01 high vs low
[d] P < .001 intermediate vs low
[e] P < .01 intermediate vs low
Probabilities are higher than reported by Stein and associates (4) because chi square probabilities previously were calculated using Yates' correction, which was unnecessarily conservative.
Modified and reproduced from Stein PD, Henry JW, Gottschalk A, with permission.

REFERENCES

1. Stein PD, Gottschalk A, Henry JW, et al. Stratification of patients according to prior cardiopulmonary disease and probability assessment based upon the number of mismatched segmental equivalent perfusion defects: approaches to strengthen the diagnostic value of ventilation/perfusion lung scans in acute pulmonary embolism. Chest 1993;104:461–1467.
2. Neumann RD, Sostman HD, Gottschalk A. Current status of ventilation/perfusion imaging. Semin Nucl Med 1980;10:198–217.
3. Stein PD, Henry JW, Gottschalk A. Mismatched vascular defects: an easy alternative to mismatched segmental equivalent defects for the interpretation of ventilation/ perfusion lung scans in pulmonary embolism. Chest 1993;104:1468–1471.
4. Stein PD, Henry JW, Gottschalk A. The addition of clinical assessment to stratification according to prior cardiopulmonary disease further optimizes the interpretation of ventilation-perfusion lung scans in pulmonary embolism. Chest 1993;104:1472–1476.
5. A collaborative study by the PIOPED Investigators. Value of the ventilation/perfusion scan in acute pulmonary embolism: results of the Prospective Investigation of Pulmonary Embolism Diagnosis (PIOPED). JAMA 1990;263:2753–2759.
6. Patil S, Henry JW, Rubenfire M, et al. Neural network in the diagnosis of acute pulmonary embolism. Chest 1993;104:1685–1698.

25

Stratification According to Age in the Interpretation of Ventilation-Perfusion Lung Scans

The only unique feature of the presentation of pulmonary embolism in the elderly in the Prospective Investigation of Pulmonary Embolism Diagnosis (PIOPED) was unexplained radiographic abnormalities as the initial manifestation of acute pulmonary embolism, which occurred in 11% (1). Pulmonary angiography among elderly patients was as safe as in other age groups (2). The sensitivity for pulmonary embolism of high probability scans using original PIOPED criteria in elderly patients was only 47% (1). This sensitivity is lower than desirable. Previous investigators reported difficulty in diagnosing pulmonary embolism in elderly patients (3,4).

Since the conclusion of PIOPED, we showed that stratification according to the presence or absence of prior cardiopulmonary disease permits the use of less restrictive criteria for a high probability interpretation in patients with no prior cardiopulmonary disease (5,6) (Chapters 22,23). In patients with no prior cardiopulmonary disease, a high positive predictive value can be achieved with fewer mismatched perfusion defects than required for a high probability interpretation in unstratified patients or patients with prior cardiopulmonary disease. In patients ≥ 70 years of age with no prior cardiopulmonary disease, such stratification was particularly useful (7). Although elderly patients with no prior cardiopulmonary disease represent only a small percentage of patients with suspected acute pulmonary embolism (Table 25–1), the ventilation-perfusion lung scan in such patients is sensitive and specific (7).

Among elderly patients with no prior cardiopulmonary disease, if the ventilation-perfusion scan showed 1 or more mismatched vascular perfusion defects, the positive predictive value for pulmonary embolism was 87% (Table 25–2, Fig. 25–1) (7). If the ventilation-perfusion scan showed 2 or more mismatched vascular perfusion defects, the positive predictive value for pulmonary embolism was 100%. With 1 or more, 2 or more, and 3 or more mismatched vascular

187

Table 25–1. NUMBER OF PATIENTS IN EACH AGE GROUP STRATIFIED ACCORDING TO THE PRESENCE OR ABSENCE OF PRIOR CARDIOPULMONARY DISEASE

Age (Years)	CPD	No CPD	Total
18–39	77	129	206
40–69	353	232	585
≥70	199	60	259
Total	626	421	1050

CPD, prior cardiopulmonary disease
No CPD, prior cardiopulmonary disease
Modified and reprinted with permission from Stein PD, Henry JD, Relyea B, et al. Elderly patients with no prior cardiopulmonary disease show ventilation-perfusion lung scan characteristics that are sensitive and specific for pulmonary embolism. Am J Geriatric Cardiol 1996;5:(Nov-Dec).

Table 25–2. POSITIVE PREDICTIVE VALUE, SENSITIVITY AND SPECIFICITY OF PULMONARY EMBOLISM IN RELATION TO THE CUMULATIVE NUMBER OF MISMATCHED VASCULAR PERFUSION DEFECTS AMONG PATIENTS ≥70 YEARS WITH AND WITHOUT PRIOR CARDIOPULMONARY DISEASE

Cumulative # of Defects	No Prior Cardiopulmonary Disease			Any Prior Cardiopulmonary Disease		
	PPV PE/Test+ (%)	Sens (%) (n = 31)	Spec (%) (n = 29)	PPV PE/Test+ (%)	Sens (%) (n = 66)	Spec (%) (n = 133)
≥1	27/31 (87)	87*	86	43/65 (66)	65	83
≥2	23/23 (100)**	74	100	37/47 (79)	56	92
≥3	19/19 (100)*	61	100	34/42 (81)	42	94
≥4	17/17 (100)	55	100	29/35 (83)	44	95
≥5	14/14 (100)	45	100	28/31 (90)	42	98
≥6	11/11 (100)	35	100	26/27 (96)	39	99

PE = pulmonary embolism; PPV = positive predictive value; Sens = sensitivity; Spec = specificity
Probability of difference: No prior cardiopulmonary disease vs prior cardiopulmonary disease
* P < .05
** P < .02
Reproduced from Stein PD, Henry JD, Relyea B, et al with permission.

perfusion defects, positive predictive values were higher among patients with no cardiopulmonary disease than among patients with cardiopulmonary disease. A mismatched vascular perfusion defect was defined as either a large or moderate-size mismatched segmental perfusion defect (6) (Chapter 23).

The sensitivity for pulmonary embolism of 1 or more mismatched vascular perfusion defects in elderly patients was 87% and the sensitivity of 2 or more mismatched vascular perfusion defects was 74% (Table 25–2) (7). The respective specificities for ≥ 1 and ≥ 2 mismatched vascular perfusion defects were 86% and 100%. The sensitivity of 1 or more mismatched vascular defects was higher

≥70 YEARS

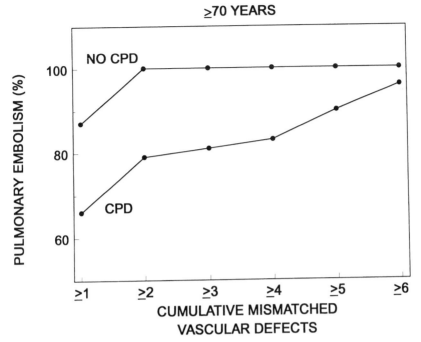

Figure 25–1. Frequency of pulmonary embolism among elderly patients (≥70 years) in relation to the cumulative number of mismatched vascular perfusion defects. Patients were stratified according to the presence or absence of prior cardiopulmonary disease (CPD). The positive predictive value for pulmonary embolism was higher in patients with ≥1 defect (P<.05), ≥2 defects (P<.02), and ≥3 defects (P<.05). (Reprinted with permission from Stein PD, Henry JD, Relyea B, et al. Elderly patients with no prior cardiopulmonary disease show ventilation-perfusion lung scan characteristics that are sensitive and specific for pulmonary embolism. Am J Geriatric Cardiol 1996;5: (Nov-Dec).)

among elderly patients with no prior cardiopulmonary disease than among elderly patients with prior cardiopulmonary disease.

Among elderly patients with prior cardiopulmonary disease, 4 or more mismatched vascular perfusion defects were required for a positive predictive value of 83%, and 5 or more mismatched vascular perfusion defects were required for a positive predictive value of 90% (Table 25–2, Fig. 25–1) (7). The respective sensitivities for pulmonary embolism were 44% and 42%, and the respective specificities were 95% and 98% (Table 25–2).

The sensitivity of a high probability ventilation-perfusion scan for elderly patients with no prior cardiopulmonary disease, using original PIOPED criteria, (8) was 55%; with prior cardiopulmonary disease, the sensitivity was 45%. Among all elderly patients, the sensitivity of a high probability ventilation-perfusion scan using PIOPED criteria was 48%. The specificities in these respective groups were 100%, 97%, and 98%.

The positive predictive values, sensitivities, and specificities of ≥1 to ≥6 cumulative mismatched vascular perfusion defects among patients 40 to 69 years of age are shown in Table 25–3. A trend showed a higher positive predictive value for ≥1, ≥2 and ≥3 mismatched vascular perfusion defects in patients with no prior cardiopulmonary diseases (7).

Table 25–3. POSITIVE PREDICTIVE VALUE, SENSITIVITY AND
SPECIFICITY OF PULMONARY EMBOLISM IN RELATION TO
THE CUMULATIVE NUMBER OF MISMATCHED VASCULAR
PERFUSION DEFECTS AMONG PATIENTS 40–69 YEARS
WITH AND WITHOUT PRIOR CARDIOPULMONARY DISEASE

Cumulative # of Defects	No Prior Cardiopulmonary Disease			Any Prior Cardiopulmonary Disease		
	PPV PE/Test+ (%)	Sens (%) (n = 96)	Spec (%) (n = 136)	PPV PE/Test+ (%)	Sens (%) (n = 116)	Spec (%) (n = 237)
≥1	68/84 (81)	71	88	72/102 (71)	62	87
≥2	52/59 (88)	54	95	72/72 (79)	49	94
≥3	47/53 (89)	49	96	48/57 (84)	41	96
≥4	39/45 (87)	41	96	45/50 (90)	39	98
≥5	33/36 (92)	34	98	40/43 (93)	34	99
≥6	32/33 (97)	33	99	34/36 (94)	29	99

PE = pulmonary embolism; PPV = positive predictive value; Sens = sensitivity; Spec = specificity
All differences between patients with and without prior cardiopulmonary disease were not significant
Reproduced from Stein PD, Henry JD, Relyea B, et al with permission.

Table 25–4. POSITIVE PREDICTIVE VALUE, SENSITIVITY AND
SPECIFICITY OF PULMONARY EMBOLISM IN RELATION TO
THE CUMULATIVE NUMBER OF MISMATCHED VASCULAR
PERFUSION DEFECTS AMONG PATIENTS 18–39 YEARS
WITH AND WITHOUT PRIOR CARDIOPULMONARY DISEASE

Cumulative # of Defects	No Prior Cardiopulmonary Disease			Any Prior Cardiopulmonary Disease		
	PPV PE/Test+ (%)	Sens (%) (n = 96)	Spec (%) (n = 136)	PPV PE/Test+ (%)	Sens (%) (n = 23)	Spec (%) (n = 54)
≥1	28/39 (72)	61	87	15/25 (60)	65	81
≥2	19/24 (79)	41	94	11/17 (65)	48	89
≥3	13/15 (87)	28	98	8/13 (62)	35	91
≥4	11/13 (85)	24	98	7/11 (64)	30	93
≥5	8/10 (80)	17	98	7/10 (70)	30	94
≥6	6/8 (75)	13	98	7/9 (78)	30	96

PE = pulmonary embolism; PPV = positive predictive value; Sens = sensitivity; Spec = specificity
All differences between patients with and without prior cardiopulmonary disease were not significant
Reproduced from Stein PD, Henry JD, Relyea B, et al with permission.

The positive predictive values, sensitivities, and specificities of ≥1 to ≥6 cumulative mismatched vascular perfusion defects among patients 18 to 39 years of age are shown in Table 25–4. A trend showed a higher positive predictive value for ≥1, ≥2 and ≥3 mismatched vascular perfusion defects in patients with no prior cardiopulmonary diseases (7).

Among patients with no prior cardiopulmonary disease, the positive predictive value of ≥2 mismatched vascular perfusion defects was higher in patients ≥ 70 years old than in patients 19 to 39 years old (Table 25–2, Table 25–4). No difference of the positive predictive value for pulmonary embolism of any number of mismatched vascular defects was shown comparing patients ≥ 70 years old with patients 40 to 69 years old (Table 25–2, Table 25–3). The sensitivities of ≥1 and ≥2 mismatched vascular perfusion defects were higher in patients ≥ 70 years old with no prior cardiopulmonary disease than in patients 18 to 39 years old with no prior cardiopulmonary disease. The sensitivity of 2 or more mismatched vascular defects in elderly patients was also higher than in patients 40 to 69 years old (Table 25–2, Table 25–4). Specificities did not differ between age groups (Table 25–2, Table 25–3, Table 25–4).

Among patients with prior cardiopulmonary disease, sensitivities and specificities did not differ between age groups, and comparisons of positive predictive values of most cumulative numbers of mismatched vascular defects did not differ to a statistically significant extent (Table 25–2, Table 25–3, Table 25–4)

The sensitivity for pulmonary embolism in elderly patients who were not stratified according to prior cardiopulmonary disease, using PIOPED criteria, was 48%. The sensitivity for pulmonary embolism in elderly patients with no prior cardiopulmonary disease, using 2 or more mismatched vascular defects as the criterion for a high probability interpretation, was 74%. This increased sensitivity was not accompanied by a reduction of specificity or positive predictive value.

In summary, stratification according to both age and the presence or absence of prior cardiopulmonary disease was useful for the evaluation of ventilation-perfusion lung scans in patients ≥ 70 years old (7). Such stratification requires no special expertise in the diagnosis of acute pulmonary embolism. In patients ≥ 70 years old with no prior cardiopulmonary disease, ventilation-perfusion scans with ≥2 mismatched vascular defects showed a 74% sensitivity, 100% specificity and 100% positive predictive value. Although only 23% of patients ≥ 70 years old had no prior cardiopulmonary disease, stratification according to age and the absence of prior cardiopulmonary disease was particularly useful in this subset of patients.

REFERENCES

1. Stein PD, Gottschalk A, Saltzman HA, et al. Diagnosis of acute pulmonary embolism in the elderly. J Amer Coll Cardiol 1991;18:1452–1457.
2. Stein PD, Henry JW. Age-related complications of pulmonary angiography for acute pulmonary embolism. Am J Geriatric Cardiol 1993;2:13–22.
3. Taubman LB, Silverstone FA. Autopsy proven pulmonary embolism among the institutionalized elderly. J Am Geriatr Soc 1986;34:752–756.
4. Morrell MT. The incidence of pulmonary embolism in the elderly. Geriatrics 1970;25:138–153.
5. Stein PD, Gottschalk A, Henry JW, et al. Stratification of patients according to prior cardiopulmonary disease and probability assessment based upon the number of mismatched segmental equivalent perfusion defects: approaches to strengthen the diagnostic value of ventilation/perfusion lung scans in acute pulmonary embolism. Chest 1993;104:1461–1467.

6. Stein PD, Henry JW, Gottschalk A. Mismatched vascular defects: an easy alternative to mismatched segmental equivalent defects for the interpretation of ventilation/perfusion lung scans in pulmonary embolism. Chest 1993; 104:1468–1472.
7. Stein PD, Henry JD, Relyea B, et al. Elderly patients with no prior cardiopulmonary disease show ventilation/perfusion lung scan characteristics that are sensitive and specific for pulmonary embolism. Am J Geriatric Cardiol 1996;5:(Nov-Dec).
8. A collaborative study by the PIOPED Investigators. Value of the ventilation/perfusion scan in acute pulmonary embolism: results of the Prospective Investigation of Pulmonary Embolism Diagnosis (PIOPED). JAMA 1990;263:2753–2759.

Pulmonary Angiography

CHAPTER 26

Complications of Pulmonary Angiography

Complications of pulmonary angiography have been reported by several groups of investigators. Mills and associates reported major complications (including death) in 43 of 1350 (3%) (1). Three deaths occurred (0.2%), and each was in a patient with cor pulmonale, elevated right ventricular end-diastolic pressure and elevated pulmonary artery pressures. Nonfatal major complications among these 1350 patients included cardiac perforation in 14 (1%), major arrhythmias in 11 (1%), successfully treated cardiac arrest in 6 (0.4%), myocardial injury in 6 (0.4%), and significant contrast reaction in 4 (0.3%).

In the Urokinase Pulmonary Embolism Trial, among 310 patients with pulmonary embolism, 6 of 310 (2%) patients had nonfatal major complications, exclusive of local complications (2). No deaths occurred. Major arrhythmias occurred in five patients, and myocardial perforation in one.

Dalen and associates reported significant complications in 13 of 367 (4%) who underwent angiography because of suspected pulmonary embolism (3). One death (0.3%) occurred. Hull and associates reported two reactions to contrast media, but no deaths among 104 patients (4). Marsh and associates reported one death and one nonfatal perforation of the right ventricle (5) among 106 patients.

Moses and associates reported major complications of pulmonary angiography in 3 of 298 (1%) patients who had suspected pulmonary embolism (6). Two deaths and one major arrhythmia occurred. Stein and associates reported non-local complications in 12 of 122 (10%) patients with suspected pulmonary embolism or other pulmonary disorders (7). Two remote deaths occurred, which probably were not a direct result of pulmonary arteriography. Ranniger and associates reported non-local complications in 8 of 241 (3%) (8). No deaths occurred. Novelline and associates reported no major complications or deaths from pulmonary angiography in 302 patients and only minor arrhythmias in 3 (1%) (9).

We evaluated the complications of pulmonary angiography in 1111 patients who underwent angiography in the Prospective Investigation of Pulmonary

195

Embolism Diagnosis (PIOPED) (10). We defined major complications as those that were life threatening, and did not respond promptly to pharmaceutical therapy, or required intensive or prolonged treatment within the hospital. Patients who required cardiopulmonary resuscitation, endotracheal intubation, dialysis, or blood transfusion were defined as having major complications. Only one complication (the most severe complication) was listed for any patient.

Comparisons of the frequency of nonfatal major complications and less severe complications are not precise, because definitions of major or serious complications varied.

Non-major or minor complications were defined as complications that spontaneously regressed with no apparent residual damage even though prolonged monitoring may have been required. Such complications, in some instances, therefore, were important and potentially dangerous events and may have prolonged the hospital stay.

The techniques of pulmonary angiography that were employed are relevant. Pulmonary angiograms were performed through a femoral vein using the Seldinger technique with a multiple side-hole, 6 French to 8 French pigtail catheter (11). Small amounts of contrast material (5 to 8 ml) were injected by hand to check the patency of the inferior vena cava by fluoroscopy. The catheter was directed into the proximal portion of the pulmonary artery of the lung with the greatest ventilation-perfusion scan abnormality. Seventy-six percent iodinated (ionic) contrast material was injected at a rate of 20 to 35 ml/sec for a total of 40 to 50 ml over 2 seconds. If emboli were not identified, injections were repeated and magnification (1.8 to 2.0 times) oblique views were obtained of the areas suspicious for pulmonary embolism.

Major Complications

Major complications, including death, occurred in 1.3% of patients (Table 26–1) (10). Most of the patients who died or suffered major non-fatal cardiopulmonary complications were in critical condition with severely compromised cardiopulmonary function before angiography. The severity of the clinical condition usually was not caused by the massive pulmonary embolism.

Death occurred in 0.5% (10). The circumstances associated with death are outlined in Table 26–2. Although five deaths were attributed to pulmonary angiography, the cause of death in patients No. 1, 3, and 5 (Table 26–2) may not have been because of the catheterization procedure or pulmonary angiography. At least one of the patients was practically moribund (patient 5) and the four others (patients 1–4) had severe underlying cardiac or respiratory diseases. The frequency of death that we reported, (0.5%), was similar to the pooled value reported by others, 9 of 3074 (0.3%) (2–10).

The circumstances associated with respiratory decompensation in the 0.4% of patients who required endotracheal intubation or cardiopulmonary resuscitation are outlined in Table 26–3.

Hematomas of the groin with bleeding severe enough to require two units of blood were observed in 0.2% of patients. One of the two patients who had such bleeding was receiving anticoagulant therapy.

Three patients (0.3%) after angiography developed renal dysfunction, presumably acute tubular necrosis, which required dialysis. Serum creatinine in one patient increased from 1.2 mg/100 ml to 6.0 mg/100 ml, and in one patient

Table 26–1.   MAJOR COMPLICATIONS OF PULMONARY ANGIOGRAPHY
AMONG 1111 PATIENTS WITH SUSPECTED ACUTE
PULMONARY EMBOLISM

Complication	# Pts (%)
Death	5 (0.5)
Respiratory distress (CPR or intubation)	4 (0.4)
Renal failure (dialysis)	3 (0.3)
Hematoma (transfusion 2 units)	2 (0.1)
Total	14 (1.3)

Only 1 complication/patient is listed
CPR = cardiopulmonary resuscitation
# Pts = number of patients
Modified and reproduced from Stein PD, Athanasoulis C, Alavi A, et al. Complications and validity of pulmonary angiography in acute pulmonary embolism. Circulation 1992;85:462–469.

it increased from 2.4 mg/100 ml to 6.0 mg/100 ml. One patient developed a serum creatinine of 2.7 mg/100 ml, which was associated with pulmonary edema owing to fluid overload. The patient required endotracheal intubation.

In addition to the patients with major renal complications, 10 patients (0.9%) developed an elevation of the serum creatinine, and were treated with fluid balance, diuretics, and in one patient, dopamine. These patients did not require dialysis, and the complications therefore were defined as minor. Among these patients, five with a previously normal serum creatinine developed levels that ranged from 2.1 to 5.9 mg/100 ml. Five patients with a previously abnormal serum creatinine, which ranged from 1.5 to 2.7 mg/100 ml, developed a further increase ≥2 mg/100 ml.

Renal insufficiency induced by contrast material was a problem, particularly among elderly patients (10, 12). All pulmonary angiograms were performed with a standard ionic, high osmolar contrast agent (11). Whether the frequency of renal insufficiency would have been lower after the using a low osmolar contrast agent is undetermined. No evidence shows that the incidence of pronounced renal toxicity is different after the intravascular use of high versus low osmolar contrast agents (13–15). Also, the potential clinical advantages in regard to cardiac function have not yet been clearly demonstrated (16, 17).

Non-Major or Minor Complications

Among the patients with less severe or minor complications, many of the complications raised serious concern, some were potentially life-threatening, and some required prolonged monitoring. Minor complications, therefore, were not necessarily trivial. Minor complications are listed in Table 26–4. Two patients had bronchospasm after the injection of contrast material that was severe enough

Table 26–2. DEATHS FROM PULMONARY ANGIOGRAPHY

Pt	Age/ Gender	Associated Diagnoses and Prior Clinical Findings	PA Mean Press (mmHg)	Event Immediately Preceding Death During Catheterization	PE	Comment
1	44 F	Adeno CA of colon with lung metastasis	ND	Chest pain Shock Electromechanical dissoc with cath in RA	0	No arrhythmia Mechanism of events unclear
2	87 F	HTN, MR, CHF	ND	VT with cath in RV	?	VT reverted, but resp arrest, and hypotension occurred soon after. Died 24 hrs after cath
3	62 M	Pneumonia Acute resp distress CHD Endotracheal tube/ ventilator	27	Cardiopulm arrest 1 hr after angio	0	Unstable patient
4	67 M	Old MI CHF, EF 15%, Recent VF	26	After angio wedge pressure 37 mmHg, shock, PaO$_2$ 35 mmHg on O$_2$	+	Cardiogenic shock. Died 12 hrs after cath
5	58 F	CA Cervix Endotracheal tube/ ventilator	25	Bradycardia, hypoxia followed by cardiopulm arrest while preparing for second angio injection	?	Unstable patient

Angio = angiogram, CA = carcinoma, Cardiopulm = cardiopulmonary, Cath = catheter or catheterization, CHD = coronary heart disease, CHF = congestive heart failure, EF = ejection fraction, HTN = hypertension, MR = mitral regurgitation, ND = not done, PA = pulmonary artery, PE = pulmonary embolism, RA = right atrium, Resp = respiratory, RV = right ventricle, VF = ventricular fibrillation, VT = ventricular tachycardia
Reproduced from Stein PD, Athanasoulis C, Alavi A, et al with permission.

to discontinue the procedure. One required subcutaneous epinephrine. Two patients developed angina during the catheterization and were transferred to the coronary care unit for monitoring. Two patients (in addition to one patient whose most prominent problem was angina) became hypotensive.

Relation of Complications to Clinical Characteristics

Major complications occurred more frequently among patients sent for angiography from medical intensive care units than among patients from else-

Table 26–3. MAJOR RESPIRATORY DISTRESS

Pt	Age/ Gender	Associated Diagnoses and Prior Clinical Findings	PA Mean Press (mmHg)	Event Immediately Preceding Distress During Catheterization	PE	Comment
1	79 F	HTN Syncope	?	Angiogram followed by shock, agonal breathing, LOC	+	Endotracheal intubation
2	36 M	Hodgkin's Lymphoma	24	Angio followed by bronchospasm, airway stridor	0	Endotracheal intubation
3	63 F	Gastric adeno CA Pleural and mediastinal metastases	25	Angio followed by respiratory arrest, then cardiac arrest	0	Endotracheal intubation
4	32 F	Obese Estrogen—birth control	45	Angio followed by respiratory arrest, seizure	+	CPR

CPR = Cardiopulmonary Resuscitation, LOC = Loss of Consciousness, PA = Pulmonary Artery, PE = Pulmonary Embolism, Press = Pressure
Reproduced from Stein PD, Athanasoulis C, Alavi A, et al with permission.

where, 5 of 122 (4%) versus 9 of 989 (1%) (10). The severity of the underlying condition rendered these patients vulnerable to the procedure. Such critically ill patients often present the most vexing diagnostic dilemmas, which require precise information for their optimal management, but face a higher risk of angiography. Clinical judgment is important in this situation.

Minor complications occurred with a similar frequency among patients sent from medical intensive care units and among those sent from elsewhere, 4 of 122 (3%) versus 56 of 989 (6%).

The frequency of complications was not related to the presence or absence of pulmonary embolism. Only 4 of 11 patients with major complications, in whom a diagnosis was established, had pulmonary embolism. Major complications occurred in 1% of patients with pulmonary embolism and in 1% of patients who did not have pulmonary embolism. Minor complications occurred in 6% of patients with pulmonary embolism and in 5% of patients with no pulmonary embolism.

Complications, in general, were not related to age, although renal complications occurred more often in elderly patients (10, 12). Patients with either major or less severe renal dysfunction, compared with patients with no renal dysfunction, were 74 ± 13 years versus 57 ± 17 years (mean $\pm$ standard deviation). Complications were unrelated to gender.

The frequency of complications was not related to pulmonary artery mean pressure (10). Pulmonary artery mean pressure was measured in patients with

Table 26–4.   NON-MAJOR OR MINOR COMPLICATIONS OF PULMONARY
ANGIOGRAPHY AMONG 1111 PATIENTS WITH SUSPECTED
ACUTE PULMONARY EMBOLISM

Complication	# Pts (%)
Respiratory distress (prompt response to drugs)	4 (0.4)
Renal dysfunction (responded to drug therapy and fluid balance)	10 (0.9)
Angina (monitored in coronary care unit)	2 (0.1)
Hypotension (prompt response to drugs/fluids)	2 (0.1)
Pulmonary Congestion (prompt response to drugs)	4 (0.4)
Urticaria, itching or periorbital edema	16 (1.4)
Hematoma (not transfused)	9 (0.8)
Arrhythmia (spontaneous conversion or prompt response to drugs)	6 (0.5)
Subintimal contrast stain	4 (0.4)
Narcotic overdose (treated with naloxone)	1 (0.1)
Nausea and vomiting	1 (0.1)
Right bundle branch block	1 (0.1)
Total	60 (5.4)

Only 1 complication is listed for each patient
Modified and reproduced from Stein PD, Athanasoulis C, Alavi A, et al with permission.

major, minor, and no complications, and it was 22 ± 14 mm Hg, 19 ± 9 mm
Hg and 23 ± 11 mm Hg, respectively. Patients with major or minor complications
had right atrial mean pressures no higher than in patients with no complications.

The volume of contrast material injected was not significantly larger in
patients with major or minor complications than in patients with no complications, 106 ± 73 ml, 185 ± 84 ml, and 181 ± 61 ml, respectively (10). Even
among the 13 patients who suffered renal dysfunction, either major or minor,
the volume of contrast material injected was not significantly greater than among
those who had no complications, 207 ± 53 ml versus 181 ± 61 ml.

The potential complication of myocardial perforation was specifically monitored and none was observed. The absence of myocardial perforation reflects the use of angiographic catheters with a "pigtail"-shaped tip. Such catheters also contributed to the reduced incidence of major cardiac arrhythmias occurring during the passage of the catheter through the right ventricle.

Pulmonary hypertension has been emphasized by previous investigators as an important risk factor (1), but procedural modifications diminished the risk in PIOPED. In the past, most deaths and serious complications were reported in patients with pulmonary hypertension and an elevated right ventricular end-diastolic pressure (1). In this setting, an injection of contrast material into the main pulmonary artery may result in death. In PIOPED, the protocol called for selective contrast injections into the right or left pulmonary artery, rather than the main pulmonary artery. Further, in patients with elevated pulmonary artery pressures, the protocol permitted a reduction of the rate of infection and the total amount of contrast material injected. Such precautions, however, cannot be viewed as a guarantee for the prevention of serious or fatal complications in patients with pulmonary hypertension. Marsh and associates (5) reported a death in a patient with severe pulmonary hypertension after a hand injection of 10 ml of contrast material.

In summary, severe underlying disease with impaired cardiopulmonary function posed the greatest risk for complications of pulmonary angiography. Clinical judgment is important in the assessment of the risk. It is also important to consider the experience of the angiographer. In PIOPED, the angiographers were experienced.

REFERENCES

1. Mills SR, Jackson DC, Older RA, et al. The incidence, etiologies, and avoidance of complications of pulmonary angiography in a large series. Radiology 1980;136:295–299.
2. The Urokinase Pulmonary Embolism Trial. A National Cooperative Study. Circulation 1973;47(SupplII):38–45.
3. Dalen JE, Brooks HL, Johnson LW, et al. Pulmonary angiography in acute pulmonary embolism: indications, techniques, and results in 367 patients. Am Heart J 1971;81:175–185.
4. Hull RD, Hirsh J, Carter CJ, et al. Pulmonary angiography ventilation lung scanning, and venography for clinically suspected pulmonary embolism with abnormal perfusion lung scan. Ann Intern Med 1983;98:891–899.
5. Marsh JD, Glynn M and Torman HA. Pulmonary angiography: application in a new spectrum of patients. Am J Med 1983;75:763–770.
6. Moses DC, Silver TM, Bookstein JJ. The complementary roles of chest radiography, lung scanning, and selective pulmonary angiography in the diagnosis of pulmonary embolism. Circulation 1974;49:179–188.
7. Stein MA, Winter J, Grollman JH Jr. The value of the pulmonary-artery-seeking catheter in percutaneous selective pulmonary arteriography. Radiology 1975;144:299–304.
8. Ranniger K. Pulmonary arteriography: a simple method for demonstration of clinically significant pulmonary emboli. Am J Roent 1969;106:558–562.
9. Novelline RA, Baltarowich OH, Athanasoulis CA, et a. The clinical course of patients with suspected pulmonary embolism and a negative pulmonary arteriogram. Radiology 1978;126:561–567.

10. Stein PD, Athanasoulis C, Alavi A, et al. Complications and validity of pulmonary angiography in acute pulmonary embolism. Circulation 1992;85:462–469.
11. A Collaborative Study by the PIOPED Investigators. Value of the ventilation-perfusion scan in acute pulmonary embolism: results of the Prospective Investigation of Pulmonary Embolism Diagnosis (PIOPED). JAMA 1990;263:2753–2759.
12. Stein PD, Henry JW. Age-related complications of pulmonary angiography for acute pulmonary embolism. Am J Geriatric Cardiol 1993;2:13–22.
13. Schwab SJ, Hlatky MA, Pieper KS, et al. Contrast nephrotoxicity: a randomized controlled trial of a nonionic and an ionic radiographic contrast agent. N Eng J Med 1989;320:149–153.
14. Taliercio CP, Vlietstra RE, Ilstrup DM, et al. A randomized comparison of the nephrotoxicity of iopamidol and diatrizoate in high risk patients undergoing cardiac angiography. J Am Coll Cardiol 1991;17:384–390.
15. Donadio C, Tramonti G, Giordani R, et al. Glomerular and tubular effects of ionic and nonionic contrast media (diatrizoate and iopamidol). Contr Nephrol 1988;68:212–219.
16. Hirshfeld JW Jr, Wieland J, Davis CA, et al. Hemodynamic and electrocardiographic effects of ioversol during cardiac angiography. Comparison with iopamidol and diatrizoate. Invest Radiol 1989;24:138–144.
17. Bettmann MA, Higgins CB. Comparison of an ionic with a nonionic contrast agent for cardiac angiography. Results of a multicenter trial. Invest Radiol 1985;20:S70–S74.

CHAPTER **27**

Standard and Augmented Techniques of Pulmonary Angiography

Pulmonary angiography is generally accepted as the definitive diagnostic test for pulmonary embolism. Pulmonary angiography has undergone evolutionary development, both in technique and in the identification of angiographic criteria for diagnosing pulmonary embolism. The validity of pulmonary angiography depends upon technique. It is usually easier to diagnose pulmonary embolism than confidently to exclude it by pulmonary angiography.

Historical Development of Pulmonary Angiography

The first attempt to investigate the appearance of the pulmonary vasculature in the presence of pulmonary embolism was made by Jesser and deTakats in 1941 (1). They described a reduction of the size of the pulmonary arterial tree and blocked main vessels after embolization of the pulmonary artery of dogs with a barium sulfate suspension. The absence of filling of the pulmonary artery beyond the site of occlusion was also observed by Liberson and Liberson (2) in 1942, in pulmonary angiograms taken after the injection into rabbits of lead filings mixed with paraffin.

The intraluminal filling defect in pulmonary embolism was first described by Lochhead, Roberts, and Dotter in 1952 in dogs embolized with autologous blood clots (3). They also described incomplete occlusion of vessels, reduced rate of flow through the region of the clot, diminished opacification of distal vessels, and dilation of the pulmonary artery proximal to the embolus.

Chrispin, Goodwin, and Steiner, in 1963, based on right atrial and pulmonary arterial injections in seven patients with clinical evidence of pulmonary embolism, categorized the angiographic signs into those of major artery occlusion and those of peripheral vessel occlusion (4). Obstruction of major arteries seemed to be associated with a reduced number of peripheral branches, areas of increased transradiency (oligemia), slow passage of contrast material into the capillaries (asymmetrical filling), and failure of the pulmonary veins to fill.

Obstruction of smaller vessels was associated with slow disappearance of contrast material from the arteries (prolonged arterial phase), peripheral pruning, and tortuous vessels.

Williams and associates, in 1963, in addition to previous observations, reported narrowing and irregularity of opacified vessels, which they attributed to circumferential organization of thromboemboli (5).

Smith, Dammin, and Dexter, using postmortem arteriography, showed reduced opacification of small vessels in the periphery of the lung when small vessels were embolized (6). Sasahara and associates mentioned plaque-like filling defects among the angiographic abnormalities noted in patients with clinical evidence of pulmonary embolism (7). They noted difficulty in interpreting pulmonary angiograms in patients with mitral stenosis or chronic lung disease. Dalen and colleagues (8) obtained selective pulmonary angiograms in dogs embolized with autologous clots (some with radiopaque autologous clots) and observed cutoffs, areas of oligemia, and filling defects as typical angiographic abnormalities.

Stein and associates divided angiographic signs into those of morphologic significance and those of physiologic significance (9). Morphologic signs were intraluminal filling defects, abrupt cutoff of an artery, and localized pruning (lack of fine branching). Physiologic signs were oligemia (areas of increased translucency), asymmetrical filling, prolongation of the arterial phase, and bilateral lower-zone filling delay. Absence of fine branching of the pulmonary vessels was subsequently shown to be nonspecific, and may reflect pulmonary vascular destruction such as occurs in emphysema (10,11). Abrupt cutoff of vessels may occur with tumor. It became apparent, therefore, that the only abnormality on the pulmonary angiogram that was diagnostic of pulmonary embolism was visualization of the intraluminal filling defect. Other angiographic abnormalities, in a patient with suspected pulmonary embolism who has no prior cardiopulmonary disease, may call attention to suspicious regions.

Observations in PIOPED

The validity of pulmonary angiograms in patients suspected of acute pulmonary embolism was evaluated in the Prospective Investigation of Pulmonary Embolism Diagnosis (PIOPED) (12). All patients underwent one year of surveillance after the pulmonary angiogram. Any rehospitalization, new investigation for pulmonary embolism, complication of anticoagulation, or death triggered a detailed review of the patient's medical records by the PIOPED outcome classification committee (13). The review used all available clinical information, including hospital and autopsy records, death certificates, and original radiographic studies. The outcome classification committee could reverse the reading of a negative pulmonary angiogram if pulmonary embolism was found at autopsy, or on repeat angiography, or if new perfusion scan defects interpreted as high probability for pulmonary embolism were observed.

Angiographic Technique

The femoral-vein Seldinger technique with a multiple side-hole 6 French size to 8 French size pigtail catheter was used (13). Small amounts of contrast material (5 ml to 8 ml) were injected by hand to check the patency of the inferior vena cava. The catheter was directed into the proximal portion of the pulmonary artery of the lung with the greatest abnormality on the ventilation-perfusion lung scan. Initial filming was in the anteroposterior projection. Seventy-six percent iodinated (ionic) contrast material was injected at a rate of 20 to 35 ml/sec for a total of 40 to 50 ml over 2 seconds. Film rates were 3 per second for 3 seconds, followed by 1 per second for 4 to 6 seconds. Depending on the size of the lungs, filming was not magnified or given a low magnification of 1.4. A 12:1 grid was used, and roentgenographic factors were in the range of 70 to 80 kilovolts (kV) (peak) and 0.025 to 0.04 seconds at 1000 mA with a focal spot of 1.2 to 1.5 mm. If emboli were not identified, injections were repeated and magnification (1.8 to 2.0 times) oblique views were obtained of the areas suspicious for pulmonary embolism. Films were obtained with an air-gap technique (i.e., no grid was used). Roentgenographic factors were in the range of 78 to 88 kV (peak) and 0.04 to 0.08 seconds at 160 mA with a focal spot of 0.3 to 0.6 mm in diameter. If no emboli were found in the first lung, or if bilateral angiography in the clinical center was routine, identical techniques were used for the second lung. Angiograms were usually completed within 24 hours of the onset of clinical symptoms.

Interpetation of Angiograms

Criteria for the diagnosis of pulmonary embolism were the identification of the trailing edge of an embolus obstructing a vessel or the outline of an embolus (filling defect) within a vessel (13). A nonfilling vessel or hypovascular area were not considered diagnostic, nor were webs, stenoses, or other vessel abnormalities. Angiograms were randomly assigned to pairs of angiographers from clinical centers other than the originating hospital. The pulmonary angiograms were interpreted with the lung scans. If two readers disagreed whether pulmonary embolism was present, absent or uncertain, the interpretations were adjudicated by readers randomly selected from the remaining clinical centers. If adjudicating readers did not agree with either of the first two readers, angiograms went to panels of angiography readers.

Table 27–1. INTERPRETATION OF PULMONARY ANGIOGRAMS IN PATIENTS WITH SUSPECTED ACUTE PULMONARY EMBOLISM (n = 1111)

	# Pts	%
Pulmonary embolism present	383	35
Pulmonary embolism absent	681	61
Pulmonary embolism uncertain	35	3
Angiogram incomplete	12	1

Data are from Stein and associates (12).

Results of Pulmonary Angiography

Among 1111 patients who underwent pulmonary angiography, 383 (35%) had positive angiograms, and 681 (61%) had negative angiograms (Table 27–1) (12). In 35 (3%), the angiogram was nondiagnostic, and in 12 (1%), the angiogram was not completed, usually because of complications. Among completed angiograms, therefore, 35 of 1099 (3%) were nondiagnostic. This percentage of nondiagnostic angiograms is similar to the 5% of poor angiograms reported by Dalen and associates after an injection in the main pulmonary artery (14). The angiographic interpretations that PIOPED reported, however, were consensus readings, adjudicated if necessary by a panel of readers. Individual angiographers in a clinical environment may not achieve the accuracy of these consensus readings.

Among the 681 patients in PIOPED with negative pulmonary angiograms, the diagnosis of no pulmonary embolism was reversed by the Outcome Classification Committee in 4 (1%). Each of these patients died within 6 days of the pulmonary angiogram, and pulmonary embolism was found in each at autopsy. The validity of positive pulmonary angiograms could not be assessed.

Table 27–2. ALL ANGIOGRAMS (n = 1099)

		Reader #1			
		PE+	PE–	PE?	Total
Reader #2	PE+	331	35	8	374
	PE–	37	544	60	641
	PE?	12	58	14	84
	Total	380	637	82	1099

PE+ = Pulmonary embolism present
PE– = Pulmonary embolism absent
PE? = Pulmonary embolism uncertain
Reproduced from Stein PD, Athanasoulis C, Alavi A, et al with permission.

Table 27–3. GOOD QUALITY ANGIOGRAMS (n = 691)

		Reader #1			
		PE+	PE–	PE?	Total
Reader #2	PE+	246	23	3	272
	PE–	20	355	20	395
	PE?	5	18	1	24
	Total	271	396	24	691

PE+ = Pulmonary embolism present
PE– = Pulmonary embolism absent
PE? = Pulmonary embolism uncertain
Reproduced from Stein PD, Athanasoulis C, Alavi A, et al with permission.

Reader Agreement

Overall agreement on all three categories of interpretation (both readers agreed pulmonary embolism was present, pulmonary embolism was absent, or pulmonary embolism was uncertain) was 81% (Table 27–2) (12). Closer agreement was found on the presence of pulmonary embolism than on the absence of pulmonary embolism. Both agreed pulmonary embolism was present or both agreed that pulmonary embolism could not be diagnosed with certainty in 92%. Both readers agreed that PE was absent or both agreed that pulmonary embolism could not be excluded with certainty in 82%.

The quality of the angiograms had a greater impact upon the agreement on negativity than on positivity (Table 27–3, Table 27–4, Table 27–5) (12). Agreement on positivity with good-, fair-, and poor-quality angiograms was 93%, 90%, and 98%, respectively. Agreement on negativity was 88%, 77%, and 54%, respectively.

Readers agreed with each other more often on angiograms with emboli in lobar arteries than on angiograms in which the largest emboli were in segmental or subsegmental arteries. Average copositivity (average agreement of reader

Table 27–4. FAIR QUALITY ANGIOGRAMS (n = 355)

		Reader #1			
		PE+	PE–	PE?	Total
Reader #2	PE+	76	11	3	90
	PE–	15	181	25	221
	PE?	7	32	5	44
	Total	98	224	33	355

PE+ = Pulmonary embolism present
PE– = Pulmonary embolism absent
PE? = Pulmonary embolism uncertain
Reproduced from Stein and associates (12) with permission.

Table 27–5. POOR QUALITY ANGIOGRAMS (n = 46)

		Reader #1			
		PE+	PE–	PE?	Total
Reader #2	PE+	9	0	0	9
	PE–	1	8	13	22
	PE?	0	7	8	15
	Total	10	15	21	46

PE+ = Pulmonary embolism present
PE– = Pulmonary embolism absent
PE? = Pulmonary embolism uncertain
Reproduced from Stein and associates (12) with permission.

Table 27–6. BLINDED INTERPRETATIONS OF PULMONARY ANGIOGRAMS BY THE SAME READER ON TWO OCCASIONS

Second Interpretations	PE	First Interpretations No PE	Uncertain	Total
PE	14	2	0	16
No PE	1	49	0	50
Uncertain	2	3	1	6
Total	17	54	1	72

PE = pulmonary embolism
Unpublished data from PIOPED.

No. 1 with reader No. 2 and of reader No. 2 with reader No. 1) was 98% with lobar pulmonary embolism, 90% with segmental PE, and 66% with subsegmental PE.

Intra-Reader Comparison

Unpublished data from PIOPED showed that the same angiographer who reread a group of pulmonary angiograms agreed with himself in 64 of 72 (89%). This indicates good reproducibility (Cohen's Kappa = 0.74), but still indicates that there is imprecision in the gold standard (Table 27–6).

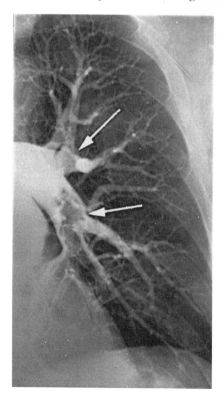

Figure 27–1. Pulmonary angiogram showing intraluminal filling defects (arrows) in left pulmonary artery and its branches.

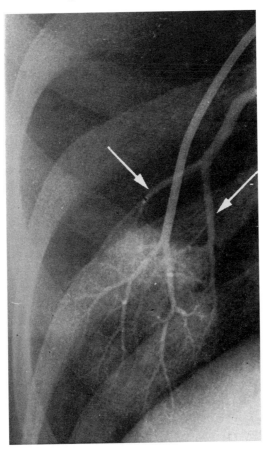

Figure 27–2.   Normal pulmonary wedge arteriogram. Vessels narrow gradually and show numerous fine branches. A background blush of capillary filling is shown. The two veins that drain this segment are also shown. Vessels 0.2 mm in diameter can be seen. The diameter of the catheter is 2.3 mm. (Reprinted with permission from Stein PD. Wedge arteriography for the identification of pulmonary emboli in small vessels. Am Heart J 1971;82:618–623.)

Techniques that Augment Standard Pulmonary Angiography

Techniques that augment standard pulmonary angiography might be employed to reduce the volume of contrast material needed and enhance the visualization of small pulmonary embolism in distal branches of the pulmonary artery. Such techniques include digital subtraction angiography (15–17), cineangiography (18), balloon-occlusion cineangiography (16, 19), and superselective angiography (20), including wedge arteriography (Fig. 27–1, Fig. 27–2, Fig. 27–3, Fig. 27–4, Fig. 27–5) (10,21). These methods might increase the diagnostic validity of angiograms in patients in whom pulmonary embolism is not apparent by standard techniques. These techniques are not routinely used, however, and some are technically difficult.

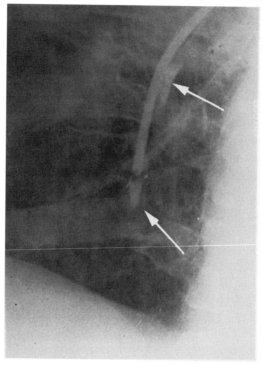

Figure 27–3. Wedge arteriogram showing a completely obstructed artery just distal to the catheter. The diameter of the occluded artery is approximately 2.0 mm. Contrast material has been forced in a retrograde direction because of the obstruction, and is seen along the side of the catheter. (Reprinted with permission from Stein PD. Wedge arteriography for the identification of pulmonary emboli in small vessels. Am Heart J 1971;82:618–623.)

Digital Subtraction Angiography

Digital subtraction angiography was evaluated during the injection of contrast material through a flow-directed balloon catheter (17). Selective or subselective pulmonary angiograms were obtained during the injection of 20 to 30 ml of iodinated contrast material at 10 to 15 ml/sec. Among 211 patients, image quality was excellent in 61.1%, adequate in 37.4% and poor in 1.4% The catheter employed was analogous to a Swan-Ganz catheter. Advantages were instant availability of images, relatively small amount of contrast material (average 65 ml), and a rapid examination, the average being 28 minutes. There were no important complications.

Computed Tomography

Contrast enhanced computed tomography may show pulmonary embolism, particularly in the lobar pulmonary arteries, although pulmonary embolism in segmental pulmonary arteries also has been identified (22). Pulmonary embo-

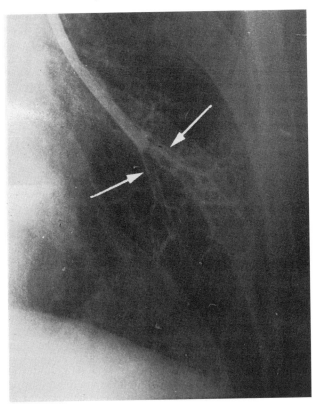

Figure 27–4.   Wedge arteriogram showing intraluminal filling defects in arteries 1.5 to 2.0 mm in diameter. (Reprinted with permission from Stein PD. Wedge arteriography for the identification of pulmonary emboli in small vessels. Am Heart J 1971;82:618–623.)

lism has been detected on rare occasions by contrast enhanced computed tomography in patients in whom the computed tomography was performed for other reasons (22).

The development of faster computed tomographic scanners and the use of well-timed intravenous injections using a contrast material injecter have shown that contrast enhanced computed tomography is a potentially effective noninvasive means of diagnosing pulmonary embolism. Contrast enhanced helical computed tomography with present technology, however, does not identify subsegmental pulmonary emboli as well as standard pulmonary angiography (23). Contrast enhanced helical computed tomography obtained during the peripheral injection of 140 ml of 30% iodinated contrast material at 4 ml/sec in patients with angiographically documented central pulmonary embolism showed the pulmonary embolism in central vessels in 6 of 7 (86%) (23). Two-dimensional multiplanar reformation of images obtained with contrast enhanced helical computed tomography in 35 patients improved the ability to exclude central pulmonary embolism, and it improved analysis of the extent of central pulmonary emboli (24). Pulmonary angiography, however, remains the study of choice (23).

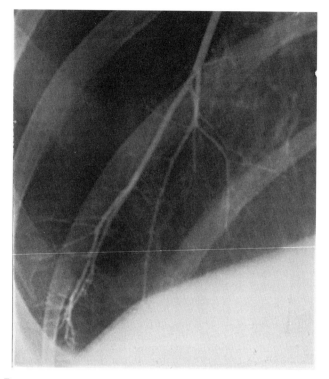

Figure 27–5. Wedge arteriogram in a patient with emphysema associated with alpha₁ antitrypsin deficiency showing diminished arborization of small arteries. (Reprinted with permission from Stein PD, Leu JD, Welch MH, et al. Patho-physiology of the pulmonary circulation in emphysema associated with alpha₁ antitrypsin deficiency. Circulation 1971:43:227–239.)

Contrast enhanced electron beam computed tomography showed pulmonary embolism in 19 of 20 (95%) patients with pulmonary embolism and showed no pulmonary embolism in 4 of 5 (80%) patients in whom pulmonary embolism was absent (25). More recently, some of these investigators showed pulmonary emolism in 15 of 23 (65%) patients with angiographically diagnosed pulmonary embolism, and contrast enhanced electron beam computed tomography was negative in 36 of 37 (97%) of patients in whom the pulmonary angiogram was negative (26). Scanning was performed after a bolus injection of 100 ml of iodinated contrast material at 1 ml/sec through an antecubital vein. Scanning required only 100 msec. This technique, therefore, seems to have potential, but has not replaced standard pulmonary angioigraphy.

Magnetic Resonance Imaging

Magnetic resonance pulmonary angiography for the detection of acute pulmonary embolism has been reported in only a few patients, but such imaging appears promising. Magnetic resonance imaging appears reliably to depict large and medium-size pulmonary embolism, regardless of infiltrates or effusion (27).

Magnetic resonance imaging enabled diagnosis of pulmonary embolism in 12 of 12 patients (100%) and enabled an exclusion of pulmonary embolism in 7 of 9 patients (78%) (27). In a study of 20 patients, magnetic resonance pulmonary angiography had a sensitivity of 92% with one reader and 100% with another (28). Specificity was 62% (28). Others showed a sensitivity of 85%, based on examination of 518 pulmonary arterial segments in eight patients (29). Pulmonary emboli larger than 1 cm in anteroposterior diameter were identified with >75% confidence.

REFERENCES

1. Jesser JH, de Takats G. Visualization of the pulmonary artery during its embolic obstruction. Arch Surg 1941;42:1034–1041.
2. Liberson F, Liberson IR. The use of Diodrast in determining the location and extent of pulmonary embolism: an experimental study. Am J Roetgenol 1942;48:352–355.
3. Lochhead RP, Roberts DJ Jr, Dotter CT. Pulmonary embolism, experimental and angiocardiographic study. Am J Roentgenol 1952;68:627–633.
4. Chrispin AR, Goodwin JR, Steiner RE. The radiology of obliterative pulmonary hypertension and thromboembolism. Brit J Radiol 1963;36:705–714.
5. Williams JR, Wilcox C, Andrews GJ, et al. Angiography in pulonary embolism. JAMA 1963;184:473–476.
6. Smith GT, Dammin GJ, Dexter L. Postmortem arteriographic studies of the human lung in pulmonary embolization. JAMA 1964;188:143–151.
7. Sasahara AA, Stein M, Simon M, et al. Pulmonary angiography in the diagnosis of thromboembolic disease. N Engl J Med 1964;270:1075–1081.
8. Dalen JE, Mathur VS, Evans H, et al. Pulmonary angiography in experimental pulmonary embolism. Am Heart J 1966;72:509–520.
9. Stein PD, O'Connor JF, Dalen JE, et al. The angiographic diagnosis of acute pulmonary embolism: evaluation of criteria. Am Heart J 1967;73:730–741.
10. Stein PD, Leu JD, Welch MH, et al. Pathophysiology of the pulmonary circulation in emphysema associated with alpha$_1$ antitrypsin deficiency. Circulation 1971;43:227–239.
11. Jacobson G, Turner AF, Balchum OJ, et al. Pulmonary arteriovenus shunts in emphysema demonstrated by wedge arteriography. Am J Roentgen 1965;93:868–878.
12. Stein PD, Athanasoulis C, Alavi A, et al. Complications and validity of pulmonary angiography in acute pulmonary embolism. Circulation 1992;85:462–469.
13. A Collaborative Study by the PIOPED Investigators. Value of the ventilation/perfusion scan in acute pulmonary embolism: results of the Prospective Investigation of Pulmonary Embolism Diagnosis (PIOPED). JAMA 1990;263:2753–2759.
14. Dalen JE, Brooks HL, Johnson LW, et al. Pulmonary angiography in acute pulmonary embolism: indications, techniques and results in 367 patients. Am Heart J 1971;81:175–185.
15. Goodman PC, Brant-Zawadzki M. Digital subtraction pulmonary angiography. Am J Roentgen 1982;139:305–309.
16. Ferris EJ, Holder JC, Lim WN, et al. Angiograpphy of pulmonary emboli: digital studies and balloon occlusion cineangiography. Am J Roentgen 1984;142:369–373.
17. van Rooij W-JJ, den Heeten GJ, Sluzewski M. Pulmonary embolism: diagnosis in 211 patients with use of selective pulmonary digital subtraction angiography with a flow- directed catheter. Radiology 1995;195:793–797.
18. Meister SG, Brooks HL, Szucs MM, et al. Pulmonary cineangiography in acute pulmonary embolism. Am Heart J 1972;84:33–37.
19. Wilson JE III, Bynum LJ. An improved pulmonary angiographic technique using a balloon-tipped catheter. Am Rev Resp Dis 1976;114:1137–1144.

20. Bookstein JJ. Segmental arteriography in pulmonary embolism. Radiology 1969;93:1007–1012.
21. Stein PD. Wedge arteriography for the identification of pulmonary emboli in small vessels. Am Heart J 1971;82:618–623.
22. Verschakelen JA, Vanwijck E, Bogaert J, et al. Detection of unsuspected central pulmonary embolism with conventional contrast-enhanced CT. Radiology 1993;188:847–850.
23. Goodman LR, Curtin JJ, Mewissen MW, et al. Detection of pulmonary embolism in patients with unresolved clinical and scintigraphic diagnosis: helical CT versus angiography. Am J Roentgen 1995;164:1369–1374.
24. Remy-Jardin M, Remy J, Cauvain O, et al. Diagnosis of central pulmonary embolism with helical CT: role of two-dimensional multiplanar reformations. Am J Roentgen 1995;165:1131–1138.
25. Teigen CL, Maus TP, Sheedy PF II, et al. Pulmonary embolism: diagnosis with electron-beam CT. Radiology 1993;188:839–845.
26. Teigen CL, Maus TP, Sheedy PF II, et al. Pulmonary embolism: diagnosis with contrast-enhanced electron-beam CT and comparison with pulmonary angiography. Radiology 1995;194:313–319.
27. Erdman WA, Peshock RM, Redman HC, et al. Pulmonary embolism: comparison of MR images with radionuclide and angiographic studies. Thorac Radiol 1994;190:499–508.
28. Grist TM, Sostman HD, MacFall JR, et al. Pulmonary angiography with MR imaging: preliminary clinical experience. Radiology 1993;189:523–530.
29. Schiebler ML, Holland GA, Hatabu H, et al. Suspected pulmonary embolism: prospective evaluation with pulmonary MR angiography. Radiology 1993;189:125–131.

Diagnosis in Particular Patient Populations

CHAPTER 28

Diagnosis in Patients with Chronic Obstructive Pulmonary Disease

The presentation of pulmonary embolism and an exacerbation of chronic obstructive pulmonary disease (COPD) often mimic each other so closely that they cannot be distinguished clinically from each other. This may result in either an overdiagnosis or an underdiagnosis of pulmonary embolism. In patients with COPD in whom pulmonary embolism was suspected, 19% had documented pulmonary embolism (1). In patients without cardiopulmonary disease in whom pulmonary embolism was suspected, 32% had documented pulmonary embolism (2). This difference reflects the difficulty of differentiating pulmonary embolism from an exacerbation of COPD.

Lippmann and Fein suggested that the diagnosis of pulmonary embolism should be suspected in patients with COPD who have precipitous worsening of their dyspnea that is unresponsive to bronchodilator therapy (3). The diagnosis is supported by a reduction of the $PaCO_2$ in a previously hypercapnic patient (3). In PIOPED, the data did not indicate whether dyspnea was worsening (4).

Comparison of Patients with COPD Who Had Pulmonary Embolism and Patients with COPD and No Pulmonary Embolism

Among 108 patients with COPD suspected of having pulmonary embolism, wheezing was less frequent in patients with pulmonary embolism and rales were more frequent in patients with pulmonary embolism (1). The predisposing factors, symptoms, other signs, chest radiographic findings, and blood gases did not differ to a statistically significant extent between patients with pulmonary embolism and patients who did not have pulmonary embolism (1).

In patients with COPD in the Prospective Investigation of Pulmonary Embolism Diagnosis (PIOPED), no difference was noted between the alveolar-arterial

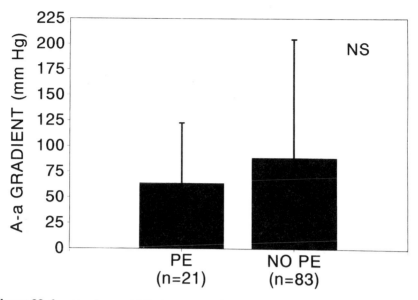

Figure 28–1. Alveolar-arterial (A-a) oxygen gradient among patients with pulmonary embolism (PE) and patients in whom pulmonary embolism was excluded (NO PE). The difference was not statistically significant (NS). N is the number of patients. (Reprinted with permission from Lesser BA, Leeper KV, Stein PD, et al. The diagnosis of pulmonary embolism in patients with chronic obstructive pulmonary disease. Chest 1992;102:17–22.)

oxygen differences (gradients) in patients with pulmonary embolism and patients with no pulmonary embolism (Fig. 28–1) (1).

In patients with COPD, a reduction of the $PaCO_2$ in a previously hypercapneic patient has been reported (3). An elevation of the $PaCO_2$ in association with pulmonary embolism also has been reported (5). The latter may reflect an inability to further increase minute ventilation in the face of a sudden increase in dead space imposed by the pulmonary embolism (6). We observed no difference of the average $PaCO_2$ in patients with pulmonary embolism and patients in whom pulmonary embolism was excluded (Fig. 28–2) (1). We also observed no change of the average $PaCO_2$ from values before the pulmonary embolism in patients with COPD (Fig. 28–3) (1). However, we saw only a small number of patients with prior measurements of the $PaCO_2$, and most of our patients were not previously hypercapnic to the extent reported by Lippman and Fein (1, 3).

Patients with COPD Compared with Patients with No Prior Cardiopulmonary Disease

The predisposing factors for pulmonary embolism in patients with COPD, compared with patients with no prior cardiopulmonary disease, are shown in Table 28–1. No statistically significant differences were noted (1,7).

The presenting syndromes of patients with COPD who had pulmonary embolism were of comparable frequency as observed in patients with no prior cardiopulmonary disease who had pulmonary embolism (Table 28–2) (1,7).

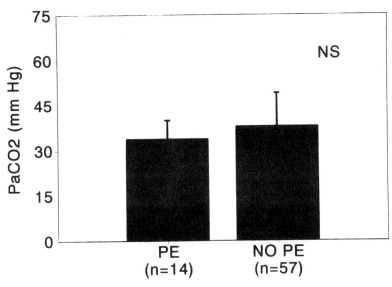

Figure 28–2.   Partial pressure of carbon dioxide in arterial blood ($PaCO_2$) while breathing room air in patients with pulmonary embolism (PE) and in patients in whom pulmonary embolism was excluded (NO PE). The difference was not statistically significant (NS). N is the number of patients. (Reprinted with permission from Lesser BA, Leeper KV, Stein PD, et al. The diagnosis of pulmonary embolism in patients with chronic obstructive pulmonary disease. Chest 1992;102:17–22.)

The symptoms of patients with COPD who had pulmonary embolism differed from patients with pulmonary embolism who had no prior cardiopulmonary disease in regard to pleuritic pain (less frequent in patients with pulmonary embolism who had COPD), cough (more frequent in patients with COPD who had pulmonary embolism), and wheezing (more frequent in patients with COPD who had pulmonary embolism) (Table 28–3) (1,7). Regarding signs, rales were also more frequent in patients with COPD who had pulmonary embolism than in patients with no prior cardiopulmonary disease who had pulmonary embolism (Table 28–4) (1,7). Whether any of these differences are meaningful is uncertain because of the possibility of a chance occurrence of a difference when large numbers of variables are tested. Cough was probably a manifestation of the COPD. The inability to hear an accentuated pulmonary component of the second sound reflects the difficulty of cardiac auscultation in patients with COPD.

Abnormalities of the plain chest radiograph in patients with COPD who had pulmonary embolism were comparable with those in patients with no prior cardiopulmonary disease who had pulmonary embolism (Table 28–5) (1,7).

Although the numbers are small, physicians, when confident of their clinical assessment of patients with COPD, were usually correct, both in making and excluding the diagnosis of pulmonary embolism (Table 28–6) (1).

The majority (60%) of ventilation-perfusion scans in patients with COPD, interpreted on the basis of the original PIOPED criteria (4), were interpreted as intermediate (indeterminate) probability for pulmonary embolism (Fig. 28–4). Only 5% of patients with COPD had high probability interpretations of the ventilation-perfusion scans, and only 5% with COPD were interpreted as near

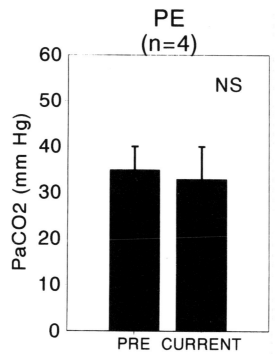

Figure 28–3. Partial pressure of carbon dioxide in arterial blood ($PaCO_2$) while breathing room air in 4 patients with pulmonary embolism (PE) who had prior assessments and measurements at the time of the PE. The difference was not statistically significant (NS). (Modified and reprinted with permission from Lesser BA, Leeper KV Jr, Stein PD, et al. The diagnosis of pulmonary embolism in patients with chronic obstructive pulmonary disease. Chest 1992;102:17–22.)

normal/normal (Table 28–7) (1). A ventilation-perfusion scan interpretation of low probability was made in 31% of patients with COPD (Fig. 28–5).

The cause of the perfusion defect, at least in patients with alpha$_1$ antitrypsin deficiency, is an absence of fine branching of the distal pulmonary arteries and a loss of the capillary bed (8). This is shown on pulmonary angiograms and wedge arteriograms as a sparsity of arborization and diminished or absent capillary filling (Fig. 28–6, Fig. 27–4). Normal arborization and capillary filling are shown in Figure 27–1.

The distribution of ventilation-perfusion scan probabilities in patients with COPD differed from patients with no prior cardiac or pulmonary disease. The distribution of ventilation-perfusion scan probabilities in patients COPD also differed from patients with any prior cardiac or pulmonary disease (Table 28–8, Fig. 28–7). Intermediate probability ventilation-perfusion scans among patients with no prior cardiac or pulmonary disease, any prior cardiac or pulmonary disease, or COPD occurred in 33%, 43%, and 60%, respectively (1,2). Fewer patients with COPD had high probability scans or near normal/normal ventilation-perfusion scans compared with patients with no cardiac or pulmonary disease. The frequency of high probability, intermediate probability and near normal/normal ventilation-perfusion scans in patients with any cardiac or

Table 28–1. PREDISPOSING FACTORS IN PATIENTS WITH PULMONARY EMBOLISM WHO HAD COPD AND IN PATIENTS WITH PULMONARY EMBOLISM WHO HAD NO PRIOR CARDIOPULMONARY DISEASE

	COPD (n = 21) Percent	No Prior Cardiopulm Dis (n = 117) Percent
Immobilization	43	56
Surgery	33	54
Malignancy	10	23
Thrombophlebitis, ever	14	14
Trauma—lower extremities	5	10
Estrogen	0	9
Stroke	1	7
Postpartum ≤ 3 mos.	0	4

Differences between patients with COPD and patients with no prior cardiopulmonary disease were not statistically significant.
COPD = chronic obstructive pulmonary disease
Cardiopulm Dis = cardiopulmonary disease
Data from Lesser and associates (1) and Stein and associates (7).

Table 28–2. SYNDROMES OF PULMONARY EMBOLISM IN PATIENTS WHO HAD COPD AND IN PATIENTS WHO HAD NO PRIOR CARDIOPULMONARY DISEASE

	COPD (n = 21) Percent	No Prior Cardiopulm Dis (n = 117) Percent
Pleuritic pain or hemoptysis (in absence of circulatory collapse)	57	65
Isolated dyspnea (in absence of hemoptysis, pleuritic pain, shock, or loss of consciousness)	38	22
Circulatory collapse (shock or loss of consciousness)	5	8

Differences between patients with COPD and patients with no prior cardiopulmonary disease were not statistically significant.
Shock = systolic pressure < 80 mm Hg
COPD = chronic obstructive pulmonary disease
Cardiopulm Dis = cardiopulmonary disease
Data from Lesser and associates (1) and Stein and associates (7).

Table 28–3. SYMPTOMS IN PATIENTS WITH PULMONARY EMBOLISM
WHO HAD COPD AND IN PATIENTS WITH PULMONARY
EMBOLISM WHO HAD NO PRIOR CARDIOPULMONARY
DISEASE

	COPD (n = 21) Percent	No Prior Cardiopulm Dis (n = 117) Percent
Dyspnea	90	73
Pleuritic pain	43	66*
Cough	62	37*
Leg swelling	43	28
Leg pain	19	26
Hemoptysis	19	13
Palpitations	10	10
Wheezing	39	9**
Angina-like pain	0	4

COPD = chronic obstructive pulmonary disease
Cardiopulm Dis = cardiopulmonary disease
* P < 0.05, **P < 0.001 COPD vs no prior cardiopulmonary disease
Data from Lesser and associates (1) and Stein and associates (7).

pulmonary disease was intermediate between those with no cardiopulmonary disease and those with COPD. (Patients with COPD were included among the patients with any prior cardiac or pulmonary disease.)

The decreased percent of high probability interpretations of ventilation-perfusion scans and of near normal/normal interpretations of ventilation-perfusion scans among patients with COPD compared with patients with no cardiopulmonary disease reflected the effect of abnormalities of airflow obstruction and lung parenchymal destruction on the distribution of radioisotope in both the ventilation and perfusion lung scans. As might be expected, no patient with moderate or severe airflow obstruction had a near normal/normal scan (1).

Each of the five patients with high probability ventilation-perfusion scans had pulmonary embolism (1). None of the five patients with near normal/normal ventilation-perfusion scans had pulmonary embolism. Alderson and associates, in patients with COPD, found pulmonary embolism in 86% of patients with high probability ventilation-perfusion scans (9). The positive predictive value of high and low probability ventilation-perfusion scans was similar in their study and our study (1). Among patients with COPD, the positive predictive value of high probability, low probability, and near normal/normal ventilation-perfusion scans was as accurate as among patients with no prior cardiopulmo-

Table 28–4. SIGNS IN PATIENTS WITH PULMONARY EMBOLISM WHO
HAD COPD AND IN PATIENTS WITH PULMONARY
EMBOLISM WHO HAD NO PRIOR CARDIOPULMONARY
DISEASE

	COPD (n = 21) Percent	No Prior Cardiopulm Dis (n = 117) Percent
Tachypnea (≥20/min)	71	70
Rales (crackles)	81	51*
Tachycardia (>100/min)	33	30
Increased pulmonary component of second sound	0	23*
Deep venous thrombosis	10	11
Diaphoresis	5	11
Temp >38.5°C	5	7
Wheezes	10	5
Homans' sign	0	4
Pleural friction rub	0	3
Third heart sound	10	3
Cyanosis	5	1

Data from Lesser and associates (1) and Stein and associates (7).
COPD = chronic obstructive pulmonary disease.
Cardiopulm Dis = cardiopulmonary disease
* P < 0.02 COPD vs No prior cardiopulmonary disease

nary disease (Table 28–7) (1). However, the frequency of high probability and near normal/normal ventilation-perfusion scans was dramatically decreased in patients with COPD.

The combination of a low probability clinical assessment and a low probability ventilation-perfusion scan occurred in 10% of patients with COPD (1) and in 10% of the general population of patients with suspected pulmonary embolism (4). None of the patients with COPD who had a low likelihood clinical assessment and a concordantly low probability ventilation-perfusion scan had pulmonary embolism (1). In the population of general hospital patients, 4% of patients with a concordant low likelihood clinical assessment and low probability ventilation-perfusion scans had pulmonary embolism (4).

The value of ventilation-perfusion scans in patients with COPD is diminished because the frequency of scan readings that clinicians rely on most heavily in making a ventilation-perfusion scan diagnosis (high probability and near normal/normal) is dramatically reduced in patients with COPD. Nevertheless,

Table 28–5.   PLAIN CHEST RADIOGRAPH IN PATIENTS WITH
PULMONARY EMBOLISM WHO HAD COPD AND IN
PATIENTS WITH PULMONARY EMBOLISM WHO HAD NO
PRIOR CARDIOPULMONARY DISEASE

	COPD (n = 21) Percent	No Prior Cardiopulm Dis (n = 117) Percent
Atelectasis or pulmonary parenchymal abnormality	76	68
Pleural effusion	52	48
Pleural based opacity	33	35
Elevated diaphragm	14	24
Decreased pulmonary vascularity	38	21
Prominent central pulmonary artery	29	15
Cardiomegaly	19	12
Westermark's sign	5	7
Pulmonary edema	14	4

Westermark's sign = prominent central pulmonary artery and decreased pulmonary vascularity
COPD = chronic obstructive pulmonary disease
Cardiopulm Dis = cardiopulmonary disease
Differences between COPD vs No prior cardiopulmonary disease were not statistically significant.
Data from Stein and associates (7) and unpublished data from PIOPED. Interpretations of the chest radiographs in patients with COPD are PIOPED readings and differ somewhat from the re-interpreted readings reported by Lesser and associates (1).

Table 28–6. CLINICAL ASSESSMENT IN PATIENTS WHO HAD COPD AND IN PATIENTS WHO HAD NO PRIOR CARDIOPULMONARY DISEASE

Clinical Assessment	Pulmonary Embolism COPD PE/n (%)	Pulmonary Embolism No Prior Cardiopulm Dis PE/n (%)
High probability	3/3 (100)	15/17 (88)
Intermediate probability	67/100 (67)	74/200 (37)*
Low probability	1/30 (3)	14/103 (14)

All assessment were by senior staff.
PE = pulmonary embolism
n = number of patients
COPD = chronic obstructive pulmonary disease
Cardioplum Dis = cardiopulmonary disease
* P < 0.001 COPD vs No prior cardiopulmonary disease
Data are from Lesser and associates (1) and Stein and associates (7).

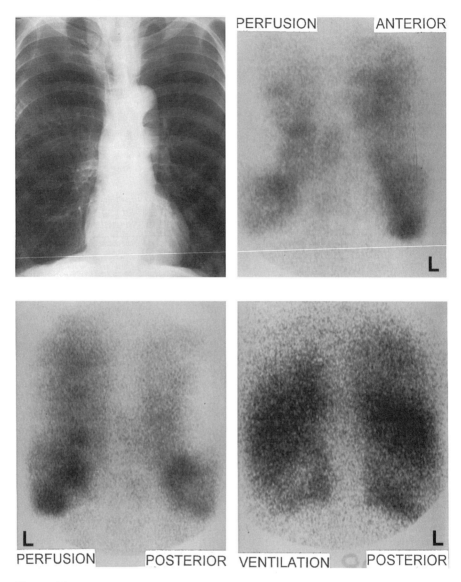

Figure 28–4. **Top left.** Plain chest radiograph in patient with chronic obstructive pulmonary disease showing no parenchymal abnormality. **Top right.** Perfusion lung scan, anterior view, showing widespread perfusion abnormalities. **Bottom left.** Perfusion scan, posterior view, showing widespread perfusion abnormalities. **Bottom right.** Ventilation scan, posterior view, showing uneven washout at 60 to 90 seconds. The ventilation-perfusion lung scan was interpreted as intermediate probability for acute pulmonary embolism, according to the original PIOPED criteria, which was also in accordance with the revised PIOPED criteria. This difficult study becomes easy if interpreted in separate portions. The right mid-lung shows a triple match associated with ventilation, perfusion, and chest radiographic abnormalities in the same region. A triple match in a middle lung zone is associated with a very low probability of pulmonary emoblism (Chapter 20). The remainder of the lung shows multiple and widespread matched ventilation-perfusion defects in regions where the chest regiograph is clear. Matched ventilation-perfusion defects in 2 or 3 zones of a single lung in the presence of a regionally normal chest radiograph are also associated with a very low probability of pulmonary embolism (Chapter 18). A pulmonary angiogram was negative in this patient.

Table 28–7.   VENTILATION-PERFUSION LUNG SCANS IN PATIENTS WHO
HAD COPD AND IN PATIENTS WHO HAD NO PRIOR
CARDIOPULMONARY DISEASE

V/Q Scan Probability	COPD PE/ Total (%)	No Prior Cardiopulm Dis PE/Total (%)
High	5/5 (100)	50/54 (93)
Intermediate	14/65 (22)	47/119 (39)*
Low	2/33 (6)	17/113 (15)
Near normal/normal	0/5 (0)	3/79 (4)

COPD = chronic obstructive pulmonary disease
Cardiopulm Dis = cardiopulmonary disease
* P < 0.02 COPD vs No prior cardiopulmonary disease
Data are from Lesser and associates (1) and Stein and associates (2).

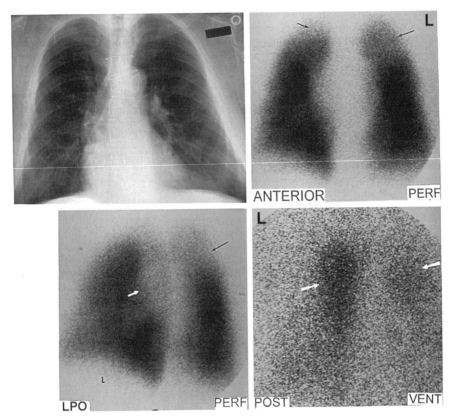

Figure 28–5. **Top left.** Plain chest radiograph in patient with chronic obstructive pulmonary disease showing no parenchymal abnormality. **Top right.** Perfusion (PERF) lung scan, anterior view, showing perfusion defects in the upper lobes, larger on the left. **Bottom left.** Perfusion scan, left posterior oblique (LPO) position, showing a larger perfusion defect in left upper lobe (white arrow) and a smaller perfusion defect in right upper lobe (black arrow). **Bottom right.** Ventilation (VENT) scan during washout phase, posterior view, showing air trapping, more extensive in the left lung. The ventilation-perfusion scan was interpreted as low probability for pulmonary embolism on the basis of matched ventilation-perfusion defects in 2 zones. A pulmonary angiogram was negative.

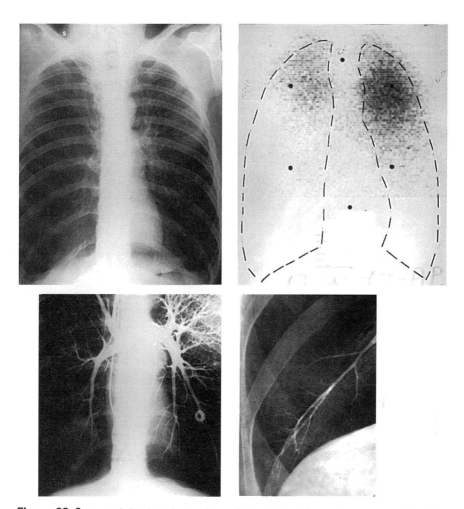

Figure 28–6. **Top left.** Plain chest radiograph in patient with emphysema caused by alpha$_1$ antitrypsin deficiency. The lower zones show hypovascularity. **Top right.** Perfusion lung scan, anterior view, showing perfusion only in the left upper lobe. **Bottom left.** Pulmonary angiogram showing a diminished number of branches in the lower lobe pulmonary arteries. Capillary hypoperfusion in the lower zones is shown, and was confirmed on later films. **Bottom right.** Wedge arteriogram in right lower lobe showing diminished arborization and capillary filling. This becomes apparent when compared with normal arborization and capillary filling, shown in Figure 27–2.(Reprinted with permission from Stein PD, Leu JD, Welch MH, et al. Pathophysiology of the pulmonary circulation in emphysema associated with alpha$_1$ antitrypsin deficiency. Circulation 1971;43:227–239.)

Table 28–8. DISTRIBUTION OF INTERPRETATION OF VENTILATION-
PERFUSION LUNG SCANS IN PATIENTS WITH NO PRIOR
CARDIOPULMONARY DISEASE, ANY PRIOR
CARDIOPULMONARY DISEASE, AND COPD

V/Q Probability	No CPD (n = 365) Percent of V/Q Scans	Any CPD (n = 526) Percent of V/Q Scans	COPD (n = 108) Percent of V/Q Scans
High	15	13	5
Intermediate	33	43	60
Low	31	35	31
Near normal/normal	22	10	5

COPD = chronic obstructive pulmonary disease
CPD = cardiopulmonary disease
V/Q = ventilation-perfusion
High prob V/Q scans were more frequent in NO CPD vs COPD (P < .01)
Intermediate prob V/Q scans were more frequent in COPD vs NO CPD (P < .001) and in COPD vs ANY CPD
(P < .01). Intermediate prob V/Q scans were also more frequent in ANY CPD vs NO CPD (P < .01)
Near normal/normal V/Q scans were frequent in NO CPD vs ANY CPD (P < .001) and in NO CPD vs COPD
(P < .001).
Modified and reproduced from Lesser BA, Leeper KV Jr., Stein PD, et al with permission.

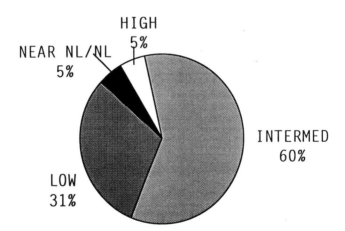

Figure 28–7. Distribution of interpretations of ventilation-perfusion lung scans using original
PIOPED criteria in patients with chronic obstructive pulmonary disease (COPD). Only 5% of patients
had high probability interpretations. NL = normal, Intermed = intermediate

in 19% of patients with COPD, the ventilation-perfusion scan was either high probability or near normal/normal or there was a concordant low probability ventilation-perfusion scan with a low probability clinical assessment, which allowed a satisfactory noninvasive diagnosis (1).

REFERENCES

1. Lesser BA, Leeper KV Jr., Stein PD, et al. The diagnosis of pulmonary embolism in patients with chronic obstructive pulmonary disease. Chest 1992;102:17–22.
2. Stein PD, Coleman RE, Gottschalk A, et al. Diagnostic utility of ventilation-perfusion lung scans in acute pulmonary embolism is not diminished by pre-existing cardiac or pulmonary disease. Chest 1991;100:604–606.
3. Lippmann M, Fein A. Pulmonary embolism in the patient with chronic obstructive pulmonary disease: a diagnostic dilemma. Chest 1981;79:39–42.
4. A Collaborative Study by the PIOPED Investigators. Value of the ventilation-perfusion scan in acute pulmonary embolism: results of the Prospective Investigation of Pulmonary Embolism Diagnosis (PIOPED). JAMA 1990;263:2753–2759.
5. Bouchama A, Curley W, Al-Dossary S, et al. Refractory hypercapnia complicating massive pulmonary embolism. Am Rev Resp Dis 1988;138:466–468.
6. D'Alonzo GE, Bower JS, DeHart P, et al. The mechanisms of abnormal gas exchange in acute massive pulmonary embolism. Am Rev Respir Dis 1983;128:170–172.
7. Stein PD, Terrin ML, Hales CA, et al. Clinical, laboratory, roentgenographic, and electrocardiographic findings inpatients with acute pulmonary embolism and no pre-existingcardiac or pulmonary disease. Chest 1991;100:598–603.
8. Stein PD, Leu JD, Welch MH, et al. Pathophysiology of the pulmonary circulation in emphysema associated with alpha$_1$ antitrypsin deficiency. Circulation 1971;43:227–239.
9. Alderson PO, Biello DR, Sachariah G, et al. Scintigraphic detection of pulmonary embolism in patients with obstructive pulmonary disease. Radiology 1981;138:661–666.

CHAPTER 29

Clinical Assessment and Ventilation-Perfusion Lung Scans in the Critically Ill

Autopsy studies have consistently shown that pulmonary embolism is frequently not considered antemortem in patients who died from pulmonary embolism (Chapter 1). It is apparent, therefore, that the clinical diagnosis of pulmonary embolism in critically ill patients is difficult. We assessed the clinical characteristics and ventilation-perfusion lung scans in several categories of critically ill patients in order to identify features that may alert physicians to the diagnosis.

Clinical Characteristics of Patients with Acute Pulmonary Embolism Who Had Loss of Consciousness

Among patients with acute pulmonary embolism who suffered loss of consciousness on the day of entry into the Prospective Investigation of Pulmonary Embolism Diagnosis (PIOPED), dyspnea or tachypnea were not universally present (Table 29–1, Table 29–2) (Stein PD, Relyea B. Unpublished data from PIOPED). The data are sparse, however. Among seven such patients, dyspnea or tachypnea, (respiratory rate ≥ 20/min) were present in only 71%, and dyspnea, tachypnea or pleuritic pain also were present in only 71%. Dyspnea, tachypnea, radiographic evidence of atelectasis, or a parenchymal abnormality was present in 86%. The PaO_2 on room air was low in all patients (Table 29–2). The chest radiograph occasionally showed cardiomegaly even in the absence of prior cardiopulmonary disease (Table 29–3). Radiographic findings generally associated with acute pulmonary embolism patients were usually absent (Table 29–3). Rhythm disturbances were rare (Table 29–4). The most frequent electrocardiographic findings were nonspecific ST segment and T wave changes.

Physicians were uncertain of the diagnosis based on clinical assessment or thought the likelihood of pulmonary embolism was low in 71% (Table 29–1).

Table 29–1. SYMPTOMS, COMBINATIONS OF SYMPTOMS AND SIGNS, AND LIKELIHOOD OF PULMONARY EMBOLISM BASED ON CLINICAL ASSESSMENT IN PATIENTS WITH ACUTE PULMONARY EMBOLISM AND LOSS OF CONSCIOUSNESS ON DAY OF STUDY

	All Patients (n = 7) Number (%)	No Prior Cardiopulm Dis (n = 5) Number (%)
Individual symptoms		
Dyspnea	4 (57)	2 (40)
Pleuritic pain	0 (0)	0 (0)
Cough	3 (43)	2 (40)
Leg swelling	3 (43)	2 (40)
Leg pain	2 (29)	2 (40)
Hemoptysis	0 (0)	0 (0)
Palpitations	0 (0)	0 (0)
Wheezing	2 (29)	1 (20)
Angina-like pain	0 (0)	0 (0)
Combination of symptoms and signs		
Dyspnea or tachypnea	5 (71)	3 (60)
Dyspnea or tachypnea or pleuritic pain	5 (71)	3 (60)
Dyspnea, tachypnea, or x-ray atelectasis/parenchymal	6 (86)	4 (80)
Likelihood of pulmonary embolism based on clinical assessment		
0–19% probability	1 (14)	0 (0)
20–79% probability	4 (57)	4 (80)
80–100% probability	2 (29)	1 (20)

Stein PD and Relyea B unpublished data from PIOPED. Tachypnea = respiratory rate ≥ 20/min.

Ventilatory Support, Intensive Care Units, Hypoxemic Not on Ventilatory Support

The clinical diagnosis of acute pulmonary embolism in an intensive care unit is generally considered exceedingly difficult (1). Even the ability to obtain a technically sound ventilation lung scan in patients who are on ventilatory support is difficult (2). Some, however, have succeeded in obtaining inhalation radioaerosol lung scans of excellent quality in such patients (3). Data from PIOPED showed that clinical assessment and ventilation-perfusion lung scans (or perfusion scans alone in patients on ventilatory support) are as accurate as in non-critically ill patients (4).

Clinical Assessment

A clinical assessment of the likelihood of pulmonary embolism was based on bedside evaluation, the plain chest radiograph, electrocardiogram, and ordi-

Table 29–2. SIGNS IN PATIENTS WITH ACUTE PULMONARY EMBOLISM
AND LOSS OF CONSCIOUSNESS ON DAY OF STUDY ENTRY

	All Patients (n = 7) Number (%)	No Prior Cardiopulm Dis (n = 5) Number (%)
Tachypnea (≥20/min)	3 (43)	2 (40)
Rales (Crackles)	3 (43)	1 (20)
Tachycardia (>100/min)	4 (57)	3 (60)
Increased pulm component of second sound	0 (0)	0 (0)
Diaphoresis	1 (14)	1 (20)
Temperature >38.5°C	0 (0)	0 (0)
Wheezes	1 (14)	0 (0)
Homans' sign	1 (14)	1 (20)
Right ventricular lift	0 (0)	0 (0)
Pleural friction rub	0 (0)	0 (0)
Third heart sound	0 (0)	0 (0)
Cyanosis	0 (0)	0 (0)
PaO_2 < 62 mm Hg (room air)	6 (100)*	5 (100)*

* Partial pressure of oxygen in arterial blood (P_aO_2) was not measured in 1 patient.
Pulm = pulmonary
Stein PD and Relyea B unpublished data from PIOPED.

Table 29–3. PLAIN CHEST RADIOGRAPH IN PATIENTS WITH ACUTE
PULMONARY EMBOLISM AND LOSS OF CONSCIOUSNESS
ON DAY OF STUDY ENTRY

	All Patients (n = 7) Number (%)	No Prior Cardiopulm Dis (n = 5) Number (%)
Normal chest radiograph	2 (29)	2 (40)
Atelectasis or parenchymal abnormality	1 (14)	1 (20)
Pleural effusion	1 (14)	0 (0)
Pleural based opacity	1 (14)	0 (0)
Elevated hemidiaphragm	2 (29)	1 (20)
Decreased pulmonary vascularity	2 (29)	0 (0)
Prominent central pulmonary artery	2 (29)	0 (0)
Cardiomegaly	3 (43)	2 (40)
Westermark's sign***	0 (0)	0 (0)
Pulmonary edema	0 (0)	0 (0)

*** Prominent central pulmonary artery and decreased pulmonary vascularity
Stein PD and Relyea B unpublished data from PIOPED.

Table 29–4.   ELECTROCARDIOGRAM IN PATIENTS WITH ACUTE
PULMONARY AND LOSS OF CONSCIOUSNESS ON DAY OF
STUDY ENTRY

	All Patients (n = 7) Number (%)	No Prior Cardiopulm Dis (n = 5) Number (%)
Normal electrocardiogram	1 (14)	1 (20)
Rhythm disturbances		
Atrial flutter	0 (0)	0 (0)
Atrial fibrillation	0 (0)	0 (0)
Atrial premature contractions	1 (14)	1 (20)
Ventricular premature contractions	0 (0)	0 (0)
P Wave		
P pulmonale	1 (14)	1 (20)
QRS abnormalities		
Incomplete RBBB	0 (0)	0 (0)
Complete RBBB	2 (29)	2 (40)
Right ventricular hypertrophy	0 (0)	0 (0)
Pseudoinfarction	0 (0)	0 (0)
Low voltage (frontal plane)	1 (14)	1 (20)
ST segment and T wave		
Nonspecific T wave	3 (43)	3 (60)
ST segment elevation	0 (0)	0 (0)
Nonspecific ST segment or T wave	3 (43)	3 (60)

Some patients had more than one abnormality.
Cardiopulm Dis = cardiopulmonary disease
RBBB = right bundle branch block
Stein PD and Relyea B unpublished data from PIOPED.

nary laboratory tests (5). Physicians were uncertain whether pulmonary embolism was present in 67% to 78% of critically ill patients (4). In non-critically ill patients, physicians were uncertain whether pulmonary embolism was present in 67%. In patients on ventilatory support, patients in intensive care units not on ventilatory support, and hypoxemic patients not on ventilatory support, when physicians assessed an 80 to 100% likelihood of pulmonary embolism, 75 to 88% of patients, in fact, had pulmonary embolism (Table 29–5. Table 29–6, Table 29–7) (4). This was comparable to the positive predictive value in non-critically ill patients (77%) (Table 29–8). In only a few critically ill patients were physicians confident enough to make a high likelihood clinical assessment. A high likelihood clinical assessment was made in only 9% of critically ill patients. However, the fraction of non-critically ill patients with a high likelihood clinical assessment was comparable, 8%. If physicians assessed a 0 to 19% clinical likelihood of pulmonary embolism in these critically ill patients, only 0 to 5% had pulmonary embolism. The number of critically ill patients with a low likelihood clinical assessment was also small. The frequency of pulmonary

Table 29–5. POSITIVE PREDICTIVE VALUE OF LUNG SCAN INTERPRETATION AND CLINICAL ASSESSMENT IN PATIENTS ON VENTILATORY SUPPORT

V/Q Scan	Clinical Probability			Total PE+/Test+ (%)
	Clin Prob 80–100% PE+/Test+ (%)	Clin Prob 20–79% PE+/Test+ (%)	Clin Prob 0–19% PE+/Test+ (%)	
High	2/2 (100)	2/2 (100)	0/0 (—)	4/4 (100)
Intermediate	1/1 (100)	5/16 (31)	0/7 (0)	6/24 (25)
Low	0/1 (0)	2/13 (15)	0/3 (0)	2/17 (12)
Near normal/normal	0/0 (—)	0/0 (—)	0/1 (0)	0/1 (0)
Total	3/4 (75)	9/31 (29)	0/11 (0)	12/46 (26)

Clin Prob = clinical probability
Reproduced from Henry JW, Stein PD, Gottschalk A, Relyea B, Leeper KV Jr with permission.

Table 29-6. POSITIVE PREDICTIVE VALUE OF VENTILATION/PERFUSION LUNG SCAN INTERPRETATION AND CLINICAL ASSESSMENT IN PATIENTS IN INTENSIVE CARE UNITS WHO WERE NOT ON VENTILATORY SUPPORT

V/Q Scan	Clinical Probability			Total PE+/Test+ (%)
	Clin Prob 80–100% PE+/Test+ (%)	Clin Prob 20–79% PE+/Test+ (%)	Clin Prob 0–19% PE+/Test+ (%)	
High	2/2 (100)	6/6 (100)	0/1 (0)	8/9 (89)
Intermediate	4/5 (80)	14/34 (41)	0/3 (0)	18/42 (43)
Low	1/1 (100)	4/22 (18)	0/7 (0)	5/30 (17)
Near normal/normal	0/0 (—)	0/4 (0)	0/0 (—)	0/4 (0)
Total	7/8 (88)	24/66 (36)	0/11 (0)	31/85 (36)

Clin Prob = clinical probability
Reproduced from Henry JW, Stein PD, Gottschalk A, Relyea B, Leeper KV Jr with permission.

237

Table 29-7. POSITIVE PREDICTIVE VALUE OF VENTILATION/PERFUSION LUNG SCAN INTERPRETATION AND CLINICAL ASSESSMENT IN HYPOXEMIC PATIENTS NOT ON VENTILATORY SUPPORT

V/Q Scan	Clin Prob 80–100% PE+/Test+ (%)	Clinical Probability Clin Prob 20–79% PE+/Test+ (%)	Clin Prob 0–19% PE+/Test+ (%)	Total PE+/Test+ (%)
High	6/6 (100)	11/13 (85)	0/0 (—)	17/19 (89)
Intermediate	0/0 (—)	6/29 (21)	0/13 (0)	6/42 (14)*
Low	0/0 (—)	3/18 (17)	1/6 (17)	4/24 (17)
Near normal/normal	0/2 (0)	0/1 (0)	0/1 (0)	0/4 (0)
Total	6/8 (75)	20/61 (33)	1/20 (5)	27/89 (30)

* P < .01 hypoxemic vs non-critically ill patients (see Table 29–8)
Clin Prob = clinical probability
Reproduced from Henry JW, Stein PD, Gottschalk A, Relyea B, Leeper KV Jr with permission.

Table 29-8. POSITIVE PREDICTIVE VALUE OF VENTILATION/PERFUSION LUNG SCAN INTERPRETATION AND CLINICAL ASSESSMENT IN PATIENTS WHO WERE NOT CRITICALLY ILL

V/Q Scan	Clinical Probability			Total PE+/Test+ (%)
	Clin Prob 80–100% PE+/Test+ (%)	Clin Prob 20–79% PE+/Test+ (%)	Clin Prob 0–19% PE+/Test+ (%)	
High	13/14 (93)	69/81 (85)	5/7 (71)	87/102 (85)
Intermediate	22/29 (76)	60/177 (34)	14/66 (21)	96/272 (35)
Low	4/8 (50)	29/122 (24)	4/62 (6)	37/192 (19)
Near normal/normal	1/1 (100)	5/38 (13)	1/22 (5)	7/61 (11)
Total	40/52 (77)	163/418 (39)	24/157 (15)	227/627 (36)

Clin Prob = clinical probability
Reproduced from Henry JW, Stein PD, Gottschalk A, Relyea B, Leeper KV Jr with permission.

239

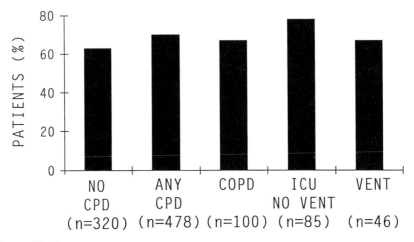

PERCENT OF PATIENTS WITH UNCERTAIN CLINICAL LIKELIHOOD OF PE

Figure 29–1.   Percent of patients in whom clinical assessment was uncertain regarding the likelihood of pulmonary embolism (PE). NO CPD, no prior cardiopulmonary disease; any CPD, any prior cardiopulmonary disease; COPD, chronic obstructive pulmonary disease; ICU NO VENT, intensive care unit not on ventilatory support; VENT, ventilatory support. NO CPD versus ICU NO VENT P<.01. All other differences were not statistically significant.

embolism in non-critically ill patients with a low likelihood clinical assessment was 15%.

Physicians in PIOPED, after making a clinical assessment, were uncertain whether pulmonary embolism was present in 63 to 78% of patients with no prior cardiopulmonary disease (6), any prior cardiopulmonary disease (Stein PD, Henry JW. Unpublished data from PIOPED), chronic obstructive pulmonary disease (COPD) (7), patients in intensive care units not on ventilatory support (4), patients on ventilatory support (4), and hypoxemic patients not on ventilatory support (Fig. 29–1) (4). However, physicians were more often uncertain whether pulmonary embolism was present in making a clinical assessment among patients in an intensive care unit not on ventilatory support than among patients with no prior cardiopulmonary disease. The percent of patients with an uncertain clinical assessment in other categories did not differ from one another to a statistically significant extent.

Among patients with no prior cardiopulmonary disease, any prior cardiopulmonary disease, COPD, patients in intensive care units not on ventilatory support, patients on ventilatory support, and hypoxemic patients not on ventilatory support, if clinical assessment indicated a high likelihood of pulmonary embolism, it was present in 75% or more of the patients in each of these categories (Fig. 29–2) (4, 6, 7) (also Stein PD, Henry JW. Unpublished data from PIOPED). Few high likelihood clinical assessments were found among patients

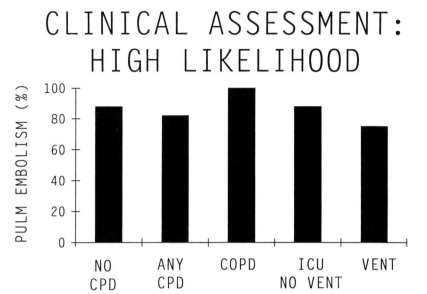

Figure 29–2. Frequency of pulmonary embolism among patients in whom a high likelihood clinical assessment was made. NO CPD, no prior cardiopulmonary disease; any CPD, any prior cardiopulmonary disease; COPD, chronic obstructive pulmonary disease; ICU NO VENT, intensive care unit not on ventilatory support; VENT, ventilatory support. No statistically significant differences of the frequency of pulmonary embolism existed between the various groups.

with COPD, those in the intensive care unit not on ventilatory support, and those on ventilatory support.

Among patients in whom physicians made a clinical assessment of pulmonary embolism as being low likelihood, pulmonary embolism was present in 0 to 14% of patients in the various categories (Fig. 29–3).

Ventilation-Perfusion Lung Scans

Among patients who suffered loss of consciousness on the day of study entry, the ventilation-perfusion lung scan was interpreted as high probability for pulmonary embolism in 5 of 7 (71%) and low probability in the 2 remaining patients (Stein PD, Relyea B. Unpublished data from PIOPED). In the patients with no prior cardiopulmonary disease, the ventilation-perfusion scan was interpreted as high probability in 4 of 5 (80%).

Twenty-two percent of patients who were on ventilatory support had perfusion lung scans without ventilation lung scans, because the ability to obtain a technically adequate ventilation lung scan is compromised in patients on ventilatory support (2). In many instances, however, a perfusion scan alone is satisfactory. In a random sample of patients from PIOPED, a high probability interpretation of a perfusion lung scan alone had a positive predictive value for pulmonary embolism of 93%, which was virtually the same as the positive

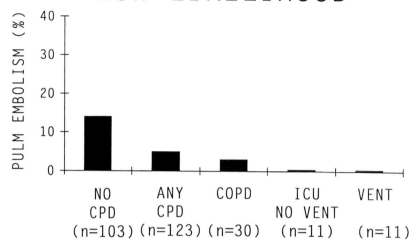

CLINICAL ASSESSMENT: LOW LIKELIHOOD

Figure 29–3. Frequency of pulmonary embolism among patients in whom the clinical assessment indicated a low likelihood of pulmonary embolism. Pulmonary embolism was more frequent among patients with no CPD than with any CPD ($P<.05$). Other differences were not statistically significant. NO CPD, no prior cardiopulmonary disease; any CPD, any prior cardiopulmonary disease; COPD, chronic obstructive pulmonary disease; ICU NO VENT, intensive care unit not on ventilatory support; VENT, ventilatory support.

predictive value of a high probability ventilation-perfusion scan, 94% (8). The sensitivity and specificity of high probability interpretations of perfusion scans alone did not differ to a statistically significant extent from sensitivity and specificity of ventilation-perfusion scans (8) (Chapter 16). However, a trend suggested that a higher percentage of patients with perfusion lung scans alone had intermediate (indeterminate) interpretations than patients who had ventilation-perfusion scans, and fewer patients with perfusion scans alone had low probability interpretations (8).

In critically ill patients, a high probability interpretation of the ventilation-perfusion lung scan (or perfusion scan alone in patients on ventilatory support) showed a sensitivity for pulmonary embolism that was not statistically significantly lower than the sensitivity in non-critically ill patients (Table 29–9) (4). The specificity of high probability lung scans among critically ill patients was also no lower than in non-critically ill patients (Table 29–9). Even patients on ventilatory support, who are likely to be difficult to study, showed a sensitivity and specificity of a high probability ventilation-perfusion scan or perfusion scan alone that was at least as high as in non-critically ill patients (4).

Among critically ill patients, the positive predictive value of a high probability interpretation of the ventilation-perfusion lung scan was as high as in non-critically ill patients (Table 29–6, Table 29–7, Table 29–8, Table 29–9). The negative predictive value of a normal/near normal ventilation-perfusion scan

Table 29–9. SENSITIVITIES AND SPECIFICITIES OF HIGH PROBABILITY
LUNG SCANS AMONG CRITICALLY ILL AND NON-
CRITICALLY ILL PATIENTS

	Sensitivity n/N (%)	Specificity n_1/N_1 (%)
Hypoxemic, not on vent	17/27 (63)*	60/62 (97)
Ventilatory support	4/12 (33)	34/34 (100)
ICU not on vent	8/31 (26)	53/54 (98)
Hypotensive, not hypoxemic	0/1 (0)	2/2 (96)
Not critically ill	87/227 (38)	385/400 (96)

ICU = intensive care unit, VENT = ventilatory support, n = number of patients with high probability V/Q scans,
N = number of patients with PE, n_1 = number of patients with non-high probability V/Q scans, N_1 = number of
patients with no PE.
* P < .02 hypoxemic vs not critically ill
Reproduced from Henry JW, Stein PD, Gottschalk A, Relyea B, Leeper KV Jr with permission.

was also as high as in non-critically ill patients (4). Few critically ill patients,
however, had normal/near normal ventilation-perfusion lung scans.

An intermediate probability interpretation of the ventilation-perfusion lung
scan was less frequent among patients with no prior cardiopulmonary disease
(9) than among patients with any prior cardiopulmonary disease (9), chronic
obstructive pulmonary disease (COPD) (7), patients in an intensive care unit
not on ventilatory support (4), and patients on ventilatory support (Fig. 29–4)
(4). An intermediate probability interpretation of the ventilation-perfusion lung
scan occurred most frequently among patients with COPD (Fig. 29–4).

If the interpretation of the ventilation-perfusion lung scan was high probability of pulmonary embolism, 83% to 100% of patients had pulmonary embolism, irrespective of the category of patients (Fig. 29–5). However, among
patients with COPD, patients in intensive care units not on ventilatory support,
and patients on ventilatory support, few had a high probability interpretation
of the ventilation-perfusion lung scan. If the interpretation of the ventilation-
perfusion lung scan was low probability for pulmonary embolism, 7% to 17% had
pulmonary embolism (Fig. 29–6). Among patients in whom the interpretation of
the ventilation-perfusion lung scan was nearly normal/normal, 4% or fewer had
pulmonary embolism among the various categories of patients (Fig. 29–7). Only
one patient on ventilatory support had a nearly normal ventilation-perfusion
lung scan and that patient did not have pulmonary embolism.

PERCENT OF PATIENTS WITH
INTERMEDIATE PROB V/Q SCANS

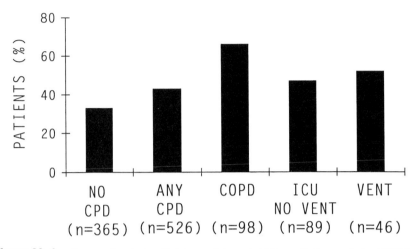

Figure 29–4. Percent of patients with intermediate probability ventilation-perfusion (V/Q) lung scans. NO CPD, no prior cardiopulmonary disease; any CPD, any prior cardiopulmonary disease; COPD, chronic obstructive pulmonary disease; ICU NO VENT, intensive care unit not on ventilatory support; VENT, ventilatory support. Fewer patients with no prior cardiopulmonary disease had intermediate probability V/Q scans than any other category (P<.01 to <.001). Patients with COPD had intermediate probability V/Q scans more frequently than any other group (P<.01 to P<.001) except in patients on ventilatory support.

V/Q HIGH PROB

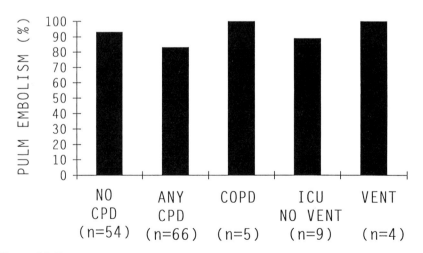

Figure 29–5. Frequency of pulmonary embolism among patients with ventilation-perfusion (V/Q) lung scans interpreted as high probability for pulmonary embolism. NO CPD, no prior cardiopulmonary disease; any CPD, any prior cardiopulmonary disease; COPD, chronic obstructive pulmonary disease; ICU NO VENT, intensive care unit not on ventilatory support; VENT, ventilatory support. No statistically significant differences existed between groups.

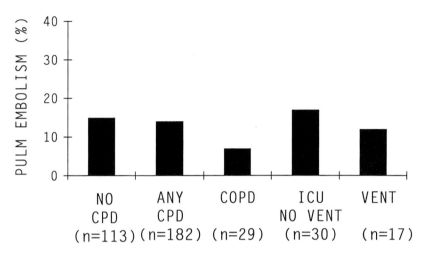

Figure 29–6. Frequency of pulmonary embolism among patients with ventilation-perfusion (V/Q) lung scans interpreted as low probability for pulmonary embolism. NO CPD, no prior cardiopulmonary disease; any CPD, any prior cardiopulmonary disease; COPD, chronic obstructive pulmonary disease; ICU NO VENT, intensive care unit not on ventilatory support; VENT, ventilatory support. No statistically significant difference existed between groups.

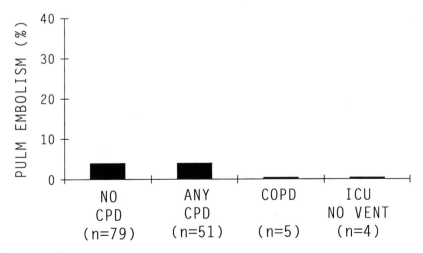

Figure 29–7. Frequency of pulmonary embolism among patients with ventilation-perfusion (V/Q) lung scans interpreted as nearly normal or normal. NO CPD, no prior cardiopulmonary disease; any CPD, any prior cardiopulmonary disease; COPD, chronic obstructive pulmonary disease; ICU NO VENT, intensive care unit not on ventilatory support; VENT, ventilatory support. Patients on ventilatory support are not shown because there was only one patient in that group. No statistically significant differences existed between groups.

REFERENCES

1. Cowen JC, Kelley MA. An organized approach to detecting pulmonary embolism in the critically ill. J Critical Illness 1994; 9:551-567.
2. Davis LP, Fink-Bennett D. Nuclear medicine in the acutely ill patient-I. Critical Care Clinics 1994; 10:365-381.
3. Butler SP, Alderson PO, Greenspan RL, Doctor DG, DeFillipi VJ. The utility of Technetium-99m DTPA inhalational scans in artificially ventilated patients. J Nucl Med 1990; 31:46-51.
4. Henry JW, Stein PD, Gottschalk A, Relyea B, Leeper KV Jr. Scintigraphic lung scans and clinical assessment in critically ill patients with suspected acute pulmonary embolism. Chest 1996;109:462-466.
5. The PIOPED investigators. Value of the ventilation/perfusion scan in acute pulmonary embolism: results of the Prospective Investigation of Pulmonary Embolism Diagnosis (PIOPED). JAMA 1990; 263:2753-2759.
6. Stein PD, Terrin ML, Hales CA, et al. Clinical, laboratory, roentgenographic and electrocardiographic findings in patients with acute pulmonary embolism and no pre-existing cardiac or pulmonary disease. Chest 1991;100:598-603.
7. Lesser BA, Leeper KV, Stein PD, et al. The diagnosis of pulmonary embolism in patients with chronic obstructive pulmonary disease. Chest 1992; 102:17-22.
8. Stein PD, Terrin ML, Gottschalk A, Alavi A, Henry JW. Value of ventilation/perfusion scans compared to perfusion scans alone in acute pulmonary embolism. Am J Cardiol 1992; 69:1239-1241.
9. Stein PD, Coleman RE, Gottschalk A, Saltzman HA, Terrin ML, Weg JG. Diagnostic utility of ventilation/perfusion lung scans in acute pulmonary embolism is not diminished by pre- existing cardiac or pulmonary disease. Chest 1991; 100:604- 606.

Diagnosis in the Elderly and Age-Related Manifestations

The diagnosis of pulmonary embolism among elderly patients has been thought to be particularly difficult because the expected signs and symptoms may be absent or ignored (1–3). This, in general, did not seem to be the case in the experience of the Prospective Investigation of Pulmonary Embolism Diagnosis (PIOPED) (4).

The nonspecific manifestations of pulmonary embolism, even among patients ≥ 70 years old, occurred with sufficient frequency to suggest the possibility of pulmonary embolism in the differential diagnosis (4). The typical signs and symptoms known to occur among younger patients were common among elderly patients, although occasional exceptions were observed. In the absence of these signs and symptoms, unexplained radiographic abnormalities were important diagnostic clues (4). When the diagnosis of pulmonary embolism is uncertain, pulmonary angiography can be performed safely in elderly patients, although renal failure was a problem (4).

Predisposing Factors According to Age

Among 72 patients ≥ 70 years old, 67% were immobilized before the pulmonary embolism, and surgery preceded the pulmonary embolism in 44% (4). Comparable percentages of patients in the younger age groups were immobilized or underwent surgery before the pulmonary embolism. Malignancy was more frequent among patients ≥ 70 years old (26%) than among the patients < 40 years old (2%), but patients 40 to 69 years had malignancy nearly as frequently as did patients ≥ 70 years old (24%). Estrogen therapy was infrequent among female patients ≥ 70 years old. Its use among female patients < 40 years of age preceded pulmonary embolism in 35%. Childbirth in these women < 40 years of age preceded pulmonary embolism in 25%.

Table 30–1. SYMPTOMS OF ACUTE PULMONARY EMBOLISM
ACCORDING TO AGE

	≥70 Years (n = 72) %	40 to 69 Years (n = 144) %	<40 Years (n = 44) %
Dyspnea	78	78	82
Pleuritic pain	51	58	70
Cough	35	42	45
Leg swelling	35	33	14
Leg pain	31	26	20
Palpitations	13	15	9
Wheezing	10	12	16
Angina-like pain	10	13	7
Hemoptysis[a]	8	4	32

[a] P < 0.01, ≥70 years versus <40 years; p < 0.001, 40 to 69 versus <40 years
Modified and reprinted with permission from Stein PD, Gottschalk A, Saltzman HA, et al. Diagnosis of acute pulmonary embolism in the elderly. J Am Col Cardiol 1991;18:1452–1457.

Syndromes of Pulmonary Embolism According to Age

The usual syndromes of pulmonary embolism, characterized by 1) pleuritic pain or hemoptysis, 2) isolated dyspnea, or 3) circulatory collapse, were observed with comparable frequency among elderly patients and younger patients (4). However, 11% of patients ≥ 70 years of age, in contrast to younger patients, did not show these syndromes (4). They were identified on the basis of unexpected radiographic abnormalities, which may have been accompanied by tachypnea or a history of thrombophlebitis. Unexplained radiographic abnormalities may be an important clue to the diagnosis of pulmonary embolism, particularly among elderly patients in whom the expected signs and symptoms are absent, as previously has been observed (1).

Symptoms According to Age

Dyspnea and pleuritic pain were the most frequent symptoms, occurring in 78% and 51% of the patients with pulmonary embolism ≥ 70 years old (4). The frequency of these symptoms was comparable among all age groups. Hemoptysis occurred less frequently among patients ≥ 70 years and among patients 40 to 69 years than among patients < 40 years of age. Other symptoms occurred with comparable frequency among all age groups (Table 30–1).

Signs According to Age

Tachypnea (respiratory rate ≥ 20/min) was the most frequent sign in all age groups with pulmonary embolism (4). Among patients ≥ 70 years of age,

Table 30–2. SIGNS OF ACUTE PULMONARY EMBOLISM ACCORDING TO AGE

	≥70 Years (n = 72) %	40 to 69 Years (n = 144) %	<40 Years (n = 44) %
Tachypnea (≥20/min)	74	69	82
Rales	65	61	41
Tachycardia$_2$ (≥100/min)	29	26	32
Increased P2	15	20	34
Deep venous thrombosis	15	17	9
Diaphoresis	8	10	18
Wheezes	8	10	5
Temperature >38.5°C	7	5	14
Third heart sound	7	6	5
Pleural friction rub	6	5	0
Homans' sign	4	2	2
Cyanosis	3	3	2

Differences among age groups were not significant
P2, pulmonary component of second heart sound.
Modified and reprinted with permission from Stein PD, Gottschalk A, Saltzman HA, et al. Diagnosis of acute pulmonary embolism in the elderly. J Am Col Cardiol 1991;18:1452–1457.

Table 30–3. CHEST RADIOGRAPH IN ACUTE PULMONARY EMBOLISM ACCORDING TO AGE

	≥70 Years (n = 72) %	40 to 69 Years (n = 144) %	<40 Years (n = 44) %
Normal	4	8	14
Atelectasis or pulmonary parenchymal abnormality	71	69	64
Pleural effusion	57	46	45
Pleural based opacity	42	34	43
Prominent central pulmonary artery	29	20	11
Elevated diaphragm	28	27	18
Cardiomegaly	22	17	14
Decreased pulmonary vascularity	19	22	20
Pulmonary edema	13	12	7
Westermark's sign	7	8	0

Westermark's sign, prominent central pulmonary artery and decreased pulmonary vascularity
Differences among age groups were not significant.
Modified and reprinted with permission from Stein PD, Gottschalk A, Saltzman HA, et al. Diagnosis of acute pulmonary embolism in the elderly. J Am Col Cardiol 1991;18:1452–1457.

tachypnea occurred in 74% and tachycardia (heart rate > 100/min) in 29%. All signs occurred with a comparable frequency among all age groups (Table 30–2).

The chest radiograph was normal in 4% of patients ≥ 70 years old (4). Atelectasis or pulmonary parenchymal abnormalities were the most frequent

Table 30–4.   COMBINATIONS OF SIGNS AND SYMPTOMS IN ACUTE
PULMONARY EMBOLISM ACCORDING TO AGE

	≥70 Years (n = 72) %	40 to 69 Years (n = 144) %	<40 Years (n = 44) %
Dyspnea or tachypnea	92	90	95
Dyspnea or tachypnea or hemoptysis	92	91	98
Dyspnea or tachypnea or pleuritic pain[a]	94	98	100
Dyspnea or tachypnea or signs of deep venous thrombosis	92	91	98
Dyspnea or tachypnea or pleuritic pain of signs of deep venous thrombosis[a]	94	99	100
Dyspnea or tachypnea or radiographic atelectasis or parenchymal abnormality[a]	100	97	98
Dyspnea or tachypnea or pleuritic pain or radiographic atelectasis or parenchymal abnormality[a]	100	99	100

[a] The addition of hemoptysis did not improve the sensitivity of the combination for the detection of pulmonary embolism.
Tachypnea, respiratory rate ≥20/min
Differences among age groups were not significant.
Modified and reprinted with permission from Stein PD, Gottschalk A, Saltzman HA, et al. Diagnosis of acute pulmonary embolism in the elderly. J Am Col Cardiol 1991;18:1452–1457.

radiographic abnormalities among all age groups. All radiographic abnormalities occurred with a comparable frequency among all age groups (Table 30–3).

Combinations of Symptoms and Signs

Even among patients ≥ 70 years old, a combination of nonspecific symptoms and signs that typically occur with pulmonary embolism was present in the great majority (4).

Dyspnea, tachypnea, or pleuritic pain occurred in 94%. Dyspnea, tachypnea, radiographic evidence of atelectasis, or a parenchymal abnormality occurred in 100% (Table 30–4).

The Electrocardiogram According to Age

Nonspecific ST segment or T wave changes were the most frequent electrocardiographic abnormalities, either or both occurring in 56% of patients ≥ 70 years old and with the same frequency in younger patients (4). With the exception of left anterior hemiblock (left axis deviation) among patients ≥ 70 years of age, other electrocardiographic abnormalities occurred in 12% or fewer patients in all age groups. No differences in the frequency of occurrence of any ECG abnormalities were apparent between patients ≥ 70 years of age and younger patients, although incomplete right bundle branch block was less

Table 30–5. ELECTROCARDIOGRAPHIC FINDINGS WITH ACUTE
PULMONARY EMBOLISM ACCORDING TO AGE

	≥70 Years (n = 72) %	40 to 69 Years (n = 113) %	<40 Years (n = 36) %
Normal	21	27	22
ST segment or T wave changes	56	51	56
Left axis deviation	18	11	8
Left ventricular hypertrophy	12	7	11
Acute myocardial infarction pattern	12	4	6
Low voltage QRS	9	5	0
Complete right bundle branch block	7	4	3
Right ventricular hypertrophy	4	3	3
Right axis deviation	2	3	8
P pulmonale	2	2	0
Incomplete right bundle branch block[a]	2	0	11

[a] P < 0.01, 40 to 69 years vs <40 years
Modified and reprinted with permission from Stein PD, Gottschalk A, Saltzman HA, et al. Diagnosis of acute pulmonary embolism in the elderly. J Am Col Cardiol 1991;13:1452–1457.

frequent among patients 40 to 69 years than among patients less than 40 years of age (Table 30–5).

Blood Gases According to Age

The partial pressure of oxygen in arterial blood (PaO_2) was lower among patients ≥ 70 years than among those < 40 years of age. Among patients 40 to 69 years, the PaO_2 was lower than in patients < 40 years, but not significantly lower than in patients ≥ 70 years of age (4). The PaO_2 among patients with pulmonary embolism ≥ 70 years of age, 40 to 69 years of age, and < 40 years of age was 61 ± 12, 67 ± 15 and 75 ± 18 mm Hg, respectively (mean ± standard deviation).

The alveolar-arterial oxygen difference (gradient) among patients with pulmonary embolism ≥ 70 years of age was 47 ± 14 mm Hg, which was higher than among patients 40 to 69 years old (40 ± 17 mm Hg), and it was higher than in patients < 40 years old (31 ± 17 mm Hg). The alveolar-arterial oxygen difference in normal adults increases with age (5–8).

Clinical Assessment According to Age

The accuracy of clinical assessment was comparable among patients in all age groups (4). When physicians were 80 to 100% confident that pulmonary embolism was present on the basis of clinical judgment and laboratory tests with the exception of ventilation-perfusion scans, they were correct in 90% of

Table 30–6. RESULTS OF VENTILATION-PERFUSION LUNG SCANS IN ACUTE PULMONARY EMBOLISM ACCORDING TO AGE OF THE PATIENT

V/Q Scan Probability	≥70 Years		40 to 69 Years		≤40 Years	
	PE/n	(%)	PE/n	(%)	PE/n	(%)
High	34/36	(94)	60/68	(99)	11/16	(69)
Intermediate	27/100	(27)	59/199	(30)	22/52	(42)
Low	10/71	(14)	24/172	(14)	8/57	(14)
Near normal/normal	1/8	(13)	1/55	(2)	3/68	(4)

Differences among age groups were not significant.
n, number of patients with the scan result shown in column
PE, pulmonary embolism
Modified and reprinted with permission from Stein PD, Gottschalk A, Saltzman HA, et al. Diagnosis of acute pulmonary embolism in the elderly. J Am Col Cardiol 1991;18:1452–1457.

10 patients ≥ 70 years old. When they believed that there was less than 20% likelihood of pulmonary embolism, it was present in 19% of 69 patients. In most patients, physicians were uncertain of the diagnosis, believing that there was a 20 to 79% chance of pulmonary embolism.

Ventilation-Perfusion Lung Scans According to Age

The use of ventilation-perfusion lung scans among patients ≥ 70 years old was comparable with that in younger patients (4). The positive predictive value of all probabilities of ventilation-perfusion lung scans, using original PIOPED criteria (9), was comparable in all age groups (4). Among patients ≥ 70 years of age with ventilation-perfusion lung scans indicating a high probability of pulmonary embolism, 94% had pulmonary embolism (Table 30–6).

The sensitivity of ventilation-perfusion scans interpreted as a high probability of pulmonary embolism among patients ≥ 70 years of age (47%) did not differ significantly from the sensitivity of such scans among younger age groups. The specificity of ventilation-perfusion scans interpreted as a high probability of pulmonary embolism among patients ≥ 70 years of age (99%) was similar among patients 40 to 69 years of age (98%) and among patients < 40 years of age (97%) (4).

Complications of Pulmonary Angiography Among Patients With and Without Pulmonary Embolism

Pulmonary angiography was not more hazardous among elderly patients, although renal failure was a more frequent sequela among patients ≥ 70 years of age than among younger patients (4). Major complications occurred in 1.0%

of 200 patients ≥ 70 years, in 1.2% in of 427 patients 40 to 69 years, and in 0.7% of 135 patients < 40 years of age. One fatal complication occurred in an 87-year-old woman who suffered from ventricular tachycardia followed by hypotension and respiratory arrest. She died 12 hours after the pulmonary angiogram.

Renal failure, either major or minor, was the most frequent complication of angiography among elderly patients. It occurred in 3% of patients ≥ 70 years of age, compared with 0.7% of patients ≤ 69 years of age. "Minor" complications of renal failure were important complications, although dialysis was not required. Patients with these complications showed either an elevation of the serum creatinine from previously normal levels to ≥ 2.1 mg/100 ml (range 2.1 to 3.5 mg/100 ml) or an increase in a previously abnormal serum creatinine level ≥ 2 mg/100 ml. All but one patient who developed renal failure after angiography was > 60 years old. The exception was a 52-year-old woman who had worsening of chronic renal failure after angiography. Among the 10 patients who developed renal failure, three required dialysis.

Among patients 40 to 69 years of age, 1.2% had a major complication, including death in two. One death was caused by cardiopulmonary arrest that occurred during angiography. The other death was a cardiopulmonary arrest that occurred 1 hour after the pulmonary angiogram. Renal failure that required dialysis occurred in two patients in the 40 to 69 year range and respiratory distress that required endotracheal intubation occurred in one patient.

Among patients < 40 years of age, 0.7% had a major complication. The major complication was a nonfatal respiratory arrest that required cardiopulmonary resuscitation.

Minor complications of prior angiography included urticaria, pulmonary edema requiring only diuretics, nausea and vomiting, arrhythmias that were not life-threatening, hematomas, interstitial staining with contrast material and narcotic overdose (4). Minor complications occurred in 7.0% of patients ≥ 70 years old, in 5.2% patients 40 to 69 years of age, and in 5.9% of patients < 40 years of age.

REFERENCES

1. Taubman LB, Silverstone FA. Autopsy proven pulmonary embolism among the institutionalized elderly. J Am Geriatr Soc 1986:34:752–756.
2. Morrell MT. The incidence of pulmonary embolism in the elderly. Geriatrics 1970;25:138–153.
3. Busby W, Bayer A, Pathy J. Pulmonary embolism in the elderly. Age Ageing 1988;17:205–209.
4. Stein PD, Gottschalk A, Saltzman HA, et al. Diagnosis of acute pulmonary embolism in the elderly. J Am Col Cardiol 1991;18:1452–1457.
5. Mellemgaard K. The alveolar-arterial oxygen difference: its size and components in normal man. Acta Physiol Scand 1966; 67:10–20.
6. Harris EA, Kenyon AM, Nisbet HD, et al. The normal alveolar-arterial oxygen-tension gradient in man. Clin Sci Molec Med 1974;46:89–104.
7. Filley GF, Gregoire F, Wright GW. Alveolar and arterial oxygen tensions and the significance of the alveolar- arterial oxygen tension difference in normal men. J Clin Invest 1954;33:517–529.

8. Kanber GJ, King FW, Eshchar YR, et al. The alveolar-arterial oxygen gradient in young and elderly men during air and oxygen breathing. Amer Review of Respir Dis 1968;97:376–381.
9. A Collaborative Study by the PIOPED Investigators. Value of the ventilation/perfusion scan in acute pulmonary embolism: results of the Prospective Investigation of Pulmonary Embolism Diagnosis (PIOPED). JAMA 1990;263:2753–2759.

CHAPTER 31

Diagnosis in Women

Women 50 years of age or under with suspected acute pulmonary embolism who were enrolled in the Prospective Investigation of Pulmonary Embolism Diagnosis (PIOPED) had a lower frequency of pulmonary embolism than men of that age (16% versus 32%), but no difference existed in patients over 50 years of age (1). The overall frequency of pulmonary embolism in women with suspected pulmonary embolism was 25% and in men, 34%.

Pulmonary embolism has been reported to occur more frequently in women than in men because of estrogen use, childbearing, and a higher frequency of deep venous thrombosis (2–6). A postmortem study of pulmonary embolism showed pulmonary embolism in 11% of women and 7% of men (7). The Tecumseh Community Health Study showed 4.5 occurrences of pulmonary embolism per 10,000 women per year, compared with 1.75 occurrences of pulmonary embolism per 10,000 men per year (5).

Most risk factors were equally prevalent among women and men (1). Myocardial infarction, coronary artery disease, and chronic obstructive pulmonary disease were more frequent in men suspected of pulmonary embolism than in women. Surgery within 3 months and estrogen use were more frequent in women suspected of pulmonary embolism.

Regarding the signs and symptoms of acute pulmonary embolism, women less frequently had hemoptysis (10% versus 21%), leg swelling (24% versus 36%) and pleural friction rub (2% versus 7%)(Table 31–1). Except for minor differences of heart rate, the prevalence of other signs and symptoms of acute pulmonary embolism did not differ significantly between women and men (1).

The sensitivity and specificity of the ventilation-perfusion scan, using original PIOPED criteria (8), were the same in women and men. The positive predictive values of a high probability ventilation-perfusion scan were similar between women (86%) and men (90%), and the negative predictive values of normal or nearly normal ventilation-perfusion scans were also similar, 93% in women and 88% in men (1).

No difference existed between women and men during 1-year follow-up in the recurrence of pulmonary embolism (1).

Table 31–1. SYMPTOMS AND SIGNS OF ACUTE PULMONARY EMBOLISM IN WOMEN AND MEN

	Women (n = 119) Percent	Men (n = 132) Percent
Dyspnea	80	78
Pleuritic pain	60	57
Cough	41	40
Leg swelling	24	36**
Leg pain	23	30
Hemoptysis	10	21***
Rales (crackles)	60	57
Pleural friction rub	2	7*

* P < .05, ** P < .04, *** P < .02, women vs men
Data are from Quinn and associates (1).

Estrogen for postmenopausal replacement did not appear to be a predisposing factor for pulmonary embolism in women who underwent surgery (1). Among women in whom pulmonary embolism was suspected, 50% of those taking estrogen for postmenopausal replacement had postoperative pulmonary embolism and 42% of those not taking estrogen for postmenopausal replacement also had postoperative pulmonary embolism.

As reviewed by Quinn and associates (1), retrospective studies found an increased risk of thromboembolic disease in women using estrogen, but this has been disputed in some prospective studies (9,10). Thromboembolic events have been linked to high estrogen content in oral contraceptives (greater than 50 µg) (11), but even this association has been questioned (12). The U.S. Food and Drug Administration in 1980 recommended the use of the lowest possible dose of estrogen for birth control.

The possibility of an increased risk of postoperative thromboembolism with oral contraceptive use was raised by Vessey and associates in 1970 (13). The majority of their patients were using oral contraceptives with more than 50 µg of estrogen.In PIOPED, among women in whom pulmonary embolism was suspected, pulmonary embolism was more frequent in women who underwent surgery if they were using oral contraceptives (1). If pulmonary embolism was suspected, and if the women who underwent surgery used oral contraceptives, 50% had pulmonary embolism. If pulmonary embolism was suspected, and if the women who underwent surgery did not use oral contraceptives, 12% had pulmonary embolism. In the PIOPED experience, however, the number of women undergoing surgery and taking oral contraceptives was small. Nevertheless, the risk of postoperative pulmonary embolism appears to be increased in women who use oral contraceptives, even in a time when oral contraceptives have a low estrogen content.

REFERENCES

1. Quinn DA, Thompson BT, Terrin ML, et al. A prospective investigation of pulmonary embolism in women and men. JAMA 1992;268:1689–1696.

2. Palevsky HI. Pulmonary hypertension and thromboembolic disease in women. Cardiovasc Clin 1989;19:267–283.

3. Bernstein D, Goupey S, Schonberg SK. Pulmonary embolism in adolescents. AJDC 1986;140:667–671.

4. Coon W. Epidemiology of venous thromboembolism. Ann Surg 1977;186:149–164.

5. Coon WW, Willis PW III, Keller JB. Venous thrombosis and other venous disease in the Tecumseh Community Study. Circulation 1973;48:839–846.

6. Breckenridge RT, Ralnoff OD. Pulmonary embolism and unexpected death in supposedly normal persons. N Engl J Med 1964;270:298–299.

7. Karwinski B, Svendsen E. Comparison of clinical and postmortem diagnosis of pulmonary embolism. J Clin Pathol 1989;42:135–139.

8. A Collaborative Study by the PIOPED Investigators.Value of the ventilation-perfusion scan in acutepulmonary embolism: results of the ProspectiveInvestigation of Pulmonary Embolism Diagnosis (PIOPED). JAMA 1990;263:2753–2759.

9. Drill VA. Oral contraceptives and thromboembolic disease. JAMA 1972;219:583–592.

10. Ramacharan S, Pellegrin FA, Ray RM, et al. The Walnut Creek contraceptive drug study. J Reprod Med 1980;25(suppl):S345–S372.

11. Inman W, Vessey M, Westerholm B, et al. Thromboembolic disease and the steroidal content of oral contraceptives: a report to the committee on safety of drugs. BMJ 1970;2:203–209.

12. Sturtevant FM. Special report: safety of oral contraceptives as related to steroidal content: a critical review. Int J Fertil 1989;34:323–332.

13. Vessey M, Doll R, Fairbain A, et al. Postoperative thromboembolism and the use of oral contraceptives. BMJ 1970;3:123–126.

Strategies of Diagnosis and Management

CHAPTER 32

Strategies for Diagnosis

It has been known for many years that at least 80% of patients with pulmonary embolism have thrombi that originate in the lower extremities (1–4). Nevertheless, pulmonary embolism traditionally has been considered a discrete syndrome that requires specific methods of diagnosis, all of which have focused on the chest. In recent years, however, because of the inaccuracy of noninvasive tests for diagnosing pulmonary embolism, Hull and associates introduced the concept that it may be sufficient to diagnose and treat deep venous thrombosis as an alternative to proving the presence of pulmonary embolism among patients in whom the diagnosis of pulmonary embolism is suspected (5–8). The combined strategy of diagnosis and treatment of pulmonary embolism and/or underlying deep venous thrombosis assumes that deep venous thrombosis is present in patients with pulmonary embolism. The strategy further assumes that the treatment of deep venous thrombosis is the same as the treatment of pulmonary embolism. Noninvasive diagnostic tests for deep venous thrombosis are accurate (7,9,10), and cost effective (11). Many are optimistic that the combined strategy is useful (12–14).

If deep venous thrombosis and pulmonary embolism are equivalent, the risk of untreated deep venous thrombosis and untreated pulmonary embolism should be the same. Otherwise, pulmonary embolism might be treated more vigorously. Evidence indicates that the risk of fatal pulmonary embolism in patients with untreated deep venous thrombosis is the same as the risk of fatal recurrent pulmonary embolism in patients with untreated pulmonary embolism (15). In an era before sensitive diagnostic tests for deep venous thrombosis, the risk of death of untreated, clinically overt deep venous thrombosis was 37% (16). The risk of fatal recurrent pulmonary embolism among untreated patients was between 26 and 36% (17,18).

Present-day sensitive diagnostic tests permit detection of mild deep venous thrombosis and have reduced the danger of pulmonary embolism from it. Based upon pooled data, the risk of fatal pulmonary embolism among untreated patients with deep venous thrombosis (usually subclinical) diagnosed by radioactive fibrinogen is approximately 5% (19). This is comparable with the risk of death from recurrent pulmonary embolism among untreated patients with pulmonary embolism in the present era of early diagnosis by sensitive methods. The risk of fatal recurrent pulmonary embolism within 1 month among patients with pulmonary embolism who escaped treatment in the Prospective Investigation of Pulmonary Embolism Diagnosis (PIOPED) was 5% (1 of 20) (20) (Chapter 2). Pulmonary embolism in these patients was mild compared with pulmonary embolism in treated patients.

The seemingly polarized approaches to the diagnosis of pulmonary embolism have been drawn together to provide practical diagnostic algorithms that considerably enhance noninvasive diagnostic methods and decrease the need for pulmonary angiography in patients with clinically suspected pulmonary embolism (15,21,22). The strategies depend on ventilation-perfusion lung scans, noninvasive objective tests of the lower extremities for deep venous thrombosis, and in some instances, assessment of the clinical likelihood of pulmonary embolism.

Clinical evaluation for the diagnosis of pulmonary embolism was described in Chapters 5 and 6, laboratory tests in Chapters 7 to 10, and ventilation-perfusion lung scans in Chapters 12 to 25. The sensitivity and specificity of physical examination for deep venous thrombosis was described in Chapter 4. Prospective studies of the diagnostic validity of noninvasive diagnostic tests for deep venous thrombosis suggest that the sensitivity and specificity of impedance plethysmography (5,23) and B-mode imaging (24,25) are sufficient in patients with suspected pulmonary embolism to be of clinical value. Impedance plethysmography in combination with leg scanning correlated well with venography (26). Using impedance plethysmography during pregnancy, however, may be a problem. Tests may be falsely positive within the third month because of outflow obstruction caused by the gravid uterus (27).

Impedance plethysmography indicated deep venous thrombosis in 94% (15 of 16) legs that showed positive venograms of both the proximal and distal leg veins (28). Impedance plethysmography, however, was positive in only 25% (7 of 28) of legs in which venography showed deep venous thrombosis only in the distal leg veins (28). Similar observations were made by Hull and associates (5). If the venogram showed proximal or distal deep venous thrombosis, impedance plethysmography was positive in 75% (30 of 40). Among those with deep venous thrombosis in the proximal veins shown by venography, 86% (30 of 35) had a positive impedance plethysmogram. Impedance plethysmography, therefore, is more sensitive (86 to 94%) in the detection of proximal (thigh vein) thrombosis than distal (calf vein) thrombosis. Thrombi in the veins of the thigh are much more likely to cause symptomatic pulmonary embolism than thrombi in the veins of the calf (28). Regarding false positive impedance plethysmography, 3% (1 of 31) were not confirmed by venography (5).

Although impedance plethysmography detects deep venous thrombosis of the thigh in 86 to 94% of patients shown to have deep venous thrombosis by venography (5, 28), and autopsy showed deep venous thrombosis as the cause of pulmonary embolism in ≥ 80% of patients (1–4), noninvasive tests for deep venous thrombosis in patients with documented pulmonary embolism are positive in only 43 to 57% of the patients (5,6). This may reflect the following possibilities: (1) the residual deep venous thrombosis may be nonobstructive, or confined to the calf and remain undetected; (2) the deep venous thrombi causing the pulmonary emboli may embolize entirely from the deep veins of the thighs leaving no residual thrombosis to detect; (3) the pulmonary emboli may be from sources other than the lower extremities such as deep pelvic veins, renal veins, subclavian veins, or the right atrium.

A high percentage of patients admitted to the hospital, particularly those who are quite ill, would be expected to have subclinical deep venous thrombosis. The incidence of deep venous thrombosis in unselected patients at autopsy is 27 to 60% (29–37). It is unlikely, however, that an abnormal impedance plethysmogram would represent residual deep venous thrombosis in patients who in the past had an acute episode. Impedance plethysmograms normalize in 95% of patients within 1 year of treatment of deep venous thrombosis with anticoagulants (38). For those who prefer B-mode imaging for the detection of deep venous thrombosis, ultrasonic tissue characterization has been used to indicate acuteness (39). The red cell-fibrin mesh of early deep venous thrombosis may be detected by characteristics of the energy of the reflected signal. However, although statistically significant differences were observed, the data overlapped.

Hull and associates, in a number of studies, focused on the diagnosis of both venous thrombosis and pulmonary embolism in patients with suspected pulmonary embolism and evaluated diagnostic strategies directed toward venous thromboembolism (5–8). Based on the pathfinding work of these investigators, strategies for the management of pulmonary embolism have been developed that combine the diagnosis and treatment of deep venous thrombosis and pulmonary embolism.

Strategy Based on Single Noninvasive Leg Tests

Stein and associates, based on the results of PIOPED and observations by Hull associates, developed a strategy that combined clinical assessment with the ventilation-perfusion lung scan, as well as single objective tests of the lower extremities for deep venous thrombosis (15). The strategy indicated the likelihood of pulmonary embolism among patients grouped according to the interpretation of the ventilation-perfusion lung scan and grouped according to the likelihood of pulmonary embolism based on clinical assessment. An advantage of this strategy is that it presents a detailed probability of pulmonary embolism when a clinical assessment of likelihood is combined with the ventilation-perfusion scan and objective leg tests. A disadvantage is that stratification according to the ventilation-perfusion scan and clinical assessment, although valid and useful in the hands of experienced physicians, is complex and relies on clinical judgment in areas where many physicians feel uncomfortable (15). A low likelihood clinical assessment seems to be more accurate than other clinical assessments. Physicians in training could more accurately exclude the diagnosis of pulmonary embolism on a clinical basis than make the diagnosis (40). The strategy assumes that 50% of patients with pulmonary embolism have identifiable proximal deep venous thrombosis detectable by impedance plethysmography or B-mode ultrasound (5, 6). The strategy, based on single noninvasive leg tests, is as follows:

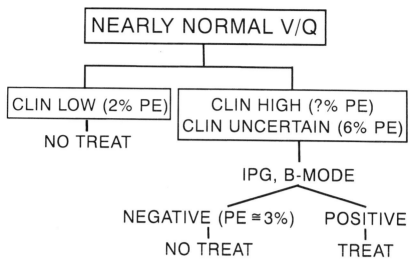

Figure 32–1. Strategy for diagnosis of patients with a nearly normal ventilation-perfusion (V/Q) scan. Clin, clinical; IPG, impedance plethysmography; Treat, treatment; B-mode, B-mode ultrasound; PE, pulmonary embolism.(Reprinted with permission from Stein PD, Hull RD, Saltzman HA, et al. Strategy for diagnosis of patients with suspected acute pulmonary embolism. Chest 1993;103:1553–1559.)

Normal Ventilation-Perfusion Lung Scan

If the ventilation-perfusion scan is normal, treatment is not indicated. Pulmonary embolism in a patient with a normal lung scan has not been documented.

Nearly Normal Ventilation-Perfusion Scan

If the ventilation-perfusion lung scan is nearly normal and the clinical likelihood of acute pulmonary embolism is low, the chance of acute pulmonary embolism is only 2% (41) (Fig. 32–1). No treatment is indicated. If the physician is uncertain based upon his clinical assessment (clinical uncertain), 6% of patients with a nearly normal ventilation-perfusion scan have pulmonary embolism. We have not encountered any patients with a nearly normal ventilation-perfusion scan in whom the physician thought there was a high clinical probability of pulmonary embolism. The likelihood of pulmonary embolism in such patients, therefore, has not been assessed. If the clinical impression is high or uncertain, impedance plethysmography or B-mode ultrasound is recommended. Approximately 50% of patients with pulmonary embolism will be detected by non-invasive leg vein studies (5,6). If the results are negative, no treatment is indicated, the estimated risk of pulmonary embolism being 3%. If the results are positive, treatment is recommended.

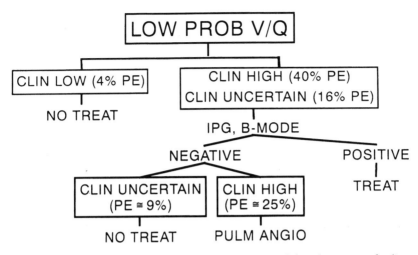

Figure 32–2. Strategy based on a single noninvasive leg test and clinical assessment for diagnosis of patients with a low probability (Low Prob) ventilation-perfusion (V/Q) scan. Pulm Angio, pulmonary angiogram; Clin, clinical; IPG, impedance plethysmography; Treat, treatment; B-mode, B-mode ultrasound; PE, pulmonary embolism. (Reprinted with permission from Stein PD, Hull RD, Saltzman HA, et al. Strategy for diagnosis of patients with suspected acute pulmonary embolism. Chest 1993;103:1553–1559.)

Low Probability Ventilation-Perfusion Scan

If clinical assessment indicates a low likelihood of pulmonary embolism in a patient with a low probability ventilation-perfusion scan, the incidence of pulmonary embolism is 4% (41) (Fig. 32–2). We suggest that the patient not be treated. If the clinical probability is uncertain or high probability, evaluation of the leg veins by impedance plethysmography or B-mode ultrasound is recommended because the likelihood of pulmonary embolism is 16 to 40%. If noninvasive studies of the leg veins are abnormal, we recommend treatment. If the results of leg vein assessment are negative, and the clinical probability was uncertain, the likelihood of pulmonary embolism is approximately 9%, and we recommend that the patient not be treated. If the results of leg vein assessment are negative, and the clinical assessment was high probability, the likelihood of pulmonary embolism is 25%. We recommend further assessment by pulmonary angiography.

Intermediate Probability Ventilation-Perfusion Scan

The likelihood of pulmonary embolism among patients with an intermediate probability ventilation-perfusion scan is 16% if the clinical assessment is low probability, 28% if the clinical assessment is uncertain, and 66% if the clinical assessment is high probability of pulmonary embolism (41) (Fig. 32–3). We recommend that all of these patients undergo noninvasive assessment of the leg veins by impedance plethysmography or B-mode ultrasound. Deep venous thrombosis will be identified in approximately half of these patients

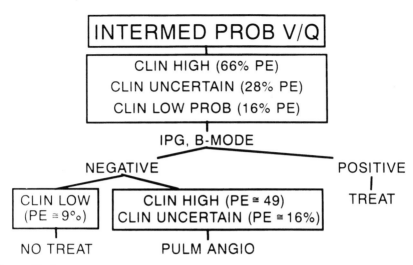

Figure 32–3. Strategy based on a single noninvasive leg test and clinical assessment for diagnosis of patients with an intermediate probability (Intermed Prob) ventilation-perfusion (V/Q) scan. Pulm Angio, pulmonary angiogram; Clin, clinical; IPG, impedance plethysmography; Treat, treatment; B-mode, B-mode ultrasound; PE, pulmonary embolism. (Reprinted with permission from Stein PD, Hull RD, Saltzman HA, et al. Strategy for diagnosis of patients with suspected acute pulmonary embolism. Chest 1993;103:1553–1559.)

(5,6). Those with positive findings in the leg veins should be treated. If the leg vein study is normal, and the clinical assessment is low probability, the probability of pulmonary embolism is reduced to 9%. We recommend observation with no treatment. If the clinical assessment is uncertain or high probability, the likelihood of pulmonary embolism, after a negative noninvasive evaluation of the leg veins, is 16% to 49%. We recommend further evaluation by pulmonary angiography.

High Probability Ventilation-Perfusion Scan

If both the ventilation-perfusion scan and clinical assessment indicate a high probability of pulmonary embolism, treatment is recommended. The likelihood of pulmonary embolism is 96% (41) (Fig. 32–4). If clinical assessment is low probability or uncertain, the likelihood of pulmonary embolism is 56% and 88%, respectively. Impedance plethysmography or B-mode ultrasound will show deep venous thrombosis in approximately half (5,6), and treatment is recommended. If the noninvasive assessment of the leg veins is negative, the likelihood of pulmonary embolism becomes 39% in patients with a low probability clinical assessment and 79% in patients with an uncertain clinical assessment. Further evaluation by pulmonary angiography is recommended.

In PIOPED, 72% of patients had either an intermediate (indeterminate) probability ventilation-perfusion scan or a clinical assessment that indicated a probability of pulmonary embolism that was discordant with the probability indicated by the ventilation-perfusion scan (41). The risk of pulmonary embo-

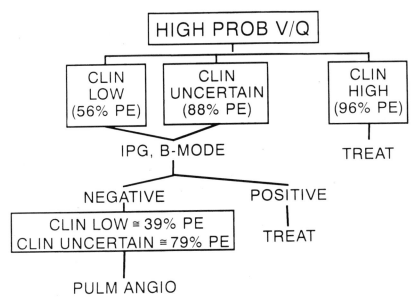

Figure 32–4.   Strategy based on a single noninvasive leg test and clinical assessment for diagnosis of patients with a high probability (High Prob) ventilation-perfusion (V/Q) scan. Pulm Angio, pulmonary angiogram; Clin, clinical; IPG, impedance plethysmography; B-mode, B-mode ultrasound; PE, pulmonary embolism. (Reprinted with permission from Stein PD, Hull RD, Saltzman HA, et al. Strategy for diagnosis of patients with suspected acute pulmonary embolism. Chest 1993;103:1553–1559.)

lism in these patients was 16 to 88% (average 34%). This strategy would reduce by 52% the need for pulmonary angiography (15).

Strategy Based on Serial Noninvasive Leg Tests

At the time of publication of this strategy for the noninvasive diagnosis of thromboembolic disease in patients with suspected acute pulmonary embolism, evaluations of serial noninvasive leg tests for deep venous thrombosis had been published (9,42), but data were insufficient for inclusion in a recommended approach. Subsequently, sufficient data were acquired to provide narrow confidence limits for the rate of recurrent pulmonary embolism among patients with suspected pulmonary embolism who had adequate cardiorespiratory reserve and who had serial noninvasive tests of the legs that were negative for proximal vein thrombosis (9,43). Among patients with adequate cardiorespiratory reserve who have a negative single noninvasive leg test, approximately 3% will show deep venous thrombosis with serial noninvasive leg tests. Although some patients with pulmonary embolism will not show deep venous thrombosis with a single noninvasive leg test or with serial noninvasive leg tests, only 0.6% of such patients suffer recurrent pulmonary embolism, and only 0.2% suffer a fatal recurrent pulmonary embolism (43).

A useful and easily followed strategy for the diagnosis of thromboembolic disease (pulmonary embolism and/or deep venous thrombosis) that incorpo-

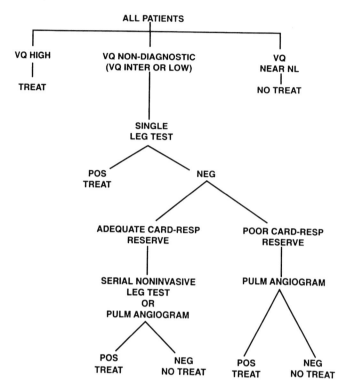

Figure 32–5. Diagram showing strategy for diagnosis of thromboembolic disease that employs serial leg tests. (Reprinted with permission from Stein PD, Hull RD, Pineo G. Strategy that includes serial noninvasive leg tests for diagnosis of thromboembolic disease in patients with suspected acute pulmonary embolism based on data from PIOPED. Arch Intern Med 1995;155:2101–2104.)

rated serial noninvasive tests of the lower extremities was suggested by Dalen (22). He recommended that patients with high probability ventilation-perfusion scans receive treatment and patients with normal ventilation-perfusion scans not receive treatment. He suggested that patients with nondiagnostic ventilation-perfusion scans undergo serial leg examinations, or perhaps pulmonary angiography, if the clinical suspicion of pulmonary embolism is very high.

We presented a strategy for diagnosing thromboembolic disease that complements the strategy recommended by Dalen (22) and adds new data related to serial noninvasive leg tests (21). Pathways in the strategy of diagnosing thromboembolic disease in patients with suspected acute pulmonary embolism are shown in Figure 32–5 (21). If the ventilation-perfusion lung scan is high probability for pulmonary embolism, treatment is recommended. If the ventilation-perfusion scan is nearly normal, it is recommended that the patient receive no treatment, and no further tests are necessary. If the ventilation-perfusion scan is nondiagnostic (intermediate probability or low probability), a single noninvasive leg test is recommended. If the single noninvasive leg test is positive, treatment is recommended. If the single noninvasive leg test is negative, we recommend serial noninvasive leg tests or pulmonary angiography, depending on the cardiorespiratory reserve of the patient. In patients with adequate cardiorespiratory reserve, we recommend serial noninvasive leg tests, although pulmonary angiography is optional. In patients with inadequate cardiorespiratory reserve, we recommend a pulmonary angiogram.

We used data from PIOPED only in patients who had a measurement of the PaO_2 to stratify according to adequate or poor cardiorespiratory reserve (21). Among such patients who had a high probability ventilation-perfusion scan, pulmonary embolism was present in 76 of 89 (85%). Although we recommend treatment if the ventilation-perfusion scan is high probability for pulmonary embolism, a single noninvasive leg test in such patients may be considered optional, and it may assist in guiding management. For example, if the single noninvasive leg test is negative in a patient with a high probability ventilation-perfusion scan, the probability of pulmonary embolism diminishes to 75%. If the risk of major bleeding with anticoagulants is high, pulmonary angiography may be considered in such patients before initiating anticoagulant therapy (42). If, however, a single noninvasive leg test is positive, therapy with anticoagulants could be initiated with confidence.

With the strategy that was based on serial noninvasive leg tests, we did not stratify patients according a clinical assessment of likelihood of pulmonary embolism (21). However, if the ventilation-perfusion scan is high probability for pulmonary embolism, but the clinical assessment is low probability, the frequency of pulmonary embolism in such patients is 56% (39). In such patients, a single noninvasive leg test might be performed and if deep venous thrombosis is not shown, a pulmonary angiogram would be recommended. If the ventilation-perfusion scan is low probability for pulmonary embolism and the clinical assessment is concordantly low likelihood, the probability of pulmonary embolism in such patients, based on data from PIOPED, is only 4% (41). Such patients perhaps require no further testing, although a single noninvasive leg test would reduce the probability of undiagnosed thromboembolic disease even further. In these instances, combined prior clinical assessment with the ventilation-perfusion reading is quite useful.

Pulmonary angiography would be required in 71% of all patients with suspected acute pulmonary embolism if no noninvasive leg tests were performed (21). If only a single noninvasive leg test were performed according to this strategy, pulmonary angiography would be required in 63%. If serial noninvasive leg tests were used where appropriate, the need for pulmonary angiography would be further reduced to 29%. The strategy was shown to be cost effective (45).

Among patients with poor cardiorespiratory reserve, the risk of even a small recurrent pulmonary embolism might be dangerous. Such patients, therefore, require pulmonary angiography for a definitive diagnosis or exclusion of acute pulmonary embolism. Serial leg tests, at the present time, are not recommended for such patients.

Even though anticoagulant treatment of proximal deep venous thrombosis and of acute pulmonary embolism is the same (46), the ventilation-perfusion lung scan is a pivotal test and should be performed as soon as possible in all patients with suspected acute pulmonary embolism (47). The reason is that if symptoms occur during anticoagulant therapy, it is important to know if there is a recurrent pulmonary embolism, which represents a failure of therapy of patients with deep venous thrombosis or pulmonary embolism.

A strategy based on the use of ventilation-perfusion lung scans and serial noninvasive leg tests is cost effective (48). However, an incalculable long-term advantage is present in management of a patient in whom there is certainty of the clinical diagnosis. In some instances, it may be advantageous to know if pulmonary embolism occurred, irrespective of the presence or absence of deep venous thrombosis.The physician should use judgment in obtaining tests that assist in the best management of the patient. Factors that affect the choice of pulmonary angiography versus serial noninvasive leg tests are their availability, reliability of the patient, the patient's ability to return for serial tests, and the risks of pulmonary angiography in the particular patient. The experience of the angiographic laboratory and of the angiographer should also be considered.

As more experience is obtained with the use of D-dimer in the exclusion of pulmonary embolism and deep venous thrombosis, algorithms may be developed that include this test (Chapter 10). One such decision analysis already has been proposed (49). It uses a negative D-dimer test result to exclude pulmonary embolism in patients with inconclusive lung scan interpretations and a low or intermediate likelihood clinical assessment (49). The investigators cautioned that a negative D-dimer result should not be interpreted to exclude pulmonary embolism in a patient with a high clinical likelihood and/or a high probability ventilation-perfusion lung scan. At the present time, extreme caution has been recommended in the use of D-dimer tests because of limited data (47, 50). Some recommended that if there is only a low level of clinical suspicion, a normal plasma D-dimer may strengthen the likelihood that no thromboembolic disease is present (47).

REFERENCES

1. Sevitt S, Gallagher N. Venous thrombosis and pulmonary embolism: a clinico-pathological study in injured and burned patients. Br J Surg 1961;48:475–489.
2. Cohn R, Walsh J. The incidence and anatomical site of origin of pulmonary emboli. Stanford Med Bull 1946;4:97–99.
3. Short DS. A survey of pulmonary embolism in a general hospital. Brit Med J 1952;1:790–796.
4. Byrne JJ, O'Neil EE. Fatal pulmonary emboli. A study of 130 autopsy-proven fatal emboli. Am J Surg 1952;83:47–54.
5. Hull RD, Hirsh J, Carter CJ, et al. Pulmonary angiography, ventilation lung scanning, and venography for clinically suspected pulmonary embolism with abnormal perfusion lung scan. Ann Intern Med 1983;98:891–899.
6. Hull RD, Hirsh J, Carter CJ, et al. Diagnostic value of ventilation-perfusion lung scanning in patients with suspected pulmonary embolism. Chest 1985;88:819–828.
7. Hull RD, Raskob GE, Coates G, et al. A new noninvasive management strategy for patients with suspected pulmonary embolism. Arch Intern Med 1989;149:2549–2555.
8. Hull RD, Raskob GE, Hirsh J. The diagnosis of clinically suspected pulmonary embolism. Practical approaches. Chest 1986;89(Suppl):417S–425S.
9. Huisman MV, Buller HR, ten Cate JW, et al. Serial impedance plethysmography for suspected deep venous thrombosis in outpatients. The Amsterdam general practitioner study. N Engl J Med 1986;314:823–828.
10. Hull RD, Hirsh J, Carter CJ, et al. Diagnostic efficacy of impedance plethysmography for clinically suspected deep-vein thrombosis. A randomized trial. Ann Intern Med 1985;102:21–28.

11. Hull R, Hirsh J, Sackett DL, et al. Cost effectiveness of clinical diagnosis, venography, and noninvasive testing in patients with symptomatic deep-vein thrombosis. N Engl J Med 1981;304:1561–1567.
12. Bone RC. Ventilation/perfusion scan in pulmonary embolism. "The emperor is incompletely attired." JAMA 1990;263:2794–2795.
13. Secker-Walker RH. On purple emperors, pulmonary embolism, and venous thrombosis. Ann Intern Med 1983;98:1006–1008.
14. Kelley MA, Carson JL, Palevsky HI, et al. Diagnosing pulmonary embolism: new facts and strategies. Ann Intern Med 1991;114:300–306.
15. Stein PD, Hull RD, Saltzman HA, et al. Strategy for diagnosis of patients with suspected acute pulmonary embolism. Chest 1993;103:1553–1559.
16. Byrne JJ. Phlebitis: a study of 748 cases at the Boston City Hospital. New Engl J Med 1955;253:579–586.
17. Barritt DW, Jordan SC. Anticoagulant drugs in the treatment of pulmonary embolism: a controlled trial. Lancet 1960;1:1309–1312.
18. Hermann RE, Davis JH, Holden WD. Pulmonary embolism: a clinical and pathologic study with emphasis on the effect of prophylactic therapy with anticoagulants. Am J Surg 1961;102:19–28.
19. Collins R, Scrimgeour A, Yusuf S, et al. Reduction in fatal pulmonary embolism and venous thrombosis by perioperative administration of subcutaneous heparin. New Engl J Med 1988;318:1162–1173.
20. Stein PD, Henry JW. Untreated patients with pulmonary embolism: outcome, clinical and laboratory assessment. Chest 1995;107:931–935.
21. Stein PD, Hull RD, Pineo G. Strategy that includes serial noninvasive leg tests for diagnosis of thromboembolic disease in patients with suspected acute pulmonary embolism based on data from PIOPED. Arch Intern Med 1995;155:2101–2104.
22. Dalen JE. When can treatment be withheld in patients with suspected pulmonary embolism? Arch Int Med 1993;153:1415–1418.
23. Hull R, Taylor DW, Hirsh J, et al. Impedance plethysmography: the relationship between venous filling and sensitivity and specificity for proximal vein thrombosis. Circulation 1978; 58:898–902.
24. White RH, McGahan JP, Daschbach MM, et al. Diagnosis of deep-vein thrombosis using duplex ultrasound. Ann Intern Med 1989;111:297–304.
25. Becker DM, Philbrick JT, Abbitt PL. Real time ultrasonography for the diagnosis of lower extremity deep venous thrombosis. Arch Intern Med 1989;149:1731–1734.
26. Hull R, Hirsh J, Sackett DL, et al. Replacement of venography in suspected venous thrombosis by impedance plethysmography and [135]I-fibrinogen leg scanning. Ann Int Med 1981;94:12–15.
27. Douketis JD, Ginsberg JS. Diagnostic problems with venous thromboembolic disease in pregnancy. Haemostasis 1995;25:58–71.
28. Moser KM, LeMoine JR. Is embolic risk conditioned by location of deep venous thrombosis? Ann Intern Med 1981;94:439–444.
29. Stein PD, Evans H. An autopsy study of leg vein thrombosis. Circulation 1967;35:671–681.
30. Rossle R. Uber die Bedeutung und die entstehung der wadenvenenthrombosen. Virchow Arch Path Anat 1937;300:180– 189.
31. Putzer R. Die wadenvenenthrombose in ihrer beziehung zur architektur der wade. Arch Gynaek 1939;169:444–452.
32. Hunter WC, Sneeden VD, Robertson TD, et al. Thrombosis of the deep veins of the leg. Arch Intern Med 1941;68:1–17.
33. Hunter WC, Krygier JJ, Kennedy JC, et al. Etiology and prevention of thrombosis of the deep leg veins: a study of 400 cases. Surgery 1945;17:178–190.
34. Neumann R. Ursprungszentren und entwicklungsformen der bein-thrombose. Virchow Arch Path Anat 1938;301:708–735.

35. Greenstein J. Thrombosis and pulmonary embolism. South Afr Med J 1945;19:350–356.
36. Raeburn C. The natural history of venous thrombosis. Brit Med J 1951;2:517–520.
37. Gibbs NM. Venous thrombosis of the lower limbs with particular reference to bedrest. Brit J Surg 1957;45:209–236.
38. Huisman MV, Buller HR, ten Cate JW. Utility of impedance plethysmography in the diagnosis of recurrent deep-vein thrombosis. Arch Int Med 1988;148:681–683.
39. Kolecki RV, Sigel B, Justin J, et al. Determining the acuteness and stability of deep venous thrombosis by ultrasonic tissue characterization. J Vasc Surg 1995;21:976–984.
40. Stein PD, Terrin ML, Hales CA, et al. Clinical, laboratory, roentgenographic and electrocardiographic findings in patients with acute pulmonary embolism and no pre-existing cardiac or pulmonary disease. Chest 1991;100:598–603.
41. A collaborative study by the PIOPED Investigators. Value of the ventilation/perfusion scan in acute pulmonary embolism: results of the Prospective Investigation of Pulmonary Embolism Diagnosis (PIOPED). JAMA 1990; 263:2753–2759.
42. Hull RD, Rascob GE, Carter CJ. Serial impedance plethysmography in pregnant patients with clinically suspected deep-vein thrombosis. Ann Intern Med 1990:112:663–667.
43. Hull RD, Raskob GE, Ginsberg JS, et al. Noninvasive strategy for the treatment of patients with suspected pulmonary embolism. Arch Int Med 1994;154:289–297.
44. Stein PD, Hull RD. Relative risks of anticoagulant treatment of acute pulmonary embolism based upon an angiographic diagnosis versus a noninvasive diagnosis. Chest 1994;106:727–730.
45. Hull RD, Feldstein W, Stein PD, et al. Cost effectiveness of pulmonary embolism diagnosis. Arch Intern Med 1996;156;68–72.
46. Hyers TM, Hull RD, Weg JG. Antithrombotic therapy for venous thromboembolic disease. Chest 1995;108(Suppl): 335S–351S.
47. ACCP Consensus Committee on Pulmonary Embolism. Opinions regarding the diagnosis and management of venous thromboembolism. Chest 1996;109:233–237.
48. Hull RD, Feldstein W, Stein PD, et al. Cost effectiveness of pulmonary embolism diagnosis. Arch Intern Med 1996;156:68–72.
49. Perrier A, Bounameaux H, Morabia A, et al. Contribution of D-dimer plasma measurement and lower-limb venous ultrasound to the diagnosis of pulmonary embolism: a decision analysis model. Am Heart J 1994;127:624–635.
50. Moser KM. Diagnosing pulmonary embolism. D-dimer needs rigorous evaluation. Brit Med J 1994;309:1525–1526.

Prevention of Deep Venous Thrombosis

The risks of deep venous thrombosis differ according to the predisposing illness or operative procedure. Risk factors for deep venous thrombosis, as reviewed in the Fourth Consensus Conference on Antithrombotic Therapy (1), are listed in Table 33–1. Pooled data indicate a risk of deep venous thrombosis of the calves ± thighs detected by fibrinogen uptake tests after general surgery of 25% (1) (Table 33–2). The risk of deep venous thrombosis is comparable after acute myocardial infarction (24%) or elective neurosurgery (24%), but nearly doubles after stroke (47%), elective hip replacement (51%), or hip fracture (48%) (Table 33–2). Studies of hip replacement and hip fracture were with venography.

Low Dose Unfractionated Heparin

Low dose unfractionated heparin (5000 U subcutaneously starting 2 hours before surgery and continuing every 8 hours or 12 hours for 7 days, or until the patient is fully ambulatory or discharged from the hospital) has been proven to reduce deep venous thrombosis after general surgery to 8% and has been shown to reduce deep venous thrombosis after acute MI to 7% (1) (Table 33–2). Low dose unfractionated heparin was only modestly effective after ischemic stroke (26% deep venous thrombosis), hip replacement (34% deep venous thrombosis), hip fracture (27% deep venous thrombosis), and knee replacement (34% deep venous thrombosis) (1) (Table 33–2).

Low dose unfractionated heparin after general surgery does not increase the incidence of major hemorrhagic complications resulting in reoperation, transfusion, or death, although the rate of wound hematoma is higher (2,3). Low dose unfractionated heparin should be used with caution in patients in whom prosthetic material is being implanted, because the risk of infection may be increased by a regional hematoma (4). Similarly, caution is advised with the use of low dose unfractionated heparin in patients with a high likelihood of wound infection (contaminated cases) or impaired healing.

Table 33–1. RISK FACTORS FOR DEEP VENOUS THROMBOSIS

Advanced age
Prolonged immobility
Paralysis
Prior deep venous thrombosis or pulmonary embolism
Cancer
Major surgery
Obesity
Varicose veins
Heart failure
Myocardial infarction
Fractures of pelvis, hip, leg
High dose estrogen (possibly)
Protein C resistance
Protein C deficiency
Antithrombin III deficiency
Protein S deficiency
Dysfibrinogenemia
Disorders of plasminogen and plasminogen activation
Antiphospholipid antibodies
Lupus anticoagulant
Heparin induced thrombocytopenia
Polycythemia vera
Hyperviscosity syndromes

Based on Clagett and associates (1).

Low Molecular Weight Heparin

Low molecular weight heparin appears slightly better than low dose unfractionated heparin in preventing deep venous thrombosis and pulmonary embolism after general surgery, and may be associated with slightly fewer bleeding problems (1) (Table 33–2). Most trials of low molecular weight heparin employed a fixed dose once or twice a day without laboratory control (4).

Low molecular weight heparin was effective in preventing deep venous thrombosis after hip replacement, but pooled data suggest that it was only modestly effective in preventing deep venous thrombosis after hip fracture and after knee replacement (Table 33–2).

Aspirin

Aspirin showed little or no benefit in preventing deep venous thrombosis after general surgery, hip replacement, hip fracture, and knee replacement (Table 33–2).

Dextran

Dextran does not prevent deep venous thrombosis as well as low dose unfractionated heparin, but it appears effective in stopping the growth and extension of thrombi, so that pulmonary embolism is prevented (5). Dextran

Table 33-2. PREVENTION OF DEEP VENOUS THROMBOSIS

	General Surgery %DVT*	Acute MI %DVT*	Stroke %DVT*	Elective Neurosurg %DVT	Hip Replace %DVT**	Hip Fracture %DVT**	Knee Replace %DnVT**
No Treatment	25	24	47	24	51	48	61
Low Dose Heparin Unfractionated	8	7	26	6	34	27	34
Adjusted Dose Heparin	—	—	—	—	11	—	—
Low Molecular Weight Heparin	5	—	10	—	15	27	30
Aspirin	20	—	—	—	56	34	79
Dextran	16	—	—	—	30	—	—
Oral Anticoagulant INR 2.0–3.0	—	—	—	—	20	24	47
Two-step Warfarin	—	—	—	—	28	—	—
Intermittent Pneumatic Compression	10	—	—	7	22	—	11
Graded Compression Elastic Stockings	9	—	—	9	38	—	—

Key: Data are pooled data obtained from (1,4)
* Fibrinogen uptake
** Venogram
Adjusted dose heparin = Partial thromboplastin time adjusted to upper range of normal

Two-step warfarin = Very low dose warfarin preoperatively, INR 2.0–3.0 postoperatively
MI = Myocardial Infarction
Replace = Replacement
Neurosurg = Neurosurgery

275

is expensive, and must be administered intravenously. It is contraindicated in patients with renal insufficiency and in patients with poor cardiac function. Anaphylactic reactions have occurred with dextran. Wound hematomas appear to be less common with dextran than with low dose unfractionated heparin (3, 5). Dextran was also only modestly effective in preventing deep venous thrombosis after general surgery and hip replacement (Table 33–2).

Oral Anticoagulants

Oral anticoagulants (INR 2.0–3.0) were more effective in preventing deep venous thrombosis in patients undergoing hip replacement than low dose unfractionated heparin. Warfarin was not as effective as low molecular heparin or adjusted dose heparin (unfractionated heparin adjusted to keep the activated partial thromboplastin time at the upper range of normal). Two-step warfarin (very low dose warfarin administered to prolong the prothrombin time only 1 or 2 sec starting 14 days before operation followed by INR 2.0 to 3.0 after operation) did not augment the effectiveness of warfarin (Table 33–2). Warfarin was not as effective as low dose unfractionated heparin or low molecular heparin after knee replacement (Table 33–2).

Intermittent Pneumatic Compression

Intermittent pneumatic compression is effective in reducing the frequency of deep venous thrombosis after general surgery and elective neurosurgery (Table 33–2). After neurosurgery, intermittent pneumatic compression is particularly useful because the procedure brings no risk of bleeding. After elective hip replacement, intermittent pneumatic compression is almost as effective as oral anticoagulants (Table 33–2). It appears to be more effective than warfarin, low molecular weight heparin, or low dose unfractionated heparin after knee replacement (Table 33–2). However, the number of patients enrolled in trials of prophylaxis using intermittent pneumatic compression (366 patients) is considerably fewer than in trials of low molecular weight heparin (1354 patients) (1). Intermittent pneumatic compression and low molecular weight heparin have not been directly compared in prospective investigations. Clagett and associates felt that the risk reductions for deep venous thrombosis are probably comparable with intermittent pneumatic compression and low molecular weight heparin, and they could not recommend one prophylaxis over the other (1).

Graded Compression Elastic Stockings

Graded compression elastic stockings after general surgery and elective neurosurgery seemed to reduce the frequency of deep venous thrombosis, but such elastic stockings failed to produce much benefit after hip replacement (Table 33–2). The data regarding elastic stockings should be interpreted guardedly, however, because high risk patients were specifically excluded in some studies (4,6,7), and patients with malignant disease have not been evaluated in sufficient numbers. Presumably, using graded compression elastic stockings with appropriate antithrombotic drugs would give better protection against deep venous thrombosis than either approach alone, but combined prophylactic measures have not been studied (1).

Recommendations for Prevention of Venous Thromboembolism

Recommendations for prevention of venous thromboembolism, made by the Fourth American College of Chest Physicians Consensus Conference on Antithrombotic Therapy (1), paraphrased, are:

1. Low-risk general surgery patients less than 40 years of age who are undergoing minor operations and have no clinical risk factors require no specific prophylaxis other than early ambulation.
2. In patients undergoing major surgery who are over 40 years of age but have no additional risk factors for venous thromboembolism, low dose unfractionated heparin (given 2 hours before and every 12 hours after operation), graded compression elastic stockings or intermittent pneumatic compression is recommended. Graded compression elastic stockings and intermittent pneumatic compression, when used, should be applied during the operation, if possible, as well as throughout the postoperative period.
3. In higher risk patients who are over the age of 40 years who are undergoing major operations and have additional risk factors, low dose unfractionated heparin (every 8 hours) or low molecular weight heparin is recommended.
4. In higher risk patients who are over the age of 40 years, undergoing major operations, have additional risk factors, and are prone to wound complications such as hematomas or infection, dextran or intermittent pneumatic compression would be a good alternative to low dose unfractionated heparin or low molecular weight heparin.
5. In very high risk general surgery patients with multiple risk factors such as previous venous thromboembolic disease, malignancy, orthopedic surgery, hip fracture, stroke or spinal cord injury, it is recommended that low dose unfractionated heparin, low molecular weight heparin, or dextran be combined with intermittent pneumatic compression. Intermittent pneumatic compression should be applied intraoperatively if possible.
6. In selected high risk general surgery patients, perioperative warfarin therapy [International Normalized Ratio (INR) 2.0 to 3.0] may be used.
7. Aspirin should not be used for prophylaxis in patients undergoing general surgery because other measures, as recommended above, are more efficacious.
8. In patients undergoing total hip replacement, postoperative subcutaneous twice daily fixed dose unmonitored low molecular weight heparin, or heparin in doses adjusted to keep the activated partial thromboplastin time (APTT) in the upper normal range, or oral anticoagulants (INR 2.0–3.0, started preoperatively or immediately after operation) are recommended for routine use. Graded compression elastic stockings or intermittent pneumatic compression may provide additional protection. Although other agents such as low dose unfractionated heparin, aspirin, and dextran reduce the overall

incidence of venous thromboembolism, they are less effective and should not be used routinely. [Note: Although Clagett and associates recommended a twice daily fixed dose, Hull and associates believe that with some preparations of low molecular weight heparin, a single daily dose is satisfactory (8).]

9. In patients undergoing total knee replacement, intermittent pneumatic compression and low molecular weight heparin (twice daily fixed dose, unmonitored) provide comparable reductions of risk, and either is recommended for routine use.

10. In patients undergoing surgery for hip fractures, either oral anticoagulant therapy (INR 2.0–3.0) or low molecular weight heparin (twice daily fixed dose, unmonitored) is recommended.

11. Placement of a prophylactic inferior vena cava filter in orthopedic surgery patients should be limited to high risk patients in whom other forms of anticoagulant-based prophylaxis are not feasible because of active bleeding.

12. In patients undergoing intracranial neurosurgery, intermittent pneumatic compression with or without graded compression elastic stockings is recommended. Low dose heparin therapy may be an acceptable alternative. A combination of intermittent pneumatic compression with low dose unfractionated heparin may be more effective than either one individually and should be considered in high risk patients.

13. In patients with acute spinal cord injury with paralysis, adjusted dose heparin or low molecular weight heparin is recommended for prophylaxis. Warfarin prophylaxis may also be effective. Intermittent pneumatic compression, graded compression elastic stockings, and low dose unfractionated heparin appear ineffective when used alone and are not recommended. However, these methods may have benefit when used together.

14. In patients with multiple trauma, intermittent pneumatic compression, warfarin, or low molecular weight heparin is recommended when feasible. Serial surveillance with duplex ultrasonography may be a successful strategy. In selected very high risk patients, prophylactic caval filter placement may be used.

15. In patients with acute myocardial infarction, low dose unfractionated heparin is recommended for prevention of deep venous thrombosis. Full dose anticoagulation is also effective. Intermittent pneumatic compression and possibly graded compression elastic stockings may be useful when heparin therapy is contraindicated.

16. In patients with ischemic stroke and lower extremity paralysis, low dose heparin or low molecular weight heparin is recommended. Intermittent pneumatic compression and graded compression elastic stockings are also probably effective, but have not been tested in such patients.

17. In general medical patients with clinical risk factors for deep venous thrombosis and pulmonary embolism, particularly patients with heart failure and patients with chest infections, low dose unfractionated heparin or low molecular weight heparin is recommended.

18. In patients with long term indwelling central venous catheters, warfarin 1 mg daily is recommended to prevent axillary-subclavian venous thrombosis.

REFERENCES

1. Clagett GP, Anderson FA, Heit J, et al.Prevention of venous thromboembolism. Chest 1995;108:312S–334S.

2. Collins R, Scrimgeour A, Yusuf S, et al. Reduction in fatal pulmonary embolism and venous thrombosis by perioperative administration of subcutaneous heparin. N Engl J Med 1988;318:1162–1173.
3. Clagett GP, Reisch JS. Prevention of venous thromboembolism in general surgical patients: results of meta-analysis. Ann Surg 1988;208:227–240.
4. Clagett GP, Anderson FA Jr, Levine MN, et al. Prevention of venous thromboembolism. Chest 1992;102:391S–407S.
5. Gruber UF, Saldeen T, Brokop T, et al. Incidences of fatal postoperative pulmonary embolism after prophylaxis with dextran 70 and low-dose heparin: an international multicentre study. Brit Med J 1980;280:69–72.
6. Turner GM, Cole SE, Brooks JH. The efficacy of graduated compression stockings in the prevention of deep vein thrombosis after major gynaecological surgery. Br J Obstet Gynaecol 1984;91:588–591.
7. Allan A, Williams JT, Bolton JP, et al. The use of graduated compression stockings in the prevention of postoperative deep vein thrombosis. Br J Surg 1983;70:172–174.
8. Hull R, Raskob G, Pineo G, et al. A comparison of subcutaneous low-molecular-weight heparin with warfarin sodium for prophylaxis against deep-vein thrombosis after hip or knee implantation. N Eng J Med 1993;329:1370–1376.

34

Antithrombotic Treatment of Deep Venous Thrombosis and Acute Pulmonary Embolism

WARFARIN

International Normalized Ratio

The prothrombin time ratio as well as the prothrombin time are dependent upon the thromboplastin reagent (1). An International Normalized Ratio (INR), based upon a World Health Organization standard thromboplastin, was defined, which permits reporting of the prothrombin time ratio in a standardized fashion. This permits comparison of the anticoagulant effect, irrespective of the local thromboplastin reagent used for measuring the prothrombin time.

The INR is calculated as follows:

$$INR = (Prothrombin\ Time\ Ratio)^{ISI}$$

where ISI is International Sensitivity Index of the thromboplastin reagent used for measuring the prothrombin time. The Prothrombin Time Ratio (the ratio of patient prothrombin time to control prothrombin time) is measured in the local laboratory. The ISI is a measure of the responsiveness of a given thromboplastin to a reduction of the vitamin K-dependent coagulation factor, compared with the international reference preparation (1). The value of the ISI for commercial thromboplastins is now indicated by many manufacturers on the reagent packages, and therefore, is easily reported by the laboratory. The INR is calculated simply by raising the prothrombin time ratio to the ISI power. For example, if the patient prothrombin time is 18 sec and the control prothrombin time is 12 sec, the prothrombin time ratio is 1.5. If the ISI is 2, then INR = 1.5^2 = 2.25.

The ISI of commercial thromboplastin reagents varies according to manufacturer, and it varies from batch to batch. Most thromboplastins used in the United States vary from 1.8 to 2.8 (2). Most thromboplastins used in the United

Kingdom, and in many parts of Scandinavia and The Netherlands, have ISI values of 1.0 to 1.1 (1).

The range of INR recommended for treatment of deep venous thrombosis or acute pulmonary embolism is 2.0 to 3.0. This is considered "less intense warfarin" compared with the range of INR recommended for preventing thrombosis in mechanical prosthetic heart valves (INR 2.5–3.5) (1,3).

Administration of Warfarin

The prothrombin time may become prolonged before a full anticoagulant effect is reached. This is a result of a rapid reduction of factor VII, which has a half-life of 6 to 7 hours (4). Full anticoagulant activity is delayed 72 to 96 hours after the administration of warfarin because the half-lives of prothrombin, factor IX, and factor X are considerably longer than the half-life of factor VII (5). Protein C and protein S are vitamin K dependent natural anticoagulants that are also affected by warfarin. The potential exists for the early anticoagulant effect of warfarin to be counteracted by a reduction of protein C, because the half life is short, similar to factor VII (1,6). Warfarin-induced skin necrosis has been attributed to this reduction in protein C (1).

Warfarin therapy should begin with a maintenance dose, or perhaps twice the predicted maintenance dose (11). Larger loading doses are not recommended (1). If there is an urgent need for antithrombotic therapy, heparin is indicated, and heparin is recommended to be continued 4 to 5 days after the prothrombin time is in the therapeutic range (1).

Warfarin should not be used during the first trimester of pregnancy because of the risk of embryopathy or fetal bleeding (1,7). If possible, it should be avoided throughout pregnancy (1). Heparin is preferred if anticoagulants are indicated in pregnancy (1). Warfarin, in nursing mothers, appears not to induce an anticoagulant effect in the breast-fed infant (8,9).

Risk of Major Hemorrhage with Warfarin

The average risk of major hemorrhagic complications among patients with thromboembolic disease treated with "less intense" warfarin (INR = 2.0–3.0) is 1.7% (10–12). Major hemorrhagic complications in general were more frequent among patients treated for thromboembolic disease with higher levels of the INR (10,13,14). Major bleeding was defined as overt bleeding associated with a reduction of hemoglobin ≥ 2 gm/dl, blood transfusion ≥ 2 units, intracerebral bleed, retroperitoneal bleed, pericardial bleed, bleeding that required a surgical intervention, bleeding into a major joint, or bleeding into the eye.

UNFRACTIONATED HEPARIN

Dosage

The unit of heparin is measured in animals using a biologic assay (15). Units of unfractionated may vary as much as 50% on a weight basis, and therefore, unfractionated heparin is properly prescribed by units, not weight (15). For the treatment of deep venous thrombosis, either intravenous (11,16) or subcutaneous (17,18) unfractionated heparin has been adequate, provided that the activated partial thromboplastin time (APPT) has been within the therapeutic range.

A blood level of heparin between 0.2 and 0.4 U/ml (protamine titration) inhibits thrombus propagation (19,20). In general, an activated partial thromboplastin time more than 1.5 times control or 1 to 5 times mean normal values corresponded to a blood level of 0.2 U/ml (15,21–23). Failure to achieve an APTT >1.5 times control in the initial treatment of proximal deep venous thrombosis was associated with a risk of recurrent deep venous thrombosis or pulmonary embolism of 20 to 25% (11). If the APTT was greater than 1.5 times control, recurrent deep venous thrombosis or pulmonary embolism was infrequent (24). Heparin requirements are usually greatest in the first few days after an acute thromboembolic event (25–27). Therapy, therefore should be monitored closely during that period. Unfortunately, the APTT does not always correlate reliably with blood heparin levels or the antithrombotic activity (15). The APTT can be shortened by increased levels of clotting factors such as factor VIII (15). The anticoagulant effect of unfractionated heparin can be suppressed by heparin binding proteins in plasma (28).

A trend suggested that patients whose blood level of unfractionated heparin was measured directly had fewer recurrences of deep venous thrombosis or pulmonary embolism and less bleeding (19). If the hospital laboratory does not measure heparin blood levels directly, it would be useful to determine the range of the APTT that corresponds to blood levels of heparin between 0.2 and 0.4 U/ml (15). With fixed blood levels of heparin, values of the APTT may change if the APTT reagent is changed or a different batch is used (15). The therapeutic range of the APTT ratio in many laboratories is higher than 1.5 to 2.5 times the mean of a normal reference range (20). No international reference APTT reagent exists that allows development of a normalized ratio for heparin analogous to the international normalized ratio (INR) for warfarin. It seems prudent, therefore, to establish a reference range in each laboratory (15).

Risk of Major Hemorrhage with Unfractionated Heparin

The risk of major hemorrhagic complications (defined as with warfarin) among patients treated with therapeutic doses of unfractionated heparin for thromboembolic disease, whether intermittent intravenous, continuous intravenous infusion or subcutaneous, in doses over 24 hours ranging from 29,180 U to 40,320 U was 3.4 to 7.8% (11,18,29,30). The average risk of major bleeding with therapeutic unfractionated heparin for thromboembolic disease in contemporary studies that used a continuous intravenous infusion or high dose subcutaneous injection was approximately 5% (31). These risks have been stratified according to whether the patients were at high risk of bleeding or low risk of bleeding (12). Among patients at high risk (surgery within previous 14 days, history of peptic ulcer disease, gastrointestinal or genitourinary tract bleeding, disorders predisposing to bleeding, thrombotic studies within 14 days, or platelet count <150 X 10^9/L), the frequency of major bleeding from heparin was 10.8%

(12). Among patients at low risk of bleeding, the frequency of major bleeding with heparin was 1.1%.

Other Complications of Therapy with Unfractionated Heparin

Although bleeding is the major complication of unfractionated heparin, thrombocytopenia is an important and frequent complication among patients receiving therapeutic doses. Frequent monitoring of the platelet count, therefore, is essential. Thrombocytopenia occurred in 15.6% of patients who received bovine unfractionated heparin and 5.8% who received porcine unfractionated heparin (32). Thrombocytopenia may occur within hours after beginning therapy with unfractionated heparin, although it usually occurs between 3 and 15 days after beginning heparin (32,33). The platelet count usually returns to baseline levels within 4 days of stopping therapy (34), but persistent thrombocytopenia may occur. Thrombocytopenia is uncommon (less than 1%) in patients who receive low dose heparin (35,36). Heparin-induced thrombocytopenia can be complicated by thrombosis caused by platelet-rich thrombi (37). An immunologic basis for heparin-induced thrombocytopenia and thrombosis has been proposed (38). Rarely, unfractionated heparin may induce skin necrosis. Histologic features are consistent with a hypersensitive angiitis (39).

Osteoporosis is unlikely in patients treated with unfractionated heparin for ≤ 3 months at doses $\leq 20,000$ U/24 hours (14). Most osteoporosis occurred in patients treated with unfractionated heparin in doses of at least 20,000 U/day for more than 6 months (39).

Low Molecular Weight Heparin

Low molecular weight heparins are used for the treatment of deep venous thrombosis and pulmonary embolism in many countries, but have not yet received regulatory approval in the United States (15). The anticoagulant response observed with a given dose was highly correlated with body weight (40). Low molecular weight heparin is effective when given in standard doses (Factor Xa units per kilogram body weight) without laboratory monitoring (15).

Low molecular weight heparin administered subcutaneously twice a day was as effective and safe as continuous intravenous unfractionated heparin in the initial treatment of deep venous thrombosis (41–44). The long-term rate of recurrent deep venous thrombosis was comparable with standard therapy and with unfractionated heparin (43). Low molecular weight heparin administered subcutaneously once a day was also shown to be as effective as continuous intravenous unfractionated heparin in the initial treatment of deep venous thrombosis (45). Low molecular weight heparin appears useful for treating patients with uncomplicated deep venous thrombosis in an outpatient setting (44).Findings of clinical trials apply only to the particular low molecular weight heparin evaluated (15). Properties of a particular low molecular weight heparin cannot be extrapolated to a different low molecular weight heparin.

Antithrombotic Treatment of Deep Venous Thrombosis and Pulmonary Embolism

The long-term outcome of patients with acute deep venous thrombosis has been assessed (46). Most patients (79%) received conventional anticoagulant therapy, and 2% had inferior vena cava filters inserted. Pulmonary embolism or deep venous thrombosis recurred in 18 of 124 (15%) patients after 6 to 8 years. Among those with recurrent thromboembolism, the majority (16 of 18) were recurrent deep venous thrombosis, 1 of 18 was pulmonary embolism and 1 of 18 was unstated. The cumulative incidence of thromboembolism was 6% at 1 year and 13% at 5 years. Recurrence was more common in patients younger than 65 years who had a history of recurrent venous thromboembolism, 34% compared with 10% among other patients.

Anticoagulant therapy of pulmonary embolism has shown excellent results. The cumulative mortality from pulmonary embolism in PIOPED among 399 patients (73% treated only with anticoagulants) was 1.3% in 1 day, 2.0% in 1 week, 2.3% in 2 weeks, and 2.5% in 1 year (47). The cumulative rate of recurrent pulmonary embolism was 4.0% in 1 week and 8.3% in 1 year. Twenty-seven percent of episodes of recurrent pulmonary embolism were fatal. Among patients who died of pulmonary embolism, 90% died of recurrent pulmonary embolism.

Acute pulmonary embolism in patients with isolated deep calf vein thrombosis has been reported (48,49). It is now generally agreed that isolated deep calf vein thrombosis should either be treated with heparin followed by oral anticoagulants, or the patient should be followed by serial noninvasive leg tests for 14 days (50). The safety of following untreated patients with serial noninvasive leg tests has been shown (51–53).

Recommendations of Fourth American College of Chest Physicians Consensus Conference on Antithrombotic Therapy

The antithrombotic treatment of pulmonary embolism is the same as the antithrombotic therapy of deep venous thrombosis. Recommendations, paraphrased from the Fourth American College of Chest Physicians Consensus Conference on Antithrombotic Therapy (15), are as follows:

1. Patients with deep venous thrombosis or pulmonary embolism should be treated with intravenous unfractionated heparin or subcutaneous unfractionated heparin sufficient to prolong the activated partial thromboplastin time (APTT) to a range that corresponds to a plasma heparin level of 0.2 to 0.4 U/mL.
2. Treatment with unfractionated heparin should be continued for 5 to 10 days and oral anticoagulation should be overlapped with heparin therapy for 4 to 5 days. For many patients, heparin and warfarin therapy can be started together and heparin therapy discontinued on day 5 or 6 if the prothrombin time is therapeutic. For massive pulmonary embolism or iliofemoral thrombosis, a longer period of therapy with unfractionated heparin may be considered.

3. In many countries, low molecular weight heparin is used in place of unfrac-tionated heparin. Dosing requirements are individualized for each product. Low molecular weight heparin should be administered for 5 to 10 days and therapy overlapped with oral anticoagulation as outlined in No. 2 above.

4. Long-term anticoagulant therapy should be continued for at least 3 months using oral anticoagulants to prolong the prothrombin time to an International Normalized Ratio (INR) of 2.0 to 3.0. When oral anticoagulants are either contraindicated or inconvenient, unfractionated heparin should be given to prolong the APTT to a time that corresponds to a plasma heparin level greater than 0.2 U/mL. This heparin level should be attained at or beyond the mid-dose interval.

5. Patients with recurrent venous thrombosis or a continuing risk factor, such as antithrombin III deficiency, protein C or S deficiency, lupus anticoagulant, or malignancy, should be treated indefinitely.

6. Symptomatic isolated deep calf vein thrombosis should be treated with anti-coagulants for 3 months. If for any reason anticoagulation cannot be given, serial noninvasive studies of the lower extremities should be performed to assess for proximal extension of deep venous thrombosis.

7. The use of thrombolytic agents in the treatment of venous thromboembolism continues to be highly individualized. Further clinical investigation is needed before more definite recommendations can be made.

8. Inferior vena caval filter placement is recommended when there is a contrain-dication or complication of anticoagulant therapy in an individual with or at high risk for proximal vein thrombosis or pulmonary embolism. It is also recommended for recurrent thromboembolism that occurs despite adequate anticoagulation, in the presence of a large free-floating vena caval thrombus, in the patient with chronic recurrent embolism with pulmonary hypertension, and during the concurrent performance of surgical pulmonary embolectomy or pulmonary endarterectomy. Whenever possible, anticoagulation should be given following placement of a vena caval filter in a patient with proximal deep vein thrombosis of the lower extremity.

Approaches to Antithrombotic Management and Follow-up That Were Not Addressed by the American College of Chest Physicians Conference on Antithrombotic Therapy

Differences of opinion exist about some aspects of the antithrombotic management and follow-up of patients with suspected acute pulmonary embo-lism not addressed by the American College of Chest Physicians Conference on Antithrombotic Therapy (15). Opinions of several physicians and a clinical epidemiologist experienced in pulmonary embolism were obtained on these issues (50). One issue is whether heparin should be administered immediately, before diagnostic studies are completed, if pulmonary embolism is suspected on the basis of clinical evaluation. Most believe that the risk of recurrent un-treated acute pulmonary embolism during the period of diagnostic tests exceeds the risks of bleeding from heparin (50). Therefore, the immediate administration of heparin is often recommended. Some reserve the immediate administration of heparin for those with poor cardiopulmonary reserve. The issue may be best resolved based upon the speed with which diagnostic tests can be obtained, the level of likelihood of suspected acute pulmonary embolism, the severity of the suspected acute pulmonary embolism, the cardiopulmonary status, and the potential risk of bleeding with heparin.

Whether bed rest is mandatory in patients with deep venous thrombosis or pulmonary embolism once therapeutic anticoagulation has been achieved is undetermined, and no data are available to guide an opinion on this subject. Concern that early ambulation may dislodge thrombi in the lower extremities led many physicians to restrict patients to bed rest after a diagnosis of deep venous thrombosis or pulmonary embolism was made. Most believe, however, that bed rest is not mandatory in patients with deep venous thrombosis or pulmonary embolism once therapeutic levels of anticoagulants have been achieved (50). Some suggest that in patients with symptomatic deep venous thrombosis, bed rest is appropriate until inflammation and swelling subside. In such patients, use of a bedside commode may be appropriate. In patients with less extensive symptoms, initiation of progressive ambulation appears reasonable after therapeutic levels of anticoagulants have been achieved (50).

Another area of difference of opinion is whether a follow-up noninvasive test of the lower extremities should be performed at the time of proposed cessation of anticoagulant therapy in patients with deep venous thrombosis or pulmonary embolism. Some believe that a follow-up study of the lower extremities would be cost effective only in patients with a continuing predisposition to pulmonary embolism and deep venous thrombosis (50). A follow-up noninvasive leg study is useful in assessing recurrent deep venous thrombosis after the initiation of therapy, particularly if it converts from negative initially to positive at the time that the recurrence of pulmonary embolism or deep venous thrombosis is suspected. The impedance plethysmogram is especially useful because it normalizes in the majority of patients (54). A 2 mm or greater increase in diameter of the thrombus on ultrasound also has been shown to indicate recurrent deep venous thrombosis (55). Magnetic resonance imaging of the legs is sensitive and specific (56), but the expense is high relative to other noninvasive leg tests.

The question of whether follow-up diagnostic studies for acute pulmonary embolism should include a repeat ventilation-perfusion scan is not entirely resolved. Some believe that a follow-up ventilation-perfusion lung scan should be performed (50). The value of a repeat ventilation-perfusion scan would be to seek an anatomic or pathologic explanation for failure of the patient to regain baseline performance or to serve as a new baseline to assess new symptomatic episodes. Sixteen percent of patients fail to achieve 90% resolution of the perfusion scan (57). Twenty-eight percent of patients with prior cardiopulmonary disease fail to show complete resolution of the perfusion scan (57). It would be useful to identify these patients.

A follow-up ventilation-perfusion scan is particularly useful at 3 months after the acute pulmonary embolism because any resolution that occurs on the ventilation-perfusion scan occurs within 3 months (57). Some prefer a ventilation-perfusion scan at the time of hospital discharge. Their primary purpose for obtaining the ventilation-perfusion scan is to serve as a new baseline to evaluate any suspected recurrent pulmonary embolism after the initial hospital discharge.

Some believe that a follow-up ventilation-perfusion scan would not be cost effective because significant recurrent pulmonary embolism is uncommon (8% in PIOPED) (47) in appropriately treated patients. Also, most patients, particularly those with no prior cardiopulmonary disease, return nearly to baseline perfusion after appropriate anticoagulant treatment for acute pulmonary embolism (57). Some, therefore, recommend a ventilation-perfusion scan only in patients who seem to have a high risk for recurrence (50). This group might include patients with coagulopathies, malignant disease, or a continuing predisposition to deep venous thrombosis, or patients in whom pulmonary embolism has already recurred.

REFERENCES

1. Hirsh J, Dalen JE, Deykin D, et al. Oral anticoagulants: mechanism of action, clinical effectiveness, and optimal therapeutic range. Chest 1992;102(Suppl):312S–326S.
2. Bussey HI, Force RW, Bianco TM, et al. Reliance on prothrombin time ratios causes significant errors in anticoagulation therapy. Arch Intern Med 1992;152:278–282.
3. Stein PD, Alpert JS, Copeland J, et al. Antithrombotic therapy in patients with mechanical and biological prosthetic heart valves. Chest 1992;102(Suppl):445S–455S.
4. O'Reilly RA, Aggeler PM. Determinants of the response to oral anticoagulant drug in man. Pharmacol Rev 1970;22:35–96.
5. Hellemans J, Vorlat M, Verstraete M. Survival time of prothrombin and factors VII, IX, and X after complete synthesis blocking doses of coumarin derivatives. Br J Haematol 1963;9:506–512.
6. Vigano S, Mannucci PM, Solinas S, et al. Decrease in protein C antigen and formation of an abnormal protein soon after starting oral anticoagulant therapy. Br J Haematol 1984;57:213–220.
7. Hall JAG, Pauli RM, Wilson KM. Maternal and fetal sequelae of anticoagulation during pregnancy. Am J Med 1980;68:122–140.
8. McKenna R, Cale ER, Vasan U. Is warfarin sodium contraindicated in the lactating mother? J Pediatr 1983;103:325–327.
9. Lao TT, DeSwiet M, Letsky SE, et al. Prophylaxis of thromboembolism in pregnancy: an alternative. Br J Obstet Gynecol 1985;92:202–206.
10. Hull R, Hirsh J, Jay R, et al. Different intensities of oral anticoagulant therapy in the treatment of proximal-vein thrombosis. N Engl J Med 1982;307:1676–1681.
11. Hull RD, Raskob GE, Hirsh J, et al. Continuous intravenous heparin compared with intermittent subcutaneous heparin in the initial treatment of proximal-vein thrombosis. N Engl J Med 1986;315:1109–1114.
12. Hull RD, Raskob GE, Rosenbloom D, et al. Heparin for 5 days versus for 10 days in the initial treatment of proximal venous thrombosis. N Engl J Med 1990;322:1260–1264.
13. Hull R, Delmore T, Genton E, et al. Warfarin sodium versus low dose heparin in the long term treatment of venous thromboembolism. N Engl J Med 1979;301:855–858.
14. Hull R, Delmore T, Carter C, et al. Adjusted subcutaneous heparin versus warfarin sodium in the long term treatment of venous thrombosis. N Engl J Med 1982;306:189–194.
15. Hyers TM, Hull RD, Weg JG. Antithrombotic therapy for venous thromboembolic disease. Chest 1995;108(Suppl):335S–351S.
16. Brandjes DPM, Heijboer H, Buller HR, et al. Acenocoumarol and heparin compared with acenocoumarol alone in the initial treatment of proximal vein thrombosis. N Eng J Med 1992;327:1485–1489.

17. Doyle DJ, Turpie AG, Hirsh J, et al. Adjusted subcutaneous heparin or continuous intravenous heparin in patients with acute deep vein thrombosis: a randomized trial. Ann Intern Med 1987;107:441–445.
18. Pini M, Pattacini C, Quintavalla R, et al. Subcutaneous vs intermittent heparin in the treatment of deep vein thrombosis—a randomized clinical trial. Thromb Haemost 1990;64:222–226.
19. Levine MN, Hirsh J, Gent M, et al. A randomized trial comparing activated thromboplastin time with heparin assay in patients with acute venous thromboembolism requiring large daily doses of heparin. Arch Intern Med 1994;154:49–56.
20. Brill-Edwards P, Ginsberg JS, Johnston M, et al. Establishing a therapeutic range for heparin therapy. Ann Intern Med 1993;119:104–109.
21. Gitel SN, Wesler S. The antithrombotic effects of warfarinand heparin following infusions of tissue thromboplastin in rabbits: clinical implication. J Lab Clin Med 1979;94:481–488.
22. Wesler S, Reimer L, Freiman R, et al. Serum-induced thrombosis: studies of its induction and evolustion under controlled conditions in vivo. Cirulation 1959;20:864–874.
23. Chiu HM, Hirsh J, Yung WL, et al. Relationship between the anticoagulant and antithrombotic effects of heparin in experimental venous thrombosis. Blood 1977;49:171–184.
24. Basu D, Gallus A, Hirsh J, et al. A prospective study of the value of monitoring heparin treatment with the activated partial thromboplastin time. N Eng J Med 1972;287:324–327.
25. Simon TL, Hyers TM, Gaston JP, et al. Heparin pharmokinetics: increased requirements in pulmonary embolism. Br J Haemotol 1978;39:111–120.
26. Hirsh J, van Aken WG, Gallus AS. Heparin kinetics in venous thrombosis and pulmonary embolism. Circulation 1976;53:691–695.
27. Cipolle RJ, Seifert RD, Neilan BA, et al. Heparin kinetics: variables related to disposition and dosage. Clin Pharmacol Ther 1982;29:387–393.
28. Young E, Pruis M, Levine MN, et al. Heparin binding to plasma proteins: and important mechanism for heparin resistance. Thromb Haemost 1992;67:639–643.
29. Doyle DJ, Turpie AGG, Hirsh J, et al. Adjusted subcutaneous heparin or continuous intravenous heparin in patients with acute deep vein thrombosis: a randomized trial. Ann Intern Med 1987;107:441–445.
30. Hull RD, Raskob GE, Pineo GF, et al. Subcutaneous low-molecular-weight heparin compared with continuous intravenous heparin in the treatment of proximal-vein thrombosis. New Engl J Med 1993;326:975–982.
31. Levine MN, Hirsh J, Landefeld S, et al. Hemorrhagic complications of anticoagulant treatment. Chest 1992;102(Suppl):352S–363S.
32. King DJ, Kelton JG. Heparin-associated thrombocytopenia. Ann Intern Med 1984;100:535–540.
33. Warkentin TE, Kelton JG. Heparin-induced thrombocytopenia. In: Creger WP, ed. Annual review in medicine. California: Annual Review Medicine Inc., 1989;40:31–44.
34. Hirsch J, Raschke R, Warkentin TE, et al. Heparin: mechanism of action, pharmacokinetics, dosing considerations, monitoring, efficacy and safety. Chest 1995;108(Suppl):258S–275S.
35. Galle PC, Muss HB, McGrath KM, et al. Thrombocytopenia in two patients treated with low-dose heparin. Obstet Gynecol 1978;52(supp):9S–11S.
36. Phillips YY, Copley JB, Stor RA. Thrombocytopenia and low-dose heparin. South Med J 1983;76:526–528.
37. Glock Y, Szmil E, Boudjema B, et al. Cardiovascular surgery and heparin-induced thrombocytopenia. Int Angio 1988;7:238–245.
38. Rhodes GR, Dixon RH, Silver D. Heparin-induced thrombocytopenia: eight cases with thrombotic-hemorrhagic complications. Ann Surg 1977;186:752–758.

39. Hirsh J, Dalen JE, Deykin D, et al. Heparin: mechanism of action, pharmacokinetics, dosing considerations, monitoring, efficacy, and safety. Chest 1992;102(Suppl): 337S–351S.
40. Matzsch T, Bergqvist D, Hedner U, et al. Effects of an enzymatically depolymerized heparin as compared with conventional heparin in healthy volunteers. Thromb Haemost 1987;57:97–101.
41. Prandoni P, Vigo M, Cattelan AM, et al. Treatment of deep venous thrombosis by fixed doses of a low-molecular-weight heparin (CY216). Haemostasis 1990;20 (Suppl1):220–223.
42. Prandoni P, Lensing AWA, Buller HR, et al. Comparison of subcutaneous low molecular weight heparin with intravenous standard heparin in proximal vein thrombosis. Lancet 1992;339:441–445.
43. Hull RD, Raskob GE, Pineo GF, et al. Subcutaneous low-molecular-weight heparin compared with continuous intravenous heparin in the treatment of proximal-vein thrombosis. New Engl J Med 1992; 326:975–982.
44. Levine M, Gent M, Hirsh J, et al. A comparison of low-molecular-weight heparin administered primarily at home with unfractionated heparin administered in the hospital for proximal deep-vein thrombosis. N Eng J Med 1996;334:677–681.
45. Simonneau G, Charbonnier B, Decousus H, et al. Subcutaneous low molecular weight heparin compared with continuous intravenous unfractionated heparin in the treatment of proximal deep vein thrombosis. Arch Intern Med 1993;153:1541–1546.
46. Beyth R, Cohen AM, Landefeld CS. Long-term outcomes of deep-vein thrombosis. Arch Intern Med. 1995;155:1031–1037.
47. Carson JL, Kelley MA, Duff A, et al. The clinical course of pulmonary embolism. N Engl J Med 1992;326:1240–1245.
48. Pellegrini VD Jr, Langhans MJ, Totterman S, et al. Embolic complications of calf thrombosis following hip arthroplasty. J Arthroplasty 1993;8:449–457.
49. Lagerstedt CI, Olsson C-G, Fagher BO, et al. Need for long term anticoagulant treatment in symptomatic calf-vein thrombosis. Lancet 1985;2:515–518.
50. ACCP Consensus Committee on Pulmonary Embolism.Opinions regarding the diagnosis and management of venous thromboembolism. Chest 1996;109:233–237.
51. Huisman MV, Buller HR, ten Cate JW, et al. Serial impedance plethysmography for suspected deep venous thrombosis in outpatients. The Amsterdam general practitioner study. New Engl J Med 1986;314:823–828.
52. Huisman MV, Buller HR, ten Cate JW. Utility of impedance plethysmography in the diagnosis of recurrent deep-vein thrombosis. Arch Intern Med 1988;148:681–683.
53. Hull RD, Raskob GE, Carter CJ. Serial impedance plethysmography in pregnant patients with clinically suspected deep-vein thrombosis. Ann Intern Med 1990;112: 663–667.
54. Huisman MV, Buller HR, ten Cate JW. Utility of impedance plethysmography in the diagnosis of recurrent deep-vein thrombosis. Arch Intern Med 1988;148:681–683.
55. Prandoni P, Cogo A, Bernardi E, et al. A simple approach for detection of recurrent proximal-vein thrombosis. Circulation 1993;88(Part1):1730–1735.
56. Evans AJ, Sostman HD, Knelson MH, et al. Detection of deep venous thrombosis: prospective comparison of MR imaging with contrast venography. Am J Roent 161:1993;131–139.
57. Urokinase Pulmonary Embolism Trial. Perfusion lung scanning. Circulation 1973;47(SupplII):46–50.

35

Relative Risks of Anticoagulant Therapy Based on an Angiographic versus a Noninvasive Diagnosis

If all patients with suspected acute pulmonary embolism underwent pulmonary angiography, those in whom the angiogram was negative would have undergone the risks of angiography, but would have been spared the risks of unnecessary treatment with anticoagulants. If all patients with suspected acute pulmonary embolism were treated on the basis of a noninvasive assessment, some who did not have pulmonary embolism would be treated unnecessarily and undergo the risks of therapy with anticoagulants, although they would be spared the risks of pulmonary angiography. If the risks of pulmonary angiography and anticoagulant therapy are known, and the probability of pulmonary embolism is also known, a physician can assess the relative risks of treatment based on an angiographic diagnosis versus a noninvasive diagnosis (1). We assessed the relative risks of pulmonary angiography and treatment with anticoagulants among patients treated on the basis of a pulmonary angiographic diagnosis versus patients treated on the basis of a noninvasive diagnosis (1). A noninvasive diagnosis could be based on a ventilation-perfusion lung scan combined with clinical assessment and a single negative test for deep venous thrombosis (2). Serial tests for deep venous thrombosis may also be used (3–6) (Chapter 32).

Risks of Pulmonary Angiography

The frequency of major complications in the Prospective Investigation of Pulmonary Embolism Diagnosis (PIOPED) was 1.3% (7) (Chapter 26). This rate of complications occurred with experienced angiographers. Major complications were death, respiratory distress requiring cardiopulmonary resuscitation or intubation, renal failure requiring dialysis, or bleeding requiring a transfusion of ≥2 units of blood.

Major Bleeding from Heparin

The risk of major hemorrhagic complications from therapy with unfractionated heparin among patients treated for thromboembolic disease, whether intermittent intravenous, continuous infusion, or subcutaneous, in doses ranging from 29,180 U to 40,320 U over 24 hours, was 4.9% (8–11). Major bleeding was defined as overt bleeding associated with a reduction of hemoglobin ≥2 gm/dl, blood transfusion ≥2 units, intracerebral bleed, retroperitoneal bleed, pericardial bleed, bleeding that required a surgical intervention, bleeding into a major joint, or bleeding into the eye. The frequency of major bleeding from unfractionated heparin in high risk patients was 10.8% (12). High risk was defined as surgery within previous 14 days, history of peptic ulcer disease, gastrointestinal or genitourinary tract bleeding, disorders predisposing to bleeding, thrombotic studies within 14 days, or platelet count <150 × 10^9/L. The frequency of major bleeding with unfractionated heparin in patients with a low risk of bleeding was 1.1% (12).

Major Bleeding from Warfarin

The risk of major hemorrhagic complications among patients with thromboembolic disease treated with "less intense" warfarin, International Normalized Ratio (INR) = 2.0–3.0, based on pooled data, was 1.7% (8,12,13). Major hemorrhagic complications in general were more frequent among patients treated for thromboembolic disease with higher levels of the INR (13–15).

Risks of Anticoagulant Therapy: Invasive versus Noninvasive Diagnosis

Knowing the risks of major complications of pulmonary angiography, the risks of major bleeding from heparin and warfarin, and the probability of pulmonary embolism, a physician can make an informed decision about the strategy of diagnosis associated with the lowest risk of major complications. A high risk of complications of pulmonary angiography favors treatment on the basis of a noninvasive diagnosis. A low risk of angiographic complications favors treatment on the basis of an angiographic diagnosis. A high risk of bleeding favors treatment on the basis of an angiographic diagnosis. A low risk of bleeding favors treatment on the basis of a noninvasive diagnosis.

Based on assumed risks of 1.3% major complications of angiography, 4.9% major bleeding with unfractionated heparin, and 1.7% major bleeding with warfarin, the relative risks of treatment on the basis of pulmonary angiography versus a noninvasive diagnosis for patients with various probabilities of pulmonary embolism are shown in Table 35–1 and Figure 35–1 (1). Among patients with a probability of pulmonary embolism higher than 81%, anticoagulant therapy on the basis of a noninvasive diagnosis would give fewer complications. Among patients with a probability of pulmonary embolism less than 80%, an angiographic diagnosis would result in fewer complications. Among patients with a probability of pulmonary embolism of 80 to 81%, the risk of treatment

Table 35–1. RISK ASSESSMENT: ANGIOGRAPHIC DIAGNOSIS VS A
VENTILATION-PERFUSION SCAN DIAGNOSIS (ALL
PATIENTS)

Prevalence of PE (%)	Major* Bleeds in Pts diagnosed by Angio (%)	Total** Complications (%)	Risk Ratio*** Angio DX/ Scan DX
90	5.9	7.2	1.1
80	5.3	6.6	1.0
70	4.6	5.9	0.9
60	4.0	5.3	0.8
50	3.3	4.6	0.7
40	2.6	3.9	0.6
30	2.0	3.3	0.5
20	1.3	2.6	0.4
10	0.7	2.0	0.3

* Assumes 4.9% major bleeds with heparin and 1.7% major bleeds with less intense warfarin
** Assumes 1.3% major angiographic complications plus 6.6% major bleeds among patients in whom PE was diagnosed by angiography.
*** Assumes 6.6% major bleeds among patients treated on basis of a V/Q diagnosis. A risk ratio >1 favors V/Q diagnosis; a risk ratio <1 favors angiography.
Key: ANGIO = Angiographim; DX = Diagnosis;
  V/Q = Ventilation/perfusion scan; PTS = Patients
  PE = Pulmonary embolism.
Reproduced with permission from Stein PD, Hull RD.

based on an invasive diagnosis is identical to the risk of treatment based on a noninvasive assessment.

Among patients with a high risk (12.5%) of bleeding, fewer complications would occur if pulmonary angiography were performed on patients with a probability of pulmonary embolism less than 90% (Table 35–2, Fig 35–2) (1). It would be safer to treat on the basis of a noninvasive diagnosis only if the probability of pulmonary embolism were higher than 90%.

Among patients with a low risk (2.8%) of bleeding, it would be safer to treat on the basis of a noninvasive diagnosis if the probability of pulmonary embolism were higher than 56% (Table 35–3, Fig. 35–3) (1). An angiographic diagnosis in such patients would be associated with fewer risks only if the probability of pulmonary embolism were less than 52%. The risks of treatment on the basis of an angiographic versus a noninvasive diagnosis are equal in patients with a probability of pulmonary embolism of 52 to 55%.

If the risk of pulmonary angiography were only 0.4% (one- third the reported risk), with a risk of major bleeding of 6.6% with heparin followed by warfarin, it would be safer to perform angiography if the probability of pulmonary embolism were less than 94% (Table 35–4) (1). If the risk of angiography were 3.9% (triple the reported risk), it would be safer to treat on the basis of an angiographic diagnosis only if the probability of pulmonary embolism were less than 41%.

Among patients with a high risk (12.5%) of bleeding, and if the risk of major complications of angiography were 0.4% (one-third the reported risk),

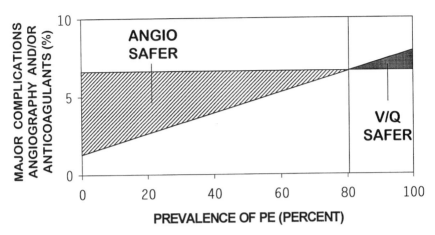

ASSUMES: 4.9% MAJOR BLEED - HEPARIN
1.7% MAJOR BLEED - WARFARIN
1.3% MAJOR COMPLICATIONS - ANGIO

Figure 35–1.   Frequency (percent) of major complications of anticoagulant therapy plus compli-cations of angiography among patients treated on the basis of an angiographic (ANGIO) diagnosis, compared with the frequency of complications among patients treated on the basis of a noninvasive (ventilation-perfusion lung scan, V/Q) diagnosis. The frequency of complications depends on the prevalence of pulmonary embolism. Calculations are based on average reported values:4.9% frequency of major bleeding with heparin,1.7% frequency of major bleeding with warfarin, and1.3% major complications from pulmonary angiography. Among patients with a probability of pulmonary embolism less than 80%, treatment on the basis of an angiographic diagnosis would be accompanied by fewer complications (cross-hatched area). Among patients with a probability of pulmonary embolism greater than 81%, treatment on the basis of a noninvasive diagnosis ventilation-perfusion scan (V/Q) diagnosis would be accompanied by fewer complications (gray area).

an angiographic diagnosis would result in fewer complications if the probability of pulmonary embolism were less than 97% (Table 35–4). If the risk of major complications of angiography were 3.9% (triple the reported risk), it would be safer to treat on the basis of an angiographic diagnosis only if the probability of pulmonary embolism were less than 69%.

Using similar logic, if the risk of major bleeding were low (2.8%), and the risk of major complications of angiography were only 0.4%, it would be safer to treat on the basis of an angiographic diagnosis if the probability of pulmonary embolism were less than 84%. If the risk of major complications of angiography were 3.9% and the risk of major bleeding only 2.8%, it would always be safer to treat the basis of a noninvasive diagnosis (Table 35–4).

Several methods can be used to calculate the probability of pulmonary embolism. The probability of pulmonary embolism can be calculated from the ventilation-perfusion scan alone, but it can be calculated with somewhat more precision if the clinical likelihood of pulmonary embolism is estimated in combi-nation with the ventilation-perfusion scan (16) (Chapter 14). Computer-based clinical assessment using neural network logic in the future may assist in reach-ing a clinical assessment (17) (Chapter 11). It is also possible to assess the

Table 35–2.   RISK ASSESSMENT FOR TREATMENT ON THE BASIS OF AN
ANGIOGRAPHIC DIAGNOSIS VS A VENTILATION-
PERFUSION SCAN DIAGNOSIS: PATIENTS WITH HIGH RISK
OF BLEEDING WITH HEPARIN

Prevalence of PE (%)	Major* Bleeds in Pts diagnosed by Angio (%)	Total** Complications (%)	Risk Ratio*** Angio DX/ Scan DX
90	11.3	12.6	1.0
80	10.0	11.3	0.8
70	8.8	10.1	0.8
60	7.5	8.8	0.7
50	6.3	7.6	0.6
40	5.0	6.3	0.5
30	3.8	5.1	0.4
20	2.5	3.8	0.3
10	1.3	2.6	0.2

* Assumes 10.8% major bleeds with heparin and 1.7% major bleeds with less intense warfarin
** Assumes 1.3% major angiographic complications plus 12.5% major bleeds among patients in whom PE was diagnosed by angiography.
*** Assumes 12.5% major bleeds among patients treated on basis of a V/Q diagnosis. A risk ratio <1 favors angiography.
Key: ANGIO = Angiographim; DX = Diagnosis;
    V/Q = Ventilation/perfusion scan; PTS = Patients;
    PE = Pulmonary embolism
Reproduced with permission from Stein PD, Hull RD.

likelihood of pulmonary embolism based upon the number of mismatched segmental defects on ventilation-perfusion lung scans (18,19) (Chapters 22,23). A more detailed likelihood of pulmonary embolism can be determined based upon stratification according to prior cardiopulmonary disease and clinical assessment (20) (Chapter 24).

These computations assess only the relative risks of major complications of angiography and anticoagulant therapy. It may be advantageous for management of the patient to know the diagnosis with certainty, as can be determined by pulmonary angiography, irrespective of the risks associated with obtaining the diagnosis. The advantages of a confident diagnosis on the basis of angiography must be balanced with the availability and convenience of obtaining a pulmonary angiogram as well as the respective costs of both diagnostic and therapeutic approaches.

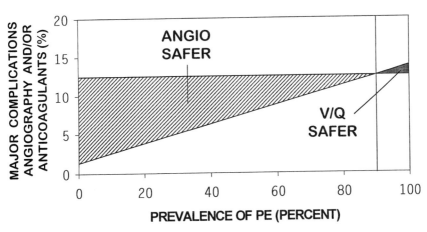

ASSUMES: 10.8% MAJOR BLEED - HEPARIN
1.7% MAJOR BLEED - WARFARIN
1.3% MAJOR COMPLICATIONS - ANGIO

Figure 35–2.   Frequency (percent) of major complications of anticoagulant therapy plus complications of angiography among patients treated on the basis of an angiographic (ANGIO) diagnosis, compared with the frequency of complications among patients treated on the basis of a noninvasive (ventilation-perfusion lung scan, V/Q) diagnosis. Calculations assume that the patient has a high risk of bleeding with heparin: 10.8% frequency of major bleeding with heparin, 1.7% frequency of major bleeding with warfarin, and 1.3% major complications from pulmonary angiography. Among patients with a probability of pulmonary embolism less than 90%, treatment on the basis of an angiographic diagnosis would be accompanied by fewer complications (cross-hatched area). Among patients with a probability of pulmonary embolism greater than 90%, treatment on the basis of a noninvasive (V/Q) diagnosis would be accompanied by fewer complications (gray area).

Table 35–3. RISK ASSESSMENT FOR TREATMENT ON THE BASIS OF AN
ANGIOGRAPHIC DIAGNOSIS VS A VENTILATION-
PERFUSION SCAN DIAGNOSIS: PATIENTS WITH LOW RISK
OF BLEEDING WITH HEPARIN

Prevalence of PE (%)	Major* Bleeds in Pts diagnosed by Angio (%)	Total** Complications (%)	Risk Ratio*** Angio DX/ Scan DX
90	2.5	3.8	1.4
80	2.2	3.5	1.3
70	2.0	3.3	1.2
60	1.7	3.0	1.1
50	1.4	2.7	1.0
40	1.1	2.4	0.9
30	0.8	2.1	0.8
20	0.6	1.9	0.7
10	0.3	1.6	0.6

* Assumes 1.1% major bleeds with heparin and 1.7% major bleeds with less intense warfarin
** Assumes 1.3% major angiographic complications plus 2.8% major bleeds among patients in whom PE was diagnosed by angiography.
*** Assumes 2.8% major bleeds among patients treated on basis of a V/Q diagnosis. A risk ratio >1 favors V/Q diagnosis; a risk ratio <1 favors angiography.
Key: ANGIO = Angiographic; DX = Diagnosis;
    V/Q = Ventilation/perfusion scan; PTS = Patients
    PE = Pulmonary embolism
Reproduced with permission from Stein PD, Hull RD.

ASSUMES: 1.1% MAJOR BLEED - HEPARIN
1.7% MAJOR BLEED - WARFARIN
1.3% MAJOR COMPLICATIONS - ANGIO

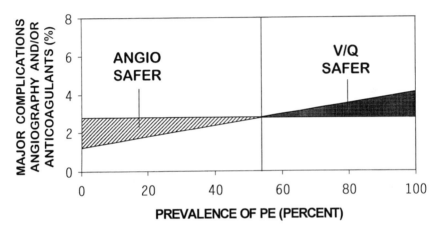

Figure 35–3.   Frequency (percent) of major complications of anticoagulant therapy plus complications of angiography among patients treated on the basis of an angiographic (ANGIO) diagnosis, compared with the frequency of complications among patients treated on the basis of a noninvasive (ventilation-perfusion lung scan, V/Q) diagnosis. Calculations assume that the patient has a low risk of bleeding with heparin:1.1% frequency of major bleeding with heparin,1.7% frequency of major bleeding with warfarin, and 1.3% major complications from pulmonary angiography. Among patients with a probability of pulmonary embolism less than 52%, treatment on the basis of an angiographic diagnosis would be accompanied by fewer complications (cross-hatched area). Among patients with a probability of pulmonary embolism greater than 55%, treatment on the basis of a noninvasive diagnosis (V/Q) diagnosis would be accompanied by fewer complications (gray area).

Table 35–4. ASSUMED RISKS OF MAJOR COMPLICATIONS OF
PULMONARY ANGIOGRAPHY AND MAJOR BLEEDING WITH
ANTICOAGULANTS AND CALCULATED PROBABILITIES OF
PULMONARY EMBOLISM WITH WHICH FEWER
COMPLICATIONS WOULD OCCUR IF TREATMENT WERE
PERFORMED ON THE BASIS OF ANGIOGRAPHY VERSUS A
VENTILATION-PERFUSION SCAN

Risk of Angiogram (%)	Risk of Bleeding (Heparin + Warfarin) (%)	Prevalence of PE Associated with Fewer Total Complications* with Angio Diagnosis (%)
0.4	2.8	<84
0.4	6.6	<94
0.4	12.5	<97
1.3	2.8	<52
1.3	6.6	<80
1.3	12.5	<90
3.9	2.8	No Patients
3.9	6.6	<41
3.9	12.5	<69

Angio = pulmonary angiogram; V/Q = ventilation/perfusion
PE = Pulmonary embolism.
* Total complications = major complications of pulmonary angiography plus major bleeds in patients in whom a diagnosis was made by angiography.
Reproduced with permission from Stein PD, Hull RD.

REFERENCES

1. Stein PD, Hull RD. Relative risks of anticoagulant treatment of acute pulmonary embolism based upon an angiographic diagnosis vs a ventilation-perfusion scan diagnosis. Chest 1994;106:727–730.
2. Stein PD, Hull RD, Saltzman HA, et al. Strategy for diagnosis of patients with suspected acute pulmonary embolism. Chest 1993;103:1553–1559.
3. Huisman MV, Buller HR, ten Cate JW, et al. Serial impedance plethysmography for suspected deep venous thrombosis in outpatients. The Amsterdam general practitioner study. N Engl J Med 1986;314:823–828.
4. Hull R, Raskob G, Coates G, et al. A new noninvasive management strategy for patients with suspected pulmonary embolism. Arch Int Med 1989;149:2549–2555.
5. Hull R, Raskob G, Ginsberg J, et al. A noninvasive strategy for the management of patients with suspected pulmonary embolism. Arch Int Med 1994;154:289–297.
6. Stein PD, Hull RD, Pineo G. Strategy that includes serial noninvasive leg tests for diagnosis of thromboembolic disease in patients with suspected acute pulmonary embolism based on data from PIOPED. Arch Intern Med 1995;155:2101–2104.
7. Stein PD, Athanasoulis C, Alavi A, et al. Complications and validity of pulmonary angiography in acute pulmonary embolism. Circulation 1992;85:462–469.
8. Hull RD, Raskob GE, Hirsh J, et al. Continuous intravenous heparin compared with intermittent subcutaneous heparin in the initial treatment of proximal-vein thrombosis. N Engl J Med 1986;315:1109–1114.

9. Doyle DJ, Turpie AG, Hirsh J, et al. Adjusted subcutaneous heparin or continuous intravenous heparin in patients with acute deep vein thrombosis: a randomized trial. Ann Intern Med 1987;107:441–445.

10. Pini M, Pattacini C, Quintavalla R, et al. Subcutaneous versus intermittent heparin in the treatment of deep vein thrombosis: a randomized clinical trial. Thromb Haemost 1990;64:222–226.

11. Hull RD, Raskob GE, Pineo GF, et al. Subcutaneous low-molecular-weight heparin compared with continuous intravenous heparin in the treatment of proximal-vein thrombosis. New Engl J Med 1992; 326:975–982.

12. Hull RD, Raskob GE, Rosenbloom D, et al. Heparin for 5 days versus for 10 days in the initial treatment of proximal venous thrombosis. N Engl J Med 1990;322:1260–1264.

13. Hull R, Hirsh J, Jay R, et al. Different intensities of oral anticoagulant therapy in the treatment of proximal-vein thrombosis. N Engl J Med 1982;307:1676–1681.

14. Hull R, Delmore T, Genton E, et al. Warfarin sodium versus low dose heparin in the long-term treatment of venous thromboembolism. N Engl J Med 1979;301:855–858.

15. Hull R, Delmore T, Carter C, et al. Adjusted subcutaneous heparin versus warfarin sodium in the long-term treatment of venous thrombosis. N Engl J Med 1982;306:189–194.

16. A collaborative study by the PIOPED Investigators. Value of the ventilation/perfusion scan in acute pulmonary embolism: results of the Prospective Investigation of Pulmonary Embolism Diagnosis (PIOPED). JAMA 1990;263:2753–2759.

17. Patil S, Henry JW, Rubenfire M, et al. Neural network in the clinical diagnosis of acute pulmonary embolism. Chest 1993;104:1685–1689.

18. Stein PD, Gottschalk A, Henry JW, et al. Stratification of patients according to prior cardiopulmonary disease and probability assessment based on the number of mismatched segmental equivalent perfusion defects: approaches to strengthen the diagnostic value of ventilation/perfusion lung scans in acute pulmonary embolism. Chest 1993;104:1461–1467.

19. Stein PD, Henry JW, Gottschalk A. Mismatched vascular defects: an easy alternative to mismatched segmental equivalent defects for the interpretation of ventilation/perfusion lung scans in pulmonary embolism. Chest 1993; 104:1468–1471.

20. Stein PD, Henry JW, Gottschalk A. The addition of clinical assessment to stratification according to prior cardiopulmonary disease further optimizes the interpretation of ventilation-perfusion lung scans in pulmonary embolism. Chest 1993;104:1472–1476.

CHAPTER

36

Thrombolytic Therapy

Early Reperfusion and Residual Impairment

A more rapid lysis of pulmonary thromboemboli occurs with thrombolytic agents than occurs spontaneously in patients treated only with anticoagulants (Fig. 36–1, Fig. 36–2) (1–3). However, pulmonary reperfusion, as shown on perfusion lung scans, was similar after 2 weeks in patients treated with thrombolytic agents and patients treated with anticoagulants (1). During the first 24 hours after therapy with urokinase, a 24% mean resolution of the perfusion lung scan occurred, whereas anticoagulants alone produced only an 8% mean resolution (1). By 14 days, a 55 to 56% resolution of the perfusion lung scan occurred in patients treated with urokinase and in patients treated with anticoagulants. At 12 months, a 77 to 79% resolution of the perfusion lung scans was seen in the two treatment groups.

Complete resolution of the perfusion lung scans occurred in 88% of patients with no prior cardiopulmonary disease by 1 year after treatment with urokinase (1). Similarly, complete resolution by 1 year occurred in 91% of patients with no prior cardiopulmonary disease who were treated with anticoagulants. Of patients who had prior cardiopulmonary disease, 77% showed complete resolution 1 year after treatment with urokinase and 72% treated only with anticoagulants showed complete resolution 1 year after the acute pulmonary embolism.

Although residual perfusion defects are comparable after 1 year among patients treated with thrombolytic agents and patients treated with anticoagulants alone, the pulmonary diffusing capacity of carbon monoxide (DLCO) after 1 year was higher among patients who received thrombolytic therapy (4). At 1 year after pulmonary embolism, among 21 patients treated with anticoagulants, compared with 19 patients treated with thrombolytic agents, the DLCO was 72% predicted versus 93% predicted (4). Others observed a continuing impairment of DLCO in 10 patients treated with anticoagulants, although the perfusion lung scan tended to return to normal (5).

Survival with Thrombolytic Therapy

In view of the accelerated dissolution of pulmonary emboli, and more rapid improvement of pulmonary perfusion and pulmonary artery pressure,

300

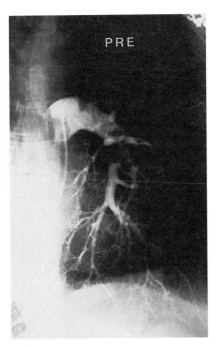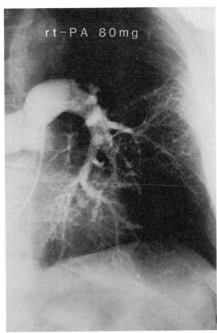

Figure 36–1. **Left.** Angiogram of the left pulmonary artery showing pulmonary embolism before thrombolytic therapy. **Right.** Angiogram 2 hours after the administration of recombinant tissue plasminogen activator (rt-PA) 80 mg. The pulmonary angiogram shows less obstruction after t-PA. (Reprinted with permission from A collaborative study by the PIOPED investigators. Tissue plasminogen activator for the treatment of acute pulmonary embolism. Chest 1990;97:528–33.)

most believe that thrombolytic therapy may be life-saving in seriously compromised patients with massive pulmonary embolism. No trials with sufficiently large numbers of patients have been conducted to prove this.

Among stable patients, the Urokinase Pulmonary Embolism Trial showed no statistically significant improvement of mortality among patients treated with urokinase and patients treated with anticoagulants (6). No significant difference in recurrence rate of pulmonary embolism was evident either. However, among patients with right ventricular dysfunction associated with pulmonary embolism, a trend suggested a lower rate of recurrent pulmonary embolism among those treated with tissue plasminogen activator (t-PA) (3).

Risk of Major Hemorrhage with Thrombolytic Therapy

The frequency of major bleeding from t-PA among patients with pulmonary embolism diagnosed by angiography, based on pooled data (3,7–10), is 12.6% (11). The definition of major bleeding was the same as with warfarin (Chapter 34). All investigators excluded patients at a high risk of bleeding, such as those who had recent surgery, recent biopsy, peptic ulcer disease, blood dyscrasia, or severe hepatic or renal disease. The reported patients, therefore, had low

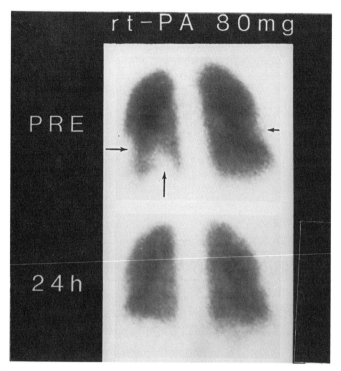

Figure 36–2. **Top.** Perfusion scan, posterior view, of a patient with pulmonary embolism before administration of recombinant tissue plasminogen activator (rt-PA) 80 mg. **Bottom.** Perfusion scan, posterior view, 24 hours after therapy. A diminution of the perfusion defections (arrows) occurred by 24 hours. (Reprinted with permission from A collaborative study by the PIOPED investigators. Tissue plasminogen activator for the treatment of acute pulmonary embolism. Chest 1990;97:528–33.)

risk of bleeding. Factors that may increase the risk of thrombolytic therapy are listed in Table 36–1 (8).

Indications for Thrombolytic Therapy

The indications for thrombolytic therapy are related to the risks, which are considerable, and the benefits, which are greatest on the first day. The established benefits of thrombolytic therapy are a more rapid lysis of thromboemboli than would occur with anticoagulants alone. Long-term benefits are uncertain. Thrombolytic therapy is not indicated for the routine treatment of pulmonary embolism. Most agree that hypotension and continuing hypoxemia, while the patient receives high fractions of inspired oxygen (FIO₂) concentration, are indications for an intervention (12). There is disagreement on the best intervention in such patients (12). Intravenous thrombolytic therapy is by far the most extensively investigated and most frequently used option. The selection of intravenous thrombolytic therapy, reduced dose thrombolytic therapy delivered by pulse spray directly into the embolus, open embolectomy, catheter-tip embo-

Table 36–1. FACTORS THAT INCREASE THE RISK OF THROMBOLYTIC THERAPY FOR ACUTE PULMONARY EMBOLISM

1. Pregnancy at any stage and the first ten days postpartum.
2. Uncontrolled hypertension, i.e., diastolic blood pressure >110 mm Hg by several measurements or hypertensive retinopathy with hemorrhages or exudates.
3. Bleeding diathesis.
4. History of major gastrointestinal bleeding within 6 months or symptoms of active gastrointestinal diseases which have a propensity to bleed.
5. Renal insufficiency (creatinine >3.0 mg/dl).
6. Severe hepatic insufficiency.
7. Evidence of a lesion known to be associated with intracranial hemorrhage including cerebral malignancy, aneurysm, abscess or head trauma.
8. History of cerebrovascular disease.
9. Neurosurgery within six months.
10. Any surgical or invasive procedure including biopsies, deep tissue aspirations, depot injections, unsuccessful attempts at central line placement or removal of successfully placed central lines (e.g., subclavian or internal jugular) within 10 days of study entry; previous arterial punctures of femoral or brachial are relative contraindications.
12. Placement of a central venous line within 48 hours.
13. Ophthalmologic surgery within six weeks.
14. Cardiopulmonary resuscitation (1 minute or more of external cardiac massage) within 2 weeks.

Reproduced with modifications from a collaborative study by the PIOPED investigators. Tissue plasminogen activator for the treatment of acute pulmonary embolism. Chest 1990;97:528–33 with permission.

lectomy, or catheter-tip fragmentation depends upon the experience of the physician and the availability of the procedure.

Many disagree whether the presence of right ventricular dysfunction on the echocardiogram is an indication for thrombolytic therapy or some other intervention (12). Interventricular septal motion, elevated right ventricular end-diastolic diameter, or tricuspid regurgitant blood velocity was abnormal by echocardiography-Doppler in the majority of patients with acute pulmonary embolism (13). Hypokinesis or asynergic motion of the right ventricular free wall was shown in 81% of patients with massive pulmonary embolism (14). Pooled data from a mixture of patients with pulmonary embolism of any severity—massive, subacute (recurrent over 6 weeks), and a few chronic—showed right ventricular dilatation in 90% and paradoxical or hypokinetic motion of the interventricular septum in 79% (15). A higher frequency of recurrent pulmonary embolism occurred in patients with right ventricular hypokinesis than in patients with normal right ventricular function (16). In patients with right ventricular hypokinesis, a trend suggested a lower rate of recurrent pulmonary embolism among those treated with thrombolytic agents (3). Most believe that these data are sparse and insufficient to make a recommendation for therapy based on the echocardiogram alone (12). Many believe that even if right ventricular dysfunction is shown, if clinical judgment, based in part upon the absence of tachypnea, tachycardia, and reliance upon supplemental oxygen, indicates that the patient is not in severe distress, an intervention is not necessary (12).

Evidence of a residual impairment of the diffusion capacity of carbon monoxide among patients treated only with anticoagulants has led to consideration of a more liberal use of thrombolytic therapy (4, 5). In the absence of further evidence that thrombolytic therapy has a long-term beneficial effect, most reserve thrombolytic therapy for patients who are hypotensive or hypoxic on high levels of oxygen (12).

Regimens of Thrombolytic Therapy

Standard regimens approved by the Food and Drug Administration (FDA) for treatment with thrombolytic therapy (17) are:

1. Streptokinase 250,000 IU over 30 minutes followed by 100,000 IU/hr for 24 hours
2. Urokinase 4,400 IU/kg/hr over 10 minutes followed by 4,400 IU/kg/hr for 12 to 24 hours
3. t-PA 100 mg (50 million IU)/2 hr

Potentially advantageous regimens of thrombolytic therapy, not fully evaluated, are:

1. Urokinase 15,000 IU/kg over 10 minutes (18)
2. t-PA 0.6 mg/kg (max 50 mg) over 2 minutes (19)

It is recommended that heparin be discontinued during thrombolytic therapy and that heparin therapy be reinstituted upon discontinuation of thrombolytic therapy. A nonsignificant increased risk of cerebral hemorrhage with heparin and thrombolytic agents in the treatment of myocardial infarction has been observed (20–22). None of the FDA-approved regimens uses concomitant heparin (17).

Low Dose Thrombolytic Therapy

Low doses of streptokinase or urokinase, administered directly into the affected pulmonary artery, particularly if administered with heparin, have shown potentially beneficial effects in small numbers of patients (23–27). This form of administration of thrombolytic therapy has not been pursued and is not standard. Even low doses of thrombolytic agents have caused major bleeding (23,24).

REFERENCES

1. National Cooperative Study. The Urokinase Pulmonary Embolism Trial: perfusion lung scanning. Circulation 1973;47(SupplII):46–50.
2. Dalla-Volta S, Palla A, Santolicandro A, et al. PAIMS-2: alteplase combined with heparin versus heparin in the treatment of acute pulmonary embolism. Plasminogen Activator Italian Multicenter Study 2. J Am Coll Cardiol 1992;20:520–526.
3. Goldhaber SZ, Haire WD, Feldstein ML, et al. Alteplase versus heparin in acute pulmonary embolism: randomised trial assessing right-ventricular function and pulmonary perfusion. Lancet 1993;341:507–511.
4. Sharma GVRK, Burleson VA, Sasahara AA. Effect of thrombolytic therapy on pulmonary-capillary blood volume in patients with pulmonary embolism. N Engl J Med 1980;303:842–845.

5. Wimalaratna HSK, Farrell J, Lee HY. Measurement of diffusing capacity in pulmonary embolism. Resp Med 1989;83:481–485.
6. National Cooperative Study. The Urokinase Pulmonary Embolism Trial. Morbidity and mortality. Circulation 1973; 47/48(SupplII):66–72.
7. Verstraete M, Miller GAH, Bounameaux H, et al. Intravenous and intrapulmonary recombinant tissue-type plasminogen activator in the treatment of acute massive pulmonary embolism. Circulation 1988;77:353–360.
8. A collaborative study by the PIOPED investigators. Tissue plasminogen activator for the treatment of acute pulmonary embolism. Chest 1990;97:528–33.
9. Goldhaber SZ, Kessler CM, Heit J, et al. Randomised controlled trial of recombinant tissue plasminogen activator versus urokinase in the treatment of acute pulmonary embolism. Lancet 1988;2:293–298.
10. Goldhaber SZ, Kessler CM, Heit JA, et al. Recombinant tissue-type plasminogen activator versus a novel dosing regimen of urokinase in acute pulmonary embolism: a randomized controlled multicenter trial. J Am Coll Cardiol 1992;20:24–30.
11. Stein PD, Hull RD, Raskob G. Risks of major bleeding in patients with acute pulmonary embolism who are candidates for thrombolytic therapy: consideration of noninvasive management. Ann Intern Med 1994;121:313–317.
12. ACCP Consensus Committee on Pulmonary Embolism. Opinion regarding the diagnosis and management of venous thromboembolism. Chest 1996;109:233–237.
13. Nazeyrollas P, Metz D, Chapoutot L, et al. Diagnostic accuracy of echocardiography-Doppler in acute pulmonary embolism. Int J Cardiol 1995;47:273–280.
14. Kasper W, Geibel A, Tiede N, et al. Distinguishing between acute and subacute massive pulmonary embolism by conventional and Doppler echocardiography. Br Heart J 1993;70:352–356.
15. Konstantinides S, Geibel A, Kasper W. Role of cardiac ultrasound in the detection of pulmonary embolism. Seminars Resp and Crit Care Med 1996;17:39–49.
16. Wolfe MW, Lee RT, Feldstein ML, et al. Prognostic significance of right ventricularhypokinesis and perfusion lung scan defects in pulmonary embolism. Am Heart J 1994;127:1371–1375.
17. Goldhaber S. Evolving concepts in thrombolytic therapy for pulmonary embolism. Chest 1992;101(Suppl):183S–185S.
18. Petipretz P, Simmoneau G, Cerrina J, et al. Effects of a single bolus of urokinase in patients with life-threatening pulmonary embolism: a descriptive trial. Circulation 1984;70:861.
19. Levine M, Hirsh J, Weitz J, et al. A randomized trial of a single bolus dosage regimen of recombinant tissue plasminogen activator in patients with acute pulmonary embolism. Chest 1990; 98:1473–1479.
20. Sleight P. Is there an age limit for thrombolytic therapy? Am J Cardiol 1993;72:30G–33G.
21. Grines CL, DeMaria AN. Optimal utilization of thrombolytic therapy for acute myocardial infarction: concepts and controversies. J Am Coll Cardiol 1990;16:223–231.
22. ISIS-3 (Third International Study of Infarct Survival) Collaborative Group. ISIS-3: a randomised comparison of streptokinase versus tissue plasminogen activator versus anistreplase and of aspirin plus heparin versus aspirin alone among 41,299 cases of suspected acute myocardial infarction. Lancet 1992;i:1–18.
23. Leeper KV, Popovich J Jr, Lesser BA, et al. Treatment of massive acute pulmonary embolism: the use of low doses of intrapulmonary arterial streptokinase combined with full doses of systemic heparin. Chest 1988;93:234–240.
24. Gallus AS, Hirsh J, Cade JF, et al. Thrombolysis with a combination of small doses of streptokinase and full doses of heparin. Semin Thromb Hemostas 1975;2:14–32.
25. Vujic I, Young JWR, Gobien RP, et al. Massive pulmonary embolism: treatment with full heparinization and topical low-dose streptokinase. Radiology 1983;148:671–675.

26. Ambrose JE, Venditto M, Dickerson WH. Local fibrinolysis for the treatment of massive pulmonary embolism: efficacy of streptokinase infusion through pulmonary arterial catheter. J Am Osteopath Assoc 1985;85:97–101.
27. Edwards IR, MacLean KS, Dow JD. Low-dose urokinase in major pulmonary embolism. Lancet 1973;2:409–413.

CHAPTER 37

Relative Risks of Thrombolytic Therapy Based on an Angiographic Versus a Noninvasive Diagnosis

Hesitancy among physicians to administer thrombolytic agents to patients with acute pulmonary embolism is because of the high frequency of major bleeding. A frequent cause of major bleeding in patients with pulmonary embolism who receive thrombolytic therapy is hemorrhage from the femoral vein at the site of insertion of the angiography catheter. Pulmonary angiography is traditionally used to confirm the diagnosis of pulmonary embolism when thrombolytic therapy is being considered, because thrombolytic therapy is thought to be so dangerous that it would be a tragic error to administer it if pulmonary embolism were not present.

We assessed the relative risks of bleeding with thrombolytic therapy in patients who are managed on the basis of a pulmonary angiogram, compared with patients managed on the basis of noninvasive tests, primarily the ventilation-perfusion lung scan (1). The average frequency of major bleeding in patients with acute pulmonary embolism who were treated with tissue plasminogen activator (t-PA) after pulmonary angiography was 14.0% (2–6) (Table 37–1). All investigations excluded patients at high risk of bleeding, such as those who had recent surgery, recent biopsy, peptic ulcer disease, blood dyscrasia or severe hepatic or renal disease.

Data are sparse on the use of thrombolytic agents for pulmonary embolism in patients in whom therapy was administered without an angiographically proven diagnosis (7,8). Among 46 patients studied by Goldhaber and associates, 87% were treated on the basis of a diagnosis made by a ventilation-perfusion lung scan (7). Among the entire group of 46, 6.5% had major bleeding with 100 mg t-PA administered over 2 hours. Among 33 patients treated by Levine and associates with a bolus regimen of t-PA, 33% were diagnosed on the basis of a ventilation-perfusion lung scan (8). No major bleeding occurred among the entire group. The mode of administration (bolus injection) differed from the mode of administration of t-PA by other investigators.

Table 37-1. MAJOR BLEEDING IN PATIENTS WITH PULMONARY EMBOLISM TREATED WITH t-PA FOLLOWING PULMONARY ANGIOGRAPHY

t-PA Dose (mg)	t-PA with Heparin	# Major Bleeds/ # Patients (%)	Bleeding Complication	Author
50–100	Yes	4/34 (11.7%)	≥2 units blood	Verstraete, et al (2)
40–80	Yes	1/9 (11.1%)	≥2 units blood	PIOPED (3)
100	Yes	4/20 (20%) ? 5/20 (25%) ?	1 intracerebral 2 pericardial 1 retroperitoneal*	Dalla-Volta, et al (4)
100	No	4/22 (18.2%)	≥10 point decreased hematocrit	Goldhaber, et al (5)
100	No	5/44 (11.4%)	2 intracerebral 3 ≥2 units blood	Goldhaber, et al (6)

* Also Melena in 1 patient, number of units transfused not stated
t-PA = tissue plasminogen activator
Reproduced from Stein PD, Hull RD, Raskob G with permission.

Because of insufficient data on the use of t-PA in patients with pulmonary embolism who were diagnosed noninvasively, the risk ratio of major bleeding with t-PA after an arteriographic diagnosis versus a noninvasive diagnosis was calculated on the basis of the risk ratio of an arteriographic diagnosis versus a noninvasive diagnosis in patients with myocardial infarction who received t-PA (1). In the Thrombolysis in Myocardial Infarction IIA (TIMI IIA) study, major bleeding (≥2 units of blood transfused or intracranial hemorrhage) occurred in 11.8% who underwent immediate coronary arteriography and 3.6% who were not invaded at the time of administration of t-PA (9). The risk ratio for major bleeding (invasive management of myocardial infarction to noninvasive management of myocardial infarction) was 11.8% divided by 3.6% = 3.3. Assuming this risk ratio of bleeding with t-PA is applicable to the invasive versus noninvasive management of pulmonary embolism, the risk of bleeding with t-PA after a noninvasive diagnosis of pulmonary embolism would be 14.0% divided by 3.3 = 4.2% (1).

The calculated risks of major complications of pulmonary angiography plus major bleeding from t-PA after pulmonary angiography are shown in Figure 37–1. These risks are based on a frequency of major complications from pulmonary angiography of 1.3% (10) (Chapter 26) and a risk of major bleeding from thrombolytic therapy of 14.0% in patients in whom an angiographic diagnosis is made.If the frequency of major bleeding with thrombolytic therapy after a noninvasive diagnosis is 4.2%, noninvasive management with thrombolytic therapy would be associated with fewer complications than invasive management if the probability of pulmonary embolism exceeds 21%. If the estimated probability of pulmonary embolism is ≤20%, it would be safer to perform a pulmonary angiogram.

Figure 37–2 shows the calculated frequency of major complications in patients treated with t-PA for risks of bleeding after angiography of 7.9%, 14.0% and 20.1%, and a risk of major complications from pulmonary angiography of 1.3% (1). Comparisons are shown for risks of bleeding of 1.4%, 4.2%, and 9.3% with t-PA administered after a noninvasive diagnosis. Assuming that the frequency of major bleeding with thrombolytic therapy after an invasive diagnosis is 14.0% and the rate of bleeding with a noninvasive diagnosis is 9.3% (the upper end of the estimated 95% confidence interval for the frequency of a major bleed with a noninvasive diagnosis), management on the basis of a noninvasive diagnosis is associated with fewer major complications if the estimated probability of pulmonary embolism is greater than 57%. Assuming that the risk of major bleeding with thrombolytic therapy after a noninvasive diagnosis is 1.4% (the lower limit of the estimated 95% confidence interval), it would always be safer to treat on the basis of a noninvasive diagnosis (Fig. 37–2).

If the risk of major bleeding with thrombolytic therapy after an angiographic diagnosis was 20.1% (the upper end of the 95% confidence interval for the frequency of major bleeding with an invasive diagnosis), and the risk of major bleeding with thrombolytic therapy after a noninvasive diagnosis was 4.2%, total complications would be fewer if thrombolytic therapy were administered on the basis of a noninvasive diagnosis if the probability of pulmonary embolism was greater than 14% (Fig. 37–2).

If the risk of major bleeding with thrombolytic therapy after an angiographic diagnosis was 7.9% (the lower end of the 95% confidence interval), and the

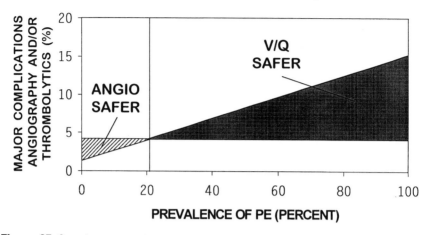

ASSUMES:
14.0% MAJOR BLEED - THROMBOLYTICS AFTER ANGIO
1.3% MAJOR COMPLICATIONS - ANGIO
4.2% MAJOR BLEED - THROMBOLYTICS, NO ANGIO

Figure 37–1. The percent of patients who would suffer major complications of thrombolytic therapy is shown in relation to the prevalence or likelihood of pulmonary embolism. The horizontal line indicates an assumed 4.2% risk of major bleeding from thrombolytic therapy administered on the basis of a noninvasive diagnosis. If the diagnosis were made noninvasively, 4.2% of patients would suffer major bleeding irrespective of the prevalence of pulmonary embolism. If all patients had pulmonary embolism and all patients underwent pulmonary angiography followed by thrombolytic therapy, the percent of patients who would develop major complications would be 15.3%, based on an assumed rate of major bleeding from thrombolytic therapy of 14.0% plus an assumed rate of major complications from angiography of 1.3%. If no patients had pulmonary embolism, and all patients underwent pulmonary angiography, none would suffer bleeding from thrombolytic therapy, but 1.3% would suffer complications of pulmonary angiography. If the prevalence of pulmonary embolism exceeds 21%, fewer patients would suffer a major complication if the diagnosis were made on the basis of a ventilation-perfusion (V/Q) lung scan (black area). If the prevalence of pulmonary embolism were 20% or less, fewer patients would suffer major complications if the diagnosis were made on the basis of a pulmonary angiogram before administering thrombolytic therapy (cross-hatched area).

risk of major bleeding with thrombolytic therapy after a noninvasive diagnosis was 4.2%, total complications would be fewer if therapy were administered on the basis of a noninvasive diagnosis if the estimated probability of pulmonary embolism was greater than 37% (Fig. 37–2).

If the risk of major bleeding with thrombolytic therapy after pulmonary angiography is only 1.0% greater than the risk of major bleeding after a noninvasive diagnosis, 5.2% compared with 4.2%, it would be safer to treat patients on a noninvasive basis if the probability of pulmonary embolism was greater than 55% (Fig. 37–2).

These calculations indicate that in many patients with suspected massive acute pulmonary embolism who definitely would require thrombolytic therapy if pulmonary embolism were diagnosed, fewer complications would occur, depending on the probability of pulmonary embolism, if treatment were initiated on the basis of a noninvasive diagnosis (1). The relatively low rate of major

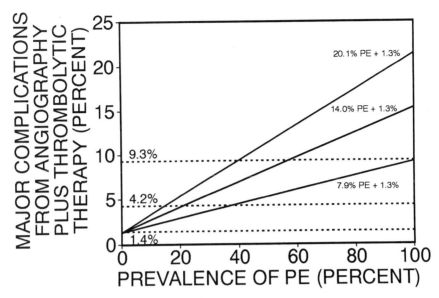

Figure 37–2. Predicted frequency of major complications from pulmonary angiography plus major bleeding from thrombolytic therapy shown as a function of the prevalence of pulmonary embolism (PE). Total major complications were major complications from angiography plus major bleeding from thrombolytic therapy. Predicted complications assume 1.3% major complications from angiography, and 20.1%, 14.0% and 7.9% major bleeding among patients treated with thrombolytic therapy after an angiographic diagnosis. The total predicted complications describe a straight line with slope=rate of major bleeding after angiography, and intercept=percent of major complications of angiography. Major bleeding from thrombolytic therapy after a noninvasive diagnosis is shown by horizontal lines at assumed rates of 9.3%, 4.2% and 1.4%. (Reprinted with permission from Stein PD, Hull RD, Raskob G. Risks for major bleeding from thrombolytic therapy in patients with acute pulmonary embolism: consideration of noninvasive management. Annals Intern Med 1994;12:313–317.)

bleeding of 6.5% after t-PA reported by Goldhaber and associates among patients with pulmonary embolism, 87% of whom were treated on the basis of a ventilation-perfusion lung scan, tends to support this conclusion (7). Unfortunately, if thrombolytic therapy is initiated on the basis of a noninvasive diagnosis, some patients who do not have pulmonary embolism will receive thrombolytic therapy and suffer bleeding complications. Overall, however, fewer patients will have major complications with the approach identified by these calculations.

Trials of thrombolytic therapy in pulmonary embolism in the 1980s and more recently showed lower rates of major bleeding than earlier studies, irrespective of the thrombolytic agent (11). Only such recent studies, therefore, were included in the analysis of the frequency of bleeding in patients with pulmonary embolism who received thrombolytic therapy (1). Studies related to bleeding with urokinase administered over 12 hours or longer were not considered in the evaluation because the improvement of hemodynamics at 2 hours with t-PA compared with urokinase could be potentially important in patients with life-threatening massive pulmonary embolism (5,6, 12). It is possible that an accelerated regimen of urokinase given over 2 hours may have a similar effectiveness to t-PA in lysis and hemodynamic improvement (6). Data related to the bleeding rate with that regimen, however, are sparse, and therefore were excluded from our evaluation (1).

In patients with pulmonary embolism, the bleeding rate after treatment with t-PA would be higher than in patients with myocardial infarction because of underlying pathology, irrespective of whether a pulmonary angiogram was obtained. Although most studies did not indicate the site of bleeding among patients who received a blood transfusion, the groin was a frequent site (2,6). Perhaps less bleeding with thrombolytic therapy may occur with catheterization of a superficial vein of the arm rather than percutaneous entrance through a femoral vein.

The risk of major bleeding with unfractionated heparin or warfarin was not considered separately in this analysis. The risk of major hemorrhagic complications from unfractionated heparin among patients treated for thromboembolic disease was 4.9% (13–16) (Chapter 34). The risk of major bleeding from unfractionated heparin in patients with a high risk of bleeding was 10.8% (17) (Chapter 34). Among patients at a low risk of bleeding, the frequency of major bleeding with unfractionated heparin was 1.1% (17). The risk of major hemorrhagic complications among patients with thromboembolic disease treated with "less intense" warfarin, International Normalized Ratio = 2.0–3.0 was 1.7% (13,17,18).

In patients who require thrombolytic therapy, it would be ideal if a noninvasive diagnosis of pulmonary embolism could be based on a high probability ventilation-perfusion lung scan, combined with a high likelihood clinical assessment. The positive predictive value of this combination is 96% (19). However, only 11% of patients with pulmonary embolism had this concordance of a high probability ventilation-perfusion lung scan and high likelihood clinical assessment (19). Among all patients with a high probability ventilation-perfusion lung scan, irrespective of the clinical assessment, pulmonary embolism was present in 87%. Only 41% of patients with pulmonary embolism had a high probability ventilation-perfusion lung scan. Among patients who do not have a high probability ventilation-perfusion lung scan, the probability of pulmonary embolism can be calculated from the ventilation-perfusion scan alone, and it can be calculated with somewhat more precision if the clinical likelihood of pulmonary embolism is estimated in combination with the ventilation-perfusion scan (19) (Chapter 14). It is also possible to assess the likelihood of pulmonary embolism based upon the number of mismatched segmental defects on ventilation-perfusion lung scans (20,21) (Chapters 22, 23). A more detailed likelihood of pulmonary embolism can be determined based upon stratification according to prior cardiopulmonary disease and clinical assessment (22) (Chapter 24). Provided that thrombolytic therapy is indicated in a patient with suspected acute pulmonary embolism, it may be safer to administer thrombolytic therapy on the basis of a noninvasive diagnosis, in spite of some uncertainty in the diagnosis.

The indications for thrombolytic therapy were discussed in Chapter 36. The calculations of major complications with thrombolytic therapy after a noninvasive diagnosis do not imply a broadening of the indications for thrombolytic therapy. This would require prospective testing.

Even if the clinical circumstances indicate the necessity of an intervention to reduce clot burden in patients with suspected acute pulmonary embolism, and if thrombolytic therapy is the intervention of choice, some believe that the risks of serious and perhaps fatal bleeding with thrombolytic therapy are so great that a pulmonary angiogram must be obtained in all patients (23). Some believe that if an intervention is clearly necessary, and if thrombolytic therapy is the intervention of choice, and if a strong clinical suspicion of acute pulmonary embolism is supported by a high probability ventilation-perfusion scan (or in an extreme emergency a noninvasive leg test showing deep venous thrombosis or an echocardiogram showing right ventricular dysfunction), then thrombolytic therapy may be administered on the basis of these noninvasive tests without a pulmonary angiogram (23). Most agree that in the absence of a pulmonary angiogram, a high probability ventilation-perfusion scan in the appropriate clinical setting offers the most useful information.

If a patient is in extremis, and an immediate intervention is necessary, and if the choice of the physician is thrombolytic therapy, most feel that if a high clinical suspicion of acute pulmonary embolism is supported by some objective evidence, either right ventricular failure shown by echocardiography or physical examination, or if a noninvasive leg test is positive for deep venous thrombosis, then that is sufficient to administer thrombolytic therapy (23). Others strongly disagree and believe that the risks of misdiagnosis are so great that a definitive diagnosis by pulmonary angiography is mandatory.

As noninvasive tests with the capability of showing pulmonary embolism, such as contrast-enhanced helical computed tomography, contrast-enhanced electron beam tomography, and magnetic resonance pulmonary angiography, become available and fully characterized (Chapter 27), these techniques may minimize or even eliminate the need for an invasive diagnosis in some patients.

REFERENCES

1. Stein PD, Hull RD, Raskob G. Risks for major bleeding from thrombolytic therapy in patients with acute pulmonary embolism: consideration of noninvasive management. Annals Intern Med 1994;121:313–317.
2. Verstraete M, Miller GAH, Bounameaux H, et al. Intravenous and intrapulmonary recombinant tissue-type plasminogen activator in the treatment of acute massive pulmonary embolism. Circulation 1988;77:353–360.
3. A collaborative study by the PIOPED investigators. Tissue plasminogen activator for the treatment of acute pulmonary embolism. Chest 1990;97:528–33.
4. Dalla-Volta S, Palla A, Santolicandro A, et al. PAIMS-2: alteplase combined with heparin versus heparin in the treatment of acute pulmonary embolism. Plasminogen Activator Italian Multicenter Study 2. J Am Coll Cardiol 1992;20:520–526.
5. Goldhaber SZ, Kessler CM, Heit J, et al. Randomised controlled trial of recombinant tissue plasminogen activator versus urokinase in the treatment of acute pulmonary embolism. Lancet 1988;2:293–298.
6. Goldhaber SZ, Kessler CM, Heit JA, et al. Recombinant tissue-type plasminogen activator versus a novel dosing regimen of urokinase in acute pulmonary embolism: a randomized controlled multicenter trial. J Am Coll Cardiol 1992;20:24–30.
7. Goldhaber SZ, Haire WD, Feldstein ML, et al. Alteplase versus heparin in acute pulmonary embolism: randomised trial assessing right-ventricular function and pulmonary perfusion. Lancet 1993;341:507–511.
8. Levine M, Hirsh J, Weitz J, et al. A randomized trial of a single bolus dosage regimen of recombinant tissue plasminogen activator in patients with acute pulmonary embolism. Chest 1990;98:1473–1479.

9. The TIMI Research Group. Immediate versus delayed catheterization and angioplasty following thrombolytic therapy for acute myocardial infarction. TIMI IIA results. JAMA 1988;260:2849–2858.
10. Stein PD, Athanasoulis C, Alavi A, et al. Complications and validity of pulmonary angiography in acute pulmonary embolism. Circulation 1992;85:462–468.
11. Levine MN, Goldhaber SZ, Califf RM, et al. Hemorrhagic complications of thrombolytic therapy in the treatment of myocardial infarction and venous thromboembolism. Chest 1992;102(Suppl):364S–373S.
12. Marini C, Di Ricco G, Rossi G, et al. Fibrinolytic effects of urokinase and heparin in acute pulmonary embolism: a randomized clinical trial. Respiration 1988;54:162–173.
13. Hull RD, Raskob GE, Hirsh J, et al. Continuous intravenous heparin compared with intermittent subcutaneous heparin in the initial treatment of proximal-vein thrombosis. N Engl J Med 1986;315:1109–1114.
14. Doyle DJ, Turpie AG, Hirsh J, et al. Adjusted subcutaneous heparin or continuous intravenous heparin in patients with acute deep vein thrombosis: a randomized trial. Ann Intern Med 1987;107:441–445.
15. Pini M, Pattacini C, Quintavalla R, et al. Subcutaneous versus intermittent heparin in the treatment of deep vein thrombosis: a randomized clinical trial. Thromb Haemost 1990;64:222–226.
16. Hull RD, Raskob GE, Pineo GF, et al. Subcutaneous low-molecular-weight heparin compared with continuous intravenous heparin in the treatment of proximal-vein thrombosis. New Engl J Med 1992; 326:975–982.
17. Hull RD, Raskob GE, Rosenbloom D, et al. Heparin for 5 days versus for 10 days in the initial treatment of proximal venous thrombosis. N Engl J Med 1990;322:1260–1264.
18. Hull R, Hirsh J, Jay R, et al. Different intensities of oral anticoagulant therapy in the treatment of proximal-vein thrombosis. N Engl J Med 1982;307:1676–1681.
19. A collaborative study by the PIOPED investigators. Value of the ventilation/perfusion scan in acute pulmonary embolism: results of the Prospective Investigation of Pulmonary Embolism Diagnosis (PIOPED). JAMA 1990; 263:2753–2759.
20. Stein PD, Gottschalk A, Henry JW, et al. Stratification of patients according to prior cardiopulmonary disease and probability assessment based upon the number of mismatched segmental equivalent perfusion defects: approaches to strengthen the diagnostic value of ventilation/perfusion lung scans in acute pulmonary embolism. Chest 1993;104:1461–1467.
21. Stein PD, Henry JW, Gottschalk A. Mismatched vascular defects: an easy alternative to mismatched segmental equivalent defects for the interpretation of ventilation/perfusion lung scans in pulmonary embolism. Chest 1993; 104:1468–1472.
22. Stein PD, Henry JW, Gottschalk A. The addition of clinical assessment to stratification according to prior cardiopulmonary disease further optimizes the interpretation of ventilation/perfusion lung scans in pulmonary embolism. Chest 1993;104:1472–1476.
23. ACCP Consensus Committee on Pulmonary Embolism. Opinions regarding the diagnosis and management of venous thromboembolism. Chest 1996;109:233–237.

CHAPTER 38

Mechanical Interventions: Inferior Vena Cava Occlusion, Catheter Embolectomy, Catheter-Tip Fragmentation, Pulmonary Embolectomy, and Thromboendarterectomy

Inferior Vena Cava Occlusion

All agree (1) that an inferior vena cava filter should be inserted in a patient with proximal deep venous thrombosis or pulmonary embolism if:

1. Anticoagulants are contraindicated.
2. Pulmonary embolism has recurred while on adequate anticoagulant therapy.
3. If pulmonary embolism is severe (right ventricular failure on physical examination, hypotension) and any recurrent pulmonary embolism may be fatal.

Insertion of an inferior vena cava filter is also strongly recommended in patients after pulmonary embolectomy (2).

It is felt that routine insertion of an inferior vena cava filter is not indicated only on the basis of a continuing predisposition for deep venous thrombosis (1). In special circumstances, however, this may be the best approach.

Some have recommended prophylactic insertion of vena cava filters for high risk patients, including those with extensive free floating thrombi in the iliac veins or vena cava (3), patients about to undergo pulmonary embolectomy (4), patients with deep venous thrombosis who have cancer (5), patients at high risk of deep venous thrombosis or pulmonary embolism who had a prior pulmonary embolism (6), patients with deep venous thrombosis, severe pulmonary hypertension, and minimal cardiopulmonary reserve (6), and patients with chronic obstructive pulmonary disease and deep venous thrombosis (7).

Table 38–1. COMPARISON BETWEEN VARIOUS CAVAL FILTERS

	PE in Spite of Filter	Significant Tilting	Caval Occlusion	Proximal Migration
Greenfield steel	+	Yes	+	+
Greenfield titanium	+	Yes	?	+
Bird's nest	+	No	+++	++[a]
Vena-Tech	+	Yes	++	++
Simon-Nitinol	+	No	+++	?
Amplatz	?	Yes	+++	−
Günther	+	Yes	++	+
Mobin-Uddin	+	Yes	+++	+

−, absent
?, not reported
+, ++, +++, increasing degrees of the presence of indicated complication
[a] No migration was reported after filter modification
Modified and reprinted with permission from Berggvist D. The role of venal caval interruption in patients with venous thromboembolism. Prog Cardiovasc Dis 1994;37:25–37.

A number of vena cava filters have been designed for percutaneous insertion. These include the stainless steel Greenfield filter (8), titanium Greenfield filter (9), Bird's nest filter (10), LGM filter (11), Simon-Nitinol filter (12), Günther filter (13), and Amplatz filter (14). They differ in outer diameter of the delivery system, maximal caval diameter into which they can be inserted, hook design, retrievability, biocompatability, and filtering efficiency. Filter migration, thrombosis, and cava wall perforation occur (15). Most authorities recommend anticoagulant therapy after insertion of a filter (16). The filter alone, however, may be effective (8).

Pulmonary embolism after insertion of an inferior vena cava filter is uncommon, and fatal pulmonary embolism is rare (9,17). Possible mechanisms that can explain pulmonary embolism after filter insertion are: 1) ineffective filtration, especially with tilting of the filter; 2) growth of trapped thrombi through the filter; 3) thrombosis on the proximal side of the filter; 4) filter migration; 5) filter retraction from the caval wall; 6) embolization through collaterals; 7) embolization from sites other than the inferior vena caval; and 8) incorrect position of the filter (17).

Complications of vena caval interruption were reviewed by Bergqvist (17) and by Webb and associates (18). Complications include filter deformation, filter fracture, insufficient opening of the filter, improper anatomic placement of the filter migration, angulation of the filter, caval stenosis, caval occlusion, erosion of the caval wall, and leg edema (17). Complications at the site of insertion of the catheter do not differ from complications observed locally with other catheter techniques (17). Deep venous thrombosis at the puncture site has been reported by most in 8 to 25% (19–22), but in one series of 17 patients, 41% development of deep venous thrombosis at the puncture site (23). Bergqvist compared the complications reported with various filters; these are shown in Table 38–1 (17).

Catheter Embolectomy

Catheter-tip devices for the extraction of pulmonary thromboemboli and for fragmentation of pulmonary thromboemboli have the potential of: 1) producing immediate relief from the deleterious effects of pulmonary embolism, and 2) offering a therapeutic option to patients with massive pulmonary embolism who have a contraindication to thrombolytic therapy. A catheter- tip device for the extraction of pulmonary embolism has been used in patients (24, 25). The present modification of the device is an 8.5 French-size catheter with a rigid cup attached to the tip and a handle with a control lever for steering (26). The tip of the catheter is advanced to the embolus. Suction is applied by withdrawing the plunger of a syringe. The thrombus, if captured, is held to the cup by suction, and the catheter, with the attached thrombus, is withdrawn. Since development of this device in the late 1960s, it has been used by Greenfield and associates in 46 patients (26). Catheter embolectomy was successful in 27 of 33 (82%) with massive pulmonary embolism and 4 of 4 (100%) with major pulmonary embolism (26). In patients with chronic pulmonary embolism, it was successful in 5 of 9 (56%).

Catheter-Tip Fragmentation

Catheter-tip devices for fragmentation of massive pulmonary embolism are being developed. Such instruments may be particularly useful in patients who have a contraindication to thrombolytic therapy. Initial studies in dogs with a Kensey flexible rotating-tip catheter, capable of 100,000 rpm, showed potential (27). Problems were difficulty in passing the catheter to the site of the embolus, difficulty in identifying the embolus, and damage of the walls of the pulmonary arteries. The release of the fragmented thromboemboli into the distal pulmonary arterial branches was not a problem, because the cross-sectional area and volume of the distal pulmonary arterey branches far exceeds the cross-sectional area and volume of the proximal branches where occlusion can cause a major hemodynamic impairment.

Some investigators simply fragmented occluding proximal thrombi using ordinary catheters and guidewires (28). Three patients with massive acute pulmonary embolism were successfully treated in this fashion by Brady and associates (28). Others used a comparable technique successfully in 29 of 36 (81%) patients with massive pulmonary embolism (28,30). Among these patients, 30 required cardiopulmonary resuscitation on presentation.

A device that appears potentially useful is a catheter with the distal tip split into four 10–15 mm strips (31). High-speed rotation at 100,000 rpm opens the distal strips by centrifugal force. The strip forms a supple helix, which is able to pulverize recent thromboemboli. In 6 of 7 (86%) patients who had life-threatening pulmonary embolism and a contraindication to thrombolytic therapy, large emboli in the main pulmonary arteries were substantially lysed.

Pulmonary Embolectomy

Most agree that a candidate for pulmonary embolectomy should meet the following criteria (16):

1. Massive pulmonary embolism, angiographically documented if possible.
2. Hemodynamic instability (shock) despite heparin therapy and resuscitative efforts.
3. Failure of thrombolytic therapy or a contraindication to its use.

Supportive medical therapy is likely to give better results (32). The operative mortality or perioperative mortality related to pulmonary embolism ranged between 28 and 38% (33–35). In patients who had cardiopulmonary arrest before the pulmonary embolectomy, the operative mortality ranged between 64 and 74% (34, 35). In spite of these statistics, this drastic measure may have life-saving potential in rare instances.

Pulmonary Thromboendarterectomy

The management of chronic thromboembolic hypertension has been reviewed (36–38). A small percentage of patients who suffer pulmonary embolism, perhaps 0.1%, are left with chronic obstruction of the pulmonary arteries resulting in pulmonary hypertension and often cor pulmonale (38). Pulmonary thromboendarterectomy reduces the pulmonary artery resistance and improves dyspnea and exercise capacity. The procedure, at this time, is performed only in specialized centers. In the hands of an experienced diagnostic and surgical team, the results can be curative (39). Early diagnosis of this condition is important because the surgical mortality in patients who have progressed to dyspnea at rest is substantially greater than among those with less severe symptoms (38). If the perfusion lung scan remains unchanged for 6 to 8 weeks after pulmonary embolism, the organized thrombotic residuals persist indefinitely and such patients merit consideration for surgical relief (38).

REFERENCES

1. ACCP Consensus Committee on Pulmonary Embolism. Opinions regarding the diagnosis and management of venous thromboembolism. Chest 1996;109:233–237.
2. Grassi CJ, Goldhaber SZ. Interruption of the inferior vena cava for prevention of pulmonary embolism: transvenous filter divices. Herz 1989;14:182–191.
3. Norris NC, Greenfield LJ, Herrmann JB. Free-floating iliofemoral thrombus. Arch Surg 1985;120:806–808.
4. Hye RJ, Mitchell AT, Dory CE, et al. Analysis of the transition to percutaneous placement of Greenfield filters.Arch Surg 1990;125:1550–1553.
5. Cohen JR, Grella L, Citron M. Greenfield filter instead of heparin as primary treatment for deep venous thrombosis or pulmonary embolism in patients with cancer. Cancer 1992;70:1993–1996.
6. Rohrer MJ, Scheidler MG, Wheeler HB, et al. Extended indications for placement of an inferior vena cava filter. J Vasc Surg 1989;10:44–50.
7. Pomper SR, Lutchman G. The role of intracaval filters in patients with COPD and DVT. Angiology 1991;42:85–89.
8. Greenfield LJ, Michna BA. Twelve-year clinical experience with the Greenfield vena caval filter. Surgery 1988;104:706–712.
9. Greenfield LJ, Cho K, Proctor M, et al. Results of a multicenter study of the modified hook–titanium Greenfield filter. J Vasc Surg 1991:14:253–257.
10. Roehm JOF, Johnsrude IS, Barth MH, et al. The bird's nest inferior vena cava filter: progress report. Radiology 1988;168:745–749.

11. Ricco JB, Crochet D, Sebilotte P, et al. Percutaneous transvenous caval interruption with the "LGM" filter: early results of a multicenter trial. Ann Vasc Surg 1988;3:242–247.
12. Simon M, Athanasoulis CA, Kim D, et al. Simon-Nitinol inferior vena cava filter: initial clinical experience. Radiology 1989;172:99–103.
13. Fobbe F, Dietzel M, Korth R, et al. Günther vena caval filter: results of long-term follow-up. Am J Roentgen 1988;151:1031–1034.
14. Epstein DH, Darcy MD, Hunter DW, et al. Experience with the Amplatz retrievable vena cava filter. Radiology 1989;172:105–110.
15. Dorfman GS. Percutaneous inferior vena caval filters. Radiology 1990;174:987–992.
16. Hyers TM, Hull RD, Weg JG. Antithrombotic therapy for venous thromboembolic disease. Chest 1995;108(Suppl):335S–351S.
17. Bergqvist D. The role of venal caval interruption in patients with venous thromboembolism. Prog Cardiovasc Dis 1994;37:25–37.
18. Webb MS, Murphy TP, Dorfman GS. Choice and selection of inferior vena cava filters. Seminars in Resp and Crit Care Med 1996;17:71–85.
19. Greenfield LJ, Tauscher JR, Marx V. Evaluation of a new percutaneous stainless steel Greenfield filter by intravascular ultrasonography. Surgery 1991;109:722–729.
20. Murphy YP, Dorfman GS, Yedlicka W, et al. LGM vena cava filter. Objective evaluation of early results. J Vasc Intervent Radio 1991;2:107–115.
21. Dorfman GS, Cronan JJ, Paolella LP, et al. Iatrogenic changes at the venotomy site after percutaneous placement of the Greenfield filter. Radiology 1989;173:159–162.
22. Hewissen MW, Erickson SJ, Foley WD, et al. Thrombosis at venous insertion sites after interior vena caval filter placement. Radiology 1989;173:155–157.
23. Kantor A, Glanz S, Gordon D, et al. Percutaneous insertion of the Kimray-Greenfield filter: incidence of femoral vein thrombosis. Am J Roent 1987;149:1065–1066.
24. Greenfield LJ, Zocco JJ. Intraluminal management of acute massive pulmonary thromboembolism. J Thorac Cardiovasc Surg 1979;77:402–410.
25. Feitelberg SP, Kahn SE, Kotler MN, et al. Transfemoral embolectomy for massive pulmonary embolus and associated myocardial infarction. Am Heart J 1987;113:819–820.
26. Greenfield LJ, Proctor MC. Role of catheter-embolectomy in treating pulmonary embolism. Seminars in Resp and Crit Care Med 1996;17:95–99.
27. Stein PD, Sabbah HN, Basha MA, et al. Mechanical disruption of pulmonary emboli in dogs with a flexible rotating-tip catheter (Kensey catheter). Chest 1990;98:994–998.
28. Brady AJB, Crake T, Oakley CM. Percutaneous catheter fragmentation and distal dispersion of proximal pulmonary embolus. Lancet 1991;338:1186–1189.
29. Essop MR, Moddlemost S, Skoularigis J, et al. Simultaneous mechanical clot fragmentation and pharmacologic thrombolysis in acute massive pulmonary embolism. Am J Cardiol 1992;69;427–430.
30. Horskotte D, Heintzen MP, Strauer BE, et al. Aggressive non-surgical management of pulmonary embolism with cardiogenic shock Eur Heart J 1991;12(Suppl):52.
31. Fourrier JL, Lefebvre JM, Gomez J, et al. Mechanical thrombolysis of severe pulmonary embolism in humans by means of a high speed rotational catheter (Angiocor Thromboembolizer). Circulation 1993;88(Suppl):I–71. Abstract.
32. Alpert JS, Smith RE, Ockene IS, et al. Treatment of massive pulmonary embolism: the role of pulmonary embolectomy. Am Heart J 1975;89:413–418.
33. Meyer G, Tamisier D, Sors H, et al. Pulmonary embolectomy: a 20-year experience at one center. Ann Thorac Surg 1991;51:232–236.
34. Gray HH, Morgan JM, Paneth M, et al. Pulmonary embolectomy for acute massive pulmonary embolism. Br Heart J 1988;60:196–200.
35. Clarke DB, Abrams LD. Pulmonary embolectomy: a 25-year experience. J Thorac Cardiovasc Surg 1986;92:442–445.

36. Shure D. Chronic thromboembolic pulmonary hypertension: diagnosis and treatment. Seminars in Resp and Crit Care Med 1996;17:7–16.
37. Viner SM, Bagg BR, Auger WR, et al. The management of pulmonary hypertension secondary to chronic thromboembolic disease. Prog Cardiovasc Dis 1994;37:79–92.
38. Moser KM: Venous thromboembolism. Am Rev Respir Dis 1990;141:235–249.
39. Moser KM, Auger WR, Fedullo PF. Chronic major-vessel thromboembolic pulmonary hypertension. Circulation 1990;81:1735–1743.

Index

References in italics denote figures; those followed by "t" denote tables.

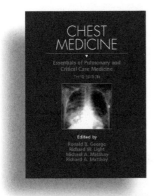
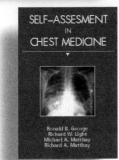
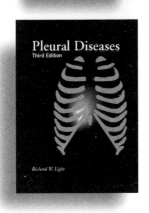